Handbook of Hysterectomy

Handbook of Hysterectomy

Editor: Molly Andrews

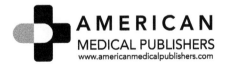

AMERICAN
MEDICAL PUBLISHERS
www.americanmedicalpublishers.com

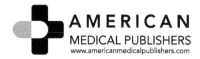

Cataloging-in-Publication Data

Handbook of hysterectomy / edited by Molly Andrews.
    p. cm.
Includes bibliographical references and index.
ISBN 978-1-63927-494-9
1. Hysterectomy. 2. Uterus--Surgery. 3. Hysterectomy--Complications. 4. Sterilization of women. I. Andrews, Molly.
RG391 .H36 2022
618.145 3--dc23

American Medical Publishers,
41 Flatbush Avenue,
1st Floor, New York,
NY 11217, USA

ISBN 978-1-63927-494-9 (Hardback)

Contents

Preface

The purpose of the book is to provide a glimpse into the dynamics and to present opinions and studies of some of the scientists engaged in the development of new ideas in the field from very different standpoints. This book will prove useful to students and researchers owing to its high content quality.

Hysterectomy is a surgical procedure for the removal of the uterus. It may also be applied for the removal of the ovaries, cervix, fallopian tubes and their surrounding structures. Hysterectomy can be total or partial. When the ovaries are removed, a woman loses her ability to bear children with associated changes to the hormonal balance. It is therefore a procedure that is performed only when other treatment modalities are not available. Hysterectomy is recommended as a treatment for intractable reproductive/uterine system conditions, such as severe endometriosis, vaginal prolapse and chronic pelvic pain. It may also be performed postpartum in order to resolve excessive obstetrical hemorrhage, or remove placenta percreta or placenta praevia. The surgical procedure of oophorectomy is often performed with hysterectomy in order to decrease the risk of ovarian cancer. This book outlines the principles and techniques of hysteretomy in detail. Also included herein is a detailed explanation of the modern methods of performing hysterectomy. This book, with its detailed analyses and data, will prove immensely beneficial to professionals and students involved in gynecology at various levels.

At the end, I would like to appreciate all the efforts made by the authors in completing their chapters professionally. I express my deepest gratitude to all of them for contributing to this book by sharing their valuable works. A special thanks to my family and friends for their constant support in this journey.

Editor

Chemoradiation with adjuvant hysterectomy for stage IB-2 cervical cancer

Glenn E. Bigsby IV · Robert W. Holloway ·
Sarfraz Ahmad · Michael D. Sombeck · George Ebra ·
Neil J. Finkler

Abstract To review outcomes of patients with stage IB-2 cervical carcinoma treated with chemoradiation therapy (CRT) followed by total abdominal hysterectomy (TAH), common iliac and para-aortic lymphadenectomy (PAL). A retrospective review of patients with stage IB-2 cervical cancer treated with CRT followed by TAH/PAL from 1999 to 2009 was performed. Brachytherapy was limited to 1,500–1,800 cGy. Sixty-nine patients were identified. The mean age was 46.7 years, tumor diameter 5.4 cm, and all patients had complete clinical response to CRT. The mean follow-up was 61.7 months. There were no central pelvic relapses and two pelvic sidewall failures (97% pelvic control). The mean time to progression was 31.6 months, and 5-year disease-specific survival was 81%. Three (4.3%) patients developed symptomatic vaginal stenosis. CRT plus adjuvant hysterectomy for stage IB-2 cervical cancer resulted in excellent pelvic control and 5-year survival. Vaginal stenosis was rare.

Keywords Chemoradiation · IB-2 cervical carcinoma · Adjuvant hysterectomy · Outcomes analyses · Survival

Background

In 2010, there were approximately 12,200 newly diagnosed cases of cervical cancer and 4,210 deaths in the USA [1].

G. E. Bigsby IV (✉) · R. W. Holloway · S. Ahmad · G. Ebra ·
N. J. Finkler
Florida Hospital Gynecologic Oncology,
Florida Hospital Cancer Institute,
2501 N. Orange Ave., Suite 800,
Orlando, FL 32804, USA
e-mail: gbigsby@mac.com

M. D. Sombeck
Radiation Oncology Program, Florida Hospital Cancer Institute,
Orlando, FL 32804, USA

The treatment of International Federation of Gynecology and Obstetrics stage IB-2 "bulky" cervical carcinoma continues to be debated. While survival for patients with IA and IB-1 tumors is generally reported greater than 90%, patients with stage IB-2 tumors have a worse prognosis with 5-year survivals ranging from 69% to 73% [2, 3] in case series collected prior to the use of cisplatin with primary or secondary radiation. More recently, Goksedef et al. reported 86% 3-year survival with chemoradiation therapy (CRT) [4]. Zivanovic et al. [5] found 55% IB-2 patients alive at 3 years with primary CRT and selected patients undergoing radical hysterectomy with secondary CRT had a 72% estimated 3-year survival.

There are four suggested therapies for stage IB-2 cervical carcinoma, three of which are included in the National Comprehensive Cancer Network (NCCN) Guidelines. Whole-pelvis radiation with cisplatin-based chemotherapy has category 1 evidence with uniform consensus. Radical hysterectomy with pelvic and para-aortic lymphadenectomy followed by tailored postoperative chemoradiation [6] has category 2B evidence with a nonuniform consensus and lower level evidence including clinical experience. A third NCCN treatment option is preoperative pelvic CRT followed by adjuvant hysterectomy and has category 3 evidence with major disagreement from panelists that the recommendation is appropriate [6]. A fourth described treatment paradigm is neoadjuvant chemotherapy followed by radical hysterectomy with or without tailored adjuvant radiation and is not recommended by the NCCN. None of these treatment regimens are uniformly considered superior, and there are no prospective randomized trials comparing the three NCCN guideline treatment options.

It has been observed that many patients with stage IB-2 cervical cancer suffer from vaginal stenosis following primary chemo/RT [7, 8]. While pelvic control is in general excellent with primary CRT [9], some patients suffer relapse and require pelvic exenteration. Furthermore, some patients develop secondary malignancy (uterine sarcoma) in the radiation field many years after radiation [10]. Primary radical hysterectomy for IB-2 lesions can be associated with considerable blood loss, may be technically difficult in morbidly obese patients, and still the majority will require adjuvant CRT for high-risk pathology [5]. Therefore, we hypothesized that chemo/RT with a reduced brachytherapy dose (in order to minimize vaginal toxicity) followed by simple hysterectomy may overcome these potential short-comings. The purpose of this study was to retrospectively analyze clinical outcomes of patients with stage IB-2 cervical carcinoma treated with concurrent CRT followed by adjuvant extrafascial total abdominal hysterectomy (TAH), common iliac and para-aortic lymphadenectomy treated at a single institution.

Materials and methods

A retrospective review of records from 69 consecutive patients with stage IB-2 cervical carcinoma who underwent CRT followed by adjuvant hysterectomy from January 1999 to January 2009 was performed. All surgeries were performed at our institution; however, 24 (35%) patients received CRT at outside facilities. A standardized treatment protocol with dosing guidelines and allowances for dose reductions was provided to radiation oncologists and medical oncologists outside our facility; however, dosing was ultimately at the discretion of the treating physician. This retrospective review of patient records was conducted with our institutional review board approval.

All patients underwent contrasted computed axial to-mography (CAT) scans of the abdomen and pelvis and were excluded from this treatment for evidence of extrapelvic disease by either physical exam or CAT scan, including para-aortic lymphadenopathy. Patients were administered cisplatin (25–40 mg/m^2 weekly) during radiation therapy with six weekly treatments, dosed to tolerance of the patient. An alternative regimen of cisplatin/5-FU (50 mg/m^2 day 1, 1,000 mg/m^2 daily × 4 days, i.e., days 1–4 and 27–30) was administered to some patients with cervical adenocarcinoma. The recommended whole pelvic radiation dose was 4,500 cGy utilizing 20 MeV X-ray in a four-field technique in 180 cGy/day fractions. The pelvic sidewall was optionally boosted utilizing anterioposterior/posterioanterior fields for an additional 540 cGy in three fractions. The total external beam dose was 4,500–5,040 cGy in 25–28 treatments and high-dose rate brachytherapy was prescribed at 1,500–1,800 cGy to point A, in three equal doses. The superior margin of the pelvic radiation field was to the mid-sacroiliac joint. Patients underwent extrafascial hysterectomy with common and para-aortic lymphadenec-

tomy. The lymphadenectomy was performed from above the radiation field, but was not taken routinely to the inferior mesenteric artery, as this was not a therapeutic lymphadenectomy. Surgery was completed 6 to 8 weeks following completion of brachytherapy.

Preoperative, intraoperative, and postoperative, demo-graphics and clinical variables were collected by reviewing the patients' hospital, office records, tumor registry entries, and the Social Security Death Index database (available at http://genealogy.rootsweb.com). Direct patient contact, telephone interviews with family, or the patient's primary care physician was used to collect patient updates. Data were collected in a standardized manner using prespecified definitions. This approach provided for standardized reporting of each patient's clinical status before and after the operation. A 100% follow-up was obtained in the present study.

Data are presented as frequency distributions and simple percentages. Patient survival was expressed by actuarial estimates according to the method of Kaplan and Meier using time zero as the start date of external beam radiation and the date of death or last follow-up as the end point (with variability expressed as the standard error of the mean). Patients alive at the last follow-up were included as right-censored values in the analysis. Data collected were analyzed using the Number Cruncher Statistical Systems, Kaysville, UT.

Findings

A total of 69 women underwent CRT followed by adjuvant hysterectomy, common iliac and para-aortic lymphadenec-tomy. The overall patient demographics and pathologic characteristics are shown in Table 1. The mean age of patients was 46.7±10.7 years (range 27–82). The mean follow-up time was 61.7 months (range 10.9–122.5). Clinical complete response determined by physical exam was documented in all patients prior to surgery.

All patients received external beam radiation. Six (9%) did not receive the recommended dose of external beam radiation; three patients received lower doses (3,980–4,140 cGy) and three were administered higher doses (5,400 cGy) than the protocol guidelines. Brachytherapy was omitted in four (6%) patients, three because of altered vaginal geometry (upper vaginal stenosis) and one for undocumented reasons. Twenty three (35%) of 65 patients receiving brachytherapy had doses outside the protocol guidelines. Fourteen patients received less brachytherapy dose (500–1,200 cGy), and nine received more doses (2,000–3,000 cGy). Cisplatin was administered weekly to all patients during pelvic radiation. Forty-nine (71%) patients received cisplatin 40 mg/m^2, 17 (25%) received

Table 1 Patient demographics and pretreatment pathologic characteristics

Variables	Mean±SD or absolute number	Range or percentage
Age (years)	46.8±10.7	27–82
Body mass index (kg/m^2)	29.5±6.0	18.2–44.8
Clinical tumor size (cm)	5.4±1.2	4.0–9.0
4–6 cm	57 (83%)	N/A
>6 cm	12 (17%)	6.5–9.0
Histology		
Squamous	55	80
Adenocarcinoma	11	16
Adenosquamous	3	4
Tumor grade		
1	4	5.8
2	24	34.8
3	19	27.5
Unknown[a]	22	31.9

[a]Biopsy reports were from several pathology departments outside our institution, and tumor grading was not always provided

SD standard deviation, *N/A* not applicable

25 mg/m^2, and 3 (4%) received cisplatin/5-FU. Nineteen (39%) patients received all 6 cycles of cisplatin at 40 mg/m^2 without dose reduction, and in the other 30 patients, chemotherapy was held for one or more weeks of therapy, or dose-reduced therapy to 25 mg/m^2. The most common reason for dose reduction or discontinuation was nausea and vomiting or fatigue. There were no dose reductions for patients who initiated therapy at 25 mg/m^2, and all received 6 cycles. Likewise, there were no reductions for patients receiving cisplatin/5-FU. There were no grade 3 or 4 hematologic toxicities related to CRT.

The mean operative time for TAH, common iliac and para-aortic lymphadenectomy was 62±15 min, and estimated blood loss (EBL) was 187±103 mL. Four (6%) patients received preoperative or intraoperative transfusions because of chronic anemia. There were no intraoperative or postoperative transfusions related to excessive blood loss. The mean LOS was 3.1 days (range 2–7). The Foley catheter was removed on the first or second postoperative day for all patients except for one patient who had a cystotomy and repair. Common iliac and para-aortic lymph node counts averaged 6.3±2.9 (range, 2–15). Despite all patients achieving a complete clinical response by exam, 35 (51%) had microscopic residual disease on pathologic exam of the cervix. Only two (3%) patients had positive cervical–vaginal surgical margins (Table 2).

Ten (14%) patients had complications potentially related to treatment, and four (6%) required surgical management (Table 3). There were no treatment-related deaths. There were no vesicovaginal or ureterovaginal fistulae. All patients requiring reoperation were greater than 12 months postadjuvant hysterectomy. There was one intraoperative cystotomy and repair that healed without further sequelae. All patients requiring surgery for treatment-related complications received radiation dosing per protocol. Only one of the four patients who required surgery for complications received additional CRT to the para-aortic nodes following adjuvant hysterectomy. Other major complications not requiring surgery are described in Table 3 and include only two (3%) cases of radiation-related vaginal stenosis.

Thirty-five (51%) patients had residual disease identified in hysterectomy or nodal specimens by hematoxylin and

Table 2 Surgical and clinico-pathologic data

Factors	Mean±SD or absolute number	Range or percentage
Operative time (min)	62±15	37–112
EBL (mL)	187±103	50–600
Transfusions (perioperative)	4	6%
Length of stay (days)	3.13±1.03	2–7
Lymph node count (common iliac/aortic)	6.32±2.94	2–15
Residual disease	35	51%
Positive margins	2	3%
Adjuvant therapy[a]	20	29%

SD standard deviation

[a]See Table 4 for details

Table 3 Treatment-related complications

Specifics	Patients ($n=10$)
Perioperative complication	
Cystotomy with repair	1
Deep venous thrombosis	1
Complete small bowel obstruction[a]	1
Vaginal vault necrosis	1
Vaginal vault necrosis/grade 4 proctitis[a]	1
Rectovaginal fistula (radiation proctitis grade 4/pSBO)[a]	1
Enterocutaneous fistula, ureteral stenosis[a]	1
Ureteral stenosis requiring temporary stent	1
Vaginal stenosis	2

[a]Required surgical intervention

eosin staining. Microscopic residual disease was identified in the cervix in 29 (42%) patients (22 cervix only, 7 cervix plus lymph nodes). Four (6%) patients had nodal metastasis and no residual cervical disease. Twenty patients with residual disease received additional therapy, including five treated with CRT to para-aortic nodes (Table 4). Fourteen patients with residual disease received additional platinum therapies, and one patient was administered additional vaginal cuff radiation. Fifteen study patients had residual disease and did not receive additional therapy, 14 of whom had residual cervical disease only. For the 22 patients who had residual cervical cancer identified in the hysterectomy specimens, there were no relapses and no deaths related to cervical cancer. Conversely, 11 (16%) patients had positive common or para-aortic lymph nodes identified at hysterectomy, and 10 died from metastatic disease. Five of the 11 patients (45%) with nodal disease had bulky lymphadenopathy identified at surgery, and their mean survival was 15 months (range 11–26). Three of these five patients with bulky nodal disease received additional chemotherapy, one received CRT, and one refused additional therapy. The other six patients with microscopic nodal metastasis all

received additional therapy; five patients had progressive disease despite therapy [mean time to progression (TTP)= 18.5 months, range 6–33], and their mean OS was 41 months (range 19–62). The remaining patient with microscopic nodal disease received 4 cycles of cisplatin with topotecan and was alive without disease at 90 months. Two (3%) patients had microscopically positive vaginal margins, and one received a brachytherapy boost of 1,500 cGy. This patient was without evidence of disease at 73.4 months. The other patient also had positive para-aortic nodes and was dead of disease at 36.8 months (included in data above), having received 1,440 cGy radiation to para-aortic nodes.

Thirty-four (49%) patients had no active carcinoma identified in the hysterectomy or nodal specimens. Twenty-nine of these patients (85%) were alive without evidence of disease, including one who relapsed in para-aortic lymph nodes, received subsequent CRT, and is currently without disease at 119 months. Two patients with no evidence of disease at surgery died from recurrent cervical cancer (one pelvic sidewall, one pulmonary) despite additional therapy. Two other patients died of breast

Table 4 Residual disease based on pathological findings

Residual disease	Total patients ($n=35$)	Alive patients (%)	Deceased patients (%)	Treatment: number of patients (% of patients treated)
Central (cervix/vaginal)	22	21 (95)	1 (5)[a]	Chemo=8/22 (36.4)
				Vaginal brachytherapy=1/22 (4.5)
Central and nodal	7	0 (0)	7 (100)	Chemo=3/7 (42.9)
				Chemo/radiation=3/7 (42.9)
Nodal	4	1 (25)	3 (75)	Chemo=2/4 (50)
				Chemo/radiation=2/4 (50)
Nonviable tumor[b]	2	1 (50)	1 (50)	Chemo=1/2 (50)

NED no evidence of disease

[a] Deceased of other causes, NED at time of death

[b] Pathology suggested necrosis; however, the treatment was at the discretion of physician

cancer, and both were free of cervical cancer at the time of death. One additional patient who relapsed in the liver at 110 months was alive on chemotherapy 118 months from initial CRT.

The mean TTP for the entire group was 31.6± 28.3 months. Kaplain–Meier estimated 5-year disease-specific survival (DSS) was 81% (Fig. 1a, b). The "pelvic control" rate was 97% with only two patients relapsing in lymph nodes of the pelvic sidewall. Specifically, no patients recurred with vaginal or parametrial disease; and no exenterative procedures were performed. Distant relapse was evident in 20% of patients (para-aortic, mediastinal, and supraclavicular lymph nodes, lung, liver, and brain). There were 13 deaths secondary to cervical cancer and three from unrelated causes (two breast cancer, one cardiovascular), and two (3%) patients remain alive with disease at the time of this analysis.

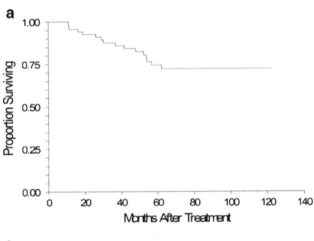

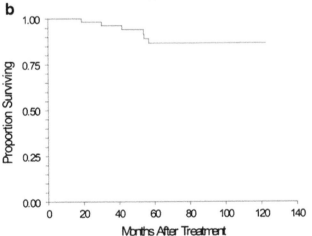

Fig. 1 **a** Actuarial 5-year overall survival ("all causes," includes three deaths from other causes in patients without evidence of active disease) curve for all 69 stage IB-2 cervical cancer patients as determined by Kaplan–Meier analysis. **b** Actuarial 5-year survival curve for 58 stage IB-2 cervical cancer patients (with negative nodes at surgery) as determined by Kaplan–Meier analysis

Discussion

Each of the NCCN guideline-supported treatment options for stage IB-2 cervical cancer has theoretical advantages and disadvantages that have not been fully compared in well-designed, prospective randomized clinical trials [6]. The GOG-71 study compared radiation therapy alone and radiation plus adjuvant hysterectomy for patients with stage IB-2 cervical cancer and reported no significant difference in overall survival between the two treatment arms [9]. However, subgroup analysis of patients with 4–6-cm lesions did benefit from adjuvant hysterectomy with unadjusted relative risk of progression at 0.58 and death 0.60, and conversely no improvement for patients with lesions greater than 6 cm [9].

In GOG-123, the effect of adding cisplatin to radiation therapy plus adjuvant hysterectomy was tested in a phase III trial. CRT using cisplatin followed by hysterectomy produced a statistically significant improvement in the OS and decreased pelvic recurrence rate compared to those treated with radiation and adjuvant hysterectomy [11]. There was no significant difference in the distant relapse rate, indicating that CRT likely had minimal affect on metastatic disease outside the radiation field. Two thirds of patients in GOG-123 had lesions ≥6 cm, and therefore, cisplatin apparently overcame some of the issues with lesion size noted in GOG-71 trial. The authors hypothesized that based on the results of the GOG-71 study, where adjuvant hysterectomy appeared to improve outcomes for patients with "small" IB-2 lesions (4–6 cm), adjuvant hysterectomy may have been of no benefit to patients in GOG-123 study. Thus, GOG-123 was designed to test the effects of cisplatin added to preoperative radiation for IB-2 lesions and perhaps the authors may have been in error suggesting that adjuvant hysterectomy was not therapeutically important without prospective randomized data [9]. Primary CRT versus radical hysterectomy was compared in the randomized GOG 201 trial; however, poor accrual lead to early termination of the trial, perhaps highlighting the polarized opinions of gynecologic and radiation oncologists regarding the best treatment of IB-2 cervical cancer.

Personal observations of our patients enrolled in the GOG-123 trial who often achieved complete clinical responses in the platinum arm and had acceptable surgical morbidity lead us to hypothesize that CRT followed by adjuvant hysterectomy was possibly the treatment of choice for stage IB-2 cervical carcinoma. Common and para-aortic lymphadenectomy was performed with hysterectomy in our protocol, recognizing the reported 10% incidence of occult para-aortic metastasis in patients with IB-2 cervix cancer [12]. Furthermore, brachytherapy dose was reduced from 30 to 15–18 Gy in order to limit radiation toxicities including vaginal stenosis. We hypothesized that the addition of cisplatin and the use of adjuvant hysterectomy likely diminish the therapeutic index of maximal brachytherapy, given that many patients were observed to have a complete clinical response prior to brachytherapy. Our bias was to avoid primary radical hysterectomy for patients with IB-2 lesions because the majority required postoperative pelvic chemoradiation [13, 14]. Furthermore, we found simple hysterectomy within 8 weeks of CRT technically easier to perform in obese patients than type III radical hysterectomy. Consequently the majority of patients with IB-2 lesions at our institution were treated on this protocol, other than a very few who were not deemed surgical candidates for medical reasons such as acute deep vein thrombosis.

This study represents one of the few investigations of patients with IB-2 carcinoma of the cervix that reports more than 5 years of median follow-up. Estimated 5-year DSS was 81% for the entire study group and 89% for the subgroup found to have no disease or only microscopic residual cervical disease and negative lymph nodes at surgery. In contrast, 10 out of 11 patients (91%) with common iliac or para-aortic nodal disease died from progressive disease. The subgroup of patients with microscopic nodal disease probably benefited from further therapy as their mean survival was 41 months, whereas those with CAT negative, but grossly bulky adenopathy at surgery had a mean survival of only 15 months. Because fluorodeoxyglucose–positron emission tomography (FDG-PET) imaging is more sensitive than CAT scanning for detecting metastatic disease [15], pretreatment screening with PET may allow exclusion of patients with occult para-aortic disease who would be less likely to benefit from adjuvant hysterectomy.

There were no central pelvic relapses and no patient required exenterative surgery in this study. In a recent retrospective investigation of primary cisplatin-based CRT, Goksedef et al. [4] reported an 86% 3-year OS. Seven of the 10 patients with recurrent disease had central pelvic recurrence, and the median TTP was only 22 months. Nevertheless, the authors concluded that completion hysterectomy was not necessary because overall patient survival was similar to the GOG-123 CRT arm. While the estimated 3-year survival may appear similar to the current study, it is possible that some patients with central relapse may have required exenterative surgery to achieve this survival, and longer follow-up would be necessary to be confident of that opinion.

Other potential disadvantages for primary CRT include short- and long-term side effects of radiation including vaginal stenosis and sexual dysfunction related to full-dose brachytherapy. Vaginal stenosis can lead to long-term sexual dysfunction, pain on examination, and difficulty diagnosing central disease recurrence. Vaginal stenosis is underreported or not quantified in the majority of studies but has been reported as high as 88% [7]. Intracavitary implants were shown to be associated with decrease in vaginal length, decreased coital

frequency and satisfaction, and increased dyspareunia [8]. A recent Cochrane review reported that there is no reliable evidence to show routine dilation during or after radiotherapy prevents late effects or improves quality of life and that treatment during radiation may be harmful [16].

The present study should be considered an exploratory analysis, and its limitations include those typically associated with observational, nonrandomized, retrospective studies. The relatively small sample size, lack of control group for comparison, and surgeon bias may have affected the findings by excluding poor surgical candidates. We could not accurately identify all patients with IB-2 lesions treated primarily with CRT or radical hysterectomy during the study period. CRT with simple hysterectomy was clearly our preferred management during the study period, and patients with severe comorbid illnesses were managed with primary CRT, undoubtedly enriching the outcomes in our study compared to what might be recognized in a multiinstitutional phase III trial. We also recognize that there were several radiation dosages outside our guidelines, which is inherent in a retrospective analysis. Chemotherapy was given postprotocol to some patients with residual disease at the discretion of the treating physician. There were not enough patients in this study to determine whether this effected survival. Strengths of the study include the mean follow-up time greater than 5 years and complete follow-up for all patients. We currently exclude patients with extrapelvic metastasis using FDG-PET scans and perform hysterectomy with aortic node dissection using robotic-assisted laparoscopic surgery. A prospective randomized trial of CRT and limited brachytherapy with adjuvant simple hysterectomy, compared to both primary CRT and primary radical hysterectomy, followed by risk-based CRT will be necessary to fully evaluate the efficacies and toxicities of these three approaches for IB-2 lesions.

Based on the observations in this study, we hypothesize that overall 5-year survival would be similar for the three treatment regimens in a phase III trial. However, we also predict that significant differences in acute and long-term morbidities, especially with respect to vaginal stenosis, bladder dysfunction, and central failure requiring pelvic exenteration, might also be recognized.

Declaration of interest The authors report no conflicts of interest. The authors alone are responsible for the content and writing of the paper.

References

1. Jemal A, Siegel R, Xu J et al (2010) Cancer statistics, 2010. CA Cancer J Clin 60:277–300
2. Eiffel PJ, Morris M, Wharton JT et al (1994) The influence of tumor size and morphology on the outcome of patients with FIGO

stage IB squamous cell carcinoma of the uterine cervix. Int J Radiat Oncol Biol Phys 29:9–16

3. Finan MA, DeCesare S, Fiorica J (1996) Radical hysterectomy for stage IB1 and IB2 carcinoma of the cervix: does the new staging system predict morbidity and survival? Gynecol Oncol 62:139–147

4. Goksedef BP, Kunos C, Belinson JL et al (2009) Concurrent cisplatin-based chemoradiation International Federation of Gynecology and Obstetrics stage IB2 cervical carcinoma. Am J Obstet Gynecol 200:175.e1–175.e5

5. Zivanovic O (2008) Treatment patterns of FIGO stage IB2 cervical cancer: a single institution experience of radical hysterectomy with individualized postoperative therapy and definitive radiation therapy. Gynecol Oncol 111:265–270

6. NCCN (2009) NCCN Clinical Practice Guidelines in Oncology™ v.1

7. Hartmann P, Diddle AW (1972) Vaginal stenosis following irradiation therapy for carcinoma of the cervix uteri. Cancer 30:426–429

8. Bruner DW, Lanciano R, Keegan M et al (1993) Vaginal stenosis and sexual function following intracavitary radiation for the treatment of cervical and endometrial cancer. Int J Radiat Oncol Biol Phys 27:825–830

9. Keys HM, Bundy BN, Stehman FB et al (1999) Cisplatin, radiation, and adjuvant hysterectomy compared with radiation and adjuvant hysterectomy for bulky stage IB cervical carcinoma. N Engl J Med 340:1154–1161

10. Ota T, Takeshima N, Tabata T et al (2007) Treatment of squamous cell carcinoma of the uterine cervix with radiation therapy alone: long-term survival, late complications, and incidence of second cancer. Br J Cancer 97:1058–1062

11. Keys HM, Bundy BN, Stehman FB et al (2003) Radiation therapy with and without extrafascial hysterectomy for bulky stage IB cervical carcinoma: a randomized trial of the Gynecologic Oncology Group. Gynecol Oncol 89:343–353

12. Averette HE, Nguyen HN, Donato DM et al (1993) Radical hysterectomy for invasive cervical cancer: a 25-year prospective experience with the Miami technique. Cancer 71(4 Suppl):1422–1437

13. Sedlis A, Bundy BN, Rotman MZ et al (1999) A randomized trial of pelvic radiation therapy versus no further therapy in selected patients with stage IB carcinoma of the cervix after radical hysterectomy and pelvic lymphadenectomy: a Gynecologic Oncology Group Study. Gynecol Oncol 73:177–183

14. Yessaian A, Magistris A, Burger RA et al (2004) Radical hysterectomy followed by tailored postoperative therapy in the treatment of stage IB-2 cervical cancer: feasibility and indications for adjuvant therapy. Gynecol Oncol 94:61–66

15. Goyal BK, Singh H, Kapur K et al (2010) Value of PET-CT in avoiding multimodality therapy in operable cervical cancer. Int J Gynecol Cancer 20:1041–1045

16. Miles T, Johnson N (2010) Vaginal dilator therapy for women receiving pelvic radiotherapy. Cochrane Database Syst Rev 9: CD007291

2

Total laparoscopic hysterectomy versus total abdominal hysterectomy with bilateral salpingo-oophorectomy for endometrial carcinoma

Kirsten B. Kluivers · Florien A. Ten Cate ·
Marlies Y. Bongers · Hans A. M. Brölmann ·
Jan C. M. Hendriks

Abstract This report is on recovery and long-term outcomes in a small-scale randomised controlled trial (RCT) after total laparoscopic hysterectomy versus total abdominal hysterectomy in (potential) endometrial carcinoma patients. An RCT was performed among women with atypical endometrial hyperplasia and endometrial carcinoma scheduled for hysterectomy in a teaching hospital in The Netherlands. Women were randomised to total laparoscopic hysterectomy versus total abdominal hysterectomy both with bilateral salpingo-oophorectomy and were followed until 5 years after the intervention. Patients completed the RAND 36-Item Short Form Health Survey (RAND-36), Quality of Recovery-40 (QoR-40) and Recovery Index-10 (RI-10) until 12 weeks after surgery. Main outcome measure was quality of life and recovery in the first 12 weeks after surgery. A linear mixed model was used for statistical analysis while accounting for baseline values where applicable. Seventeen women were included, of whom 11 allocated to the laparoscopic arm and 6 to the abdominal arm. Laparoscopic hysterectomy performed better on all scales and subscales used in the study. A statistically significant treatment effect, favouring laparoscopic hysterectomy, was found in the total RAND-36 (difference between groups 142 units, 95% confidence interval 46; 236). Clinical follow-up was completed after median 60 months, but this study was too small for conclusions regarding the safety and survival. Laparoscopic hysterectomy results in better postoperative quality of life in the first 12 weeks after surgery when compared with abdominal hysterectomy.

Keywords Abdominal hysterectomy · Endometrial carcinoma · Laparoscopic hysterectomy · Randomised · Recovery · Quality of life

K. B. Kluivers (✉)
Department of Obstetrics & Gynaecology,
Radboud University Nijmegen Medical Centre,
PO Box 9101, 6500 HB Nijmegen, The Netherlands
e-mail: K.Kluivers@obgyn.umcn.nl

F. A. Ten Cate · M. Y. Bongers
Department of Obstetrics & Gynaecology,
Máxima Medical Centre,
De Run 4600,
5504 DB Veldhoven, The Netherlands

H. A. M. Brölmann
Department of Obstetrics & Gynaecology,
VU University Medical Centre,
De Boelelaan 1117,
1081 HV Amsterdam, The Netherlands

J. C. M. Hendriks
Department of Epidemiology and Biostatistics,
Radboud University Nijmegen Medical Centre,
PO Box 9101, 6500 HB Nijmegen, The Netherlands

Background

Different approaches to hysterectomy have been extensively studied for the benign indications, and randomised controlled trials (RCTs) have been summarized in systematic review and meta-analysis [1]. One of the important results was a significant 2.6-fold increased risk of urinary tract injury. Recovery and quality of life were shown to be better after laparoscopic hysterectomy [2, 3]. In malignant disease, however, clinical outcomes such as complication rates or postoperative recovery may be different from the benign indications. The women are generally older, and the uterus is mostly smaller and less vascularised. And recurrence rate and survival rate are probably the most important long-term outcomes in these women.

At this moment, there are eight RCTs [4–12] available comparing laparoscopic and abdominal hysterectomy in (potential) endometrial carcinoma patients. Four RCTs [4–7] have been summarized in a systematic review in 2008 [13] and four further RCTs are available since then [8–12].

Quality of life was an outcome measure in four studies on 1,526 women [5, 9–11]. The laparoscopic approach was favourable in all studies, although this difference proved to be not clinically relevant in one study [9]. Better quality-of-life scores were found up till 3 months in one study [10] and up till 6 months after surgery in two further studies [5, 11].

Only two study groups on previous RCTs have already analysed the recurrence and survival rates by treatment group with 3 [4] and 6 years [12] median follow-up. These studies showed similar rates after laparoscopic and abdominal hysterectomy among 206 women. Data on recurrence and survival from the three large RCTs that have recently closed the inclusion on another 1,442 women are awaited with interest [9–11]. Future systematic review and meta-analysis of RCTs will provide a reliable answer to the question whether laparoscopic hysterectomy is a safe approach in women with endometrial cancer.

In the present paper, the results of a small RCT comparing total laparoscopic hysterectomy and total abdominal hysterectomy in women with atypical endometrial hyperplasia and endometrial carcinoma are presented. Postoperative quality of life as measured by the RAND-36 health survey and long-term clinical outcomes, including recurrence rates until 5 years after the intervention, have been assessed.

Methods

Participants

This study was performed in the Maxima Medical Centre, a large teaching hospital in the south of The Netherlands, from August 2002 through January 2005. The gynaecologic department is experienced in minimal invasive surgery, with 10 years experience in laparoscopic hysterectomy before the start of the study.

Patients were eligible for the study in case there was no suspicion of endometrial carcinoma beyond FIGO stage 1, and the size of the uterus did not exceed 18 weeks of gestation. Chest X-ray was performed in all women, but no routine hysteroscopy was performed for preoperative staging. Exclusion criteria were a previous lower abdominal midline incision, the need for simultaneous interventions and inability to speak Dutch. Approval for the study was obtained from the ethics committee of the Maxima Medical Centre on July 25, 2002 under number 0217. There is no overlap of the population with other published Dutch studies [3, 10]. Written informed consent was required for participation. The study was performed in line with the CONSORT statement.

Peritoneal fluid or cytological washing from the abdominal cavity was sent for pathology, but no standard peritoneal biopsies or lymphadenectomy was carried out in either group. No frozen sections were planned or performed. The laparoscopic procedures were total laparoscopic hysterectomies (TLH), where the operation of the vaginal part was restricted to the removal of the laparoscopically freed uterus, and the vaginal vault was sutured laparoscopically [2]. In laparoscopic hysterectomy, the uterus was manipulated by the Karl Storz Clermont-Ferrand manipulator (Karl Storz, Tuttlingen, Germany) after cauterization of the fallopian tubes to avoid spillage of cancer cells. In abdominal hysterectomy, the uterus was manipulated with the use of two Heaney clamps placed over the fallopian tube–ovarian ligament complex on both sides. There was an equal dissection of pelvic tissues in the laparoscopic as compared with the open technique.

The primary outcome of this study was quality of life. Three questionnaires have been used in the study: the RAND-36 health survey (RAND-36), Quality of Recovery-40 (QoR-40) and Recovery Index-10 (RI-10). The three questionnaires have previously been validated for the Dutch language [14, 15]. The RAND-36 is a generic health-related quality-of-life questionnaire. The questionnaire measures subjective health in eight scales, which range from 0 to 100. Thus, the total score ranges from 0 to 800, where 0 is the poorest quality of life and 800 the best imaginable. Summated ratings and standardized scoring algorithms were used to assess the eight scales [14]. The QoR-40 and RI-10 are postoperative recovery-specific questionnaires [15]. The QoR-40 consists of 40 items in five subscales: emotional state, physical comfort, psychological support, physical independence and pain. Each item was answered on a five-point Likert scale, ranging from none of the time to all the time. The QoR-40 score was defined as the sum of the scores of all items. The QoR-40 score ranged from 40 to 200, in which 200 indicates a perfect recovery. The items referred to the past 24 h and aimed at patients during hospital stay, but could be filled out at home as well. The RI-10 is a ten-item questionnaire measuring postoperative recovery on five-point Likert scales ranging from full disagreement to full agreement. The instrument has no separate subscales, and the score ranges from 10 to 50, where 50 indicates a perfect recovery. The items referred to the past week. Since most of the items in the RI-10 referred to the postoperative situation, no baseline measurement was available. The items suited best for recently discharged patients, but could be filled out in hospital as well.

Patients filled out the questionnaires without assistance of the researcher and returned the questionnaires by mail. The baseline measurement was completed after randomisation. Measurement moments were as proposed for surgical studies in the previous validation study [15].

The surgical outcome (peri and postoperative clinical outcome) and oncological outcome (recurrence and survival rates) were secondary outcome measures of the study. FIGO nomenclature (Rio de Janeiro 1988) was used to describe surgical cancer stages. The decision for postoperative external beam pelvic radiotherapy was made as based on the PORTEC trial [16]. Data were collected by completion of a standardized case record form. At the end of follow-up in the present study (June 2008), all patients were interviewed on any adverse outcomes or events from the condition or surgery. In case no written reply was received, telephone calls were made to complete these data.

Sample size and randomisation

The study has been performed parallel to a larger study on laparoscopic versus abdominal hysterectomy in benign conditions [2]. For that study, the sample size was calculated for the quality of life as measured by the questionnaire RAND-36. A difference of 15 per scale was considered as clinically relevant. With a standard deviation of 20, a type I error of 0.05, and 80% power, 28 patients were needed per arm.

After obtaining written informed consent, randomisation took place by opening numbered, sealed opaque envelopes. For concealment, an independent person had randomly assigned an equal number of 38 papers with either intervention to the envelopes. The closed envelopes were shuffled before numbering, and were used for both patients with benign and malignant disease. The patients and medical team were not blinded to the intervention.

Statistical methods

The data are presented on intention-to-treat basis. The medians with the range are presented in case of continuous data and absolute numbers with percentages in case of dichotomous variables. Differences in medical outcome between the two treatment groups were tested for statistical significance using the Mann–Whitney U test in case of continuous data, and the Fisher's exact test in case of two by two tables. A linear mixed model was used to study the differences in scores on the questionnaires between the laparoscopic and abdominal group over time while accounting for the baseline values for each of the scales and subscales separately [17]. The dependent variable was the (sub)scale of RAND-36, QoR-40 or RI-10. The independent class variables were patient and treatment (laparoscopic and abdominal hysterectomy, respectively) and time since surgery, and the independent regression variables was the baseline level. Both the intercept and the regression in time of each patient were treated as random variables in the model. This way differences between treatments are estimated given the baseline value, while differences in recovery among patients are allowed. Initially, interaction terms and quadratic terms in time were included in the linear part of the model; but as the inclusion did not significantly (likelihood-ratio test) improve the fit to the data, these terms were not included in the final model used [17]. Note that excluding the interaction term of group with time, results in a parallel line model, (i.e. the differences between groups are identical at each point of measurement). The estimated regression parameters with standard errors of each score are used to calculate the average level per week of the patients in each group. These levels with confidence bands are further presented in figures.

The quality-of-life data were analysed by SAS 8.2 software (SAS Institute, Inc., Chicago, IL, USA), all other data in SPSS 16.0 software (SPSS, Inc., Chicago, IL, USA), with p values <0.05 considered statistically significant.

Findings

Seventeen women were randomised, of whom 11 were allocated to the laparoscopic arm and 6 were allocated to the abdominal arm. Patient characteristics and surgical indications are shown in Table 1. A flowchart of the study is presented in Fig. 1. Overall median clinical follow-up after the operation was 60 months (range 18–81 months) until the last gynaecological examination. The interviews on any adverse outcomes were minimum 45 months after surgery (median 65 months, range 45–81 months). No women were lost to follow-up.

The surgical and oncological outcome

Data on the procedures including histological findings are presented in Table 2. There was one intra-operative conversion from laparoscopy to laparotomy, which was related to difficult access due to adiposity and 300 mL blood loss during laparoscopy. Her recovery and follow-up were uneventful. All other laparoscopic hysterectomies were performed as TLH. There was no macroscopically visible or palpable tumour extra-uterine tumour in either group. All final histologies showed endometroid type adenocarcinoma, except in a woman with FIGO

Table 1 Patient characteristics and surgical indications by treatment group

	LH (*n*=11)	AH (*n*=6)
Age (years)	59 [49–69]	64 [59–73]
BMI (kg/m^2)	27 [21–50]	27 [21–32]
Parity	2 [0–4]	2 [0–6]
ASA score	2 [1–3]	1 [1–2]
Uterine weight (g)	100 [50–175]	75 [50–280]
Indication for surgery		
Atypical hyperplasia	3 (27%)	2 (33%)
Endometrial carcinoma	8 (73%)	4 (66%)
Baseline RAND-36	581 [366–744]	670 [278–726]
QoR-40	183 [147–200]	184 [157–200]
RI-10	n.a.	n.a.

Data presented as median [range] or absolute numbers (percentage)]

AH abdominal hysterectomy, *ASA* American Society of Anesthesiologists, *BMI* body mass index, *LH* laparoscopic hysterectomy, *RAND-36* RAND 36-Item Short Form Health Survey, *QoR-40* Quality of Recovery-40, *RI-10* Recovery Index-10, *n.a.* not applicable

stage 3a grade 2 in the laparoscopic hysterectomy group, who had a mixed-cell type tumour (endometroid and serous adenocarcinoma).

Complications by treatment group are presented in Table 3. In one patient, randomised to abdominal hysterectomy, final histology demonstrated that the cervix had not been removed completely in a woman with atypical endometrial hyperplasia. It has been decided not to perform a reoperation. Her follow-up has been uneventful, besides a tension-free vaginal tape (TVT)] procedure, which has been performed due to deterioration of stress urinary incontinence 2 years postoperatively. Other complications in the abdominal hysterectomy group were: 1,450 mL blood loss during surgery, one woman with temporary atrial flutter, one woman with temporary low oxygenation, a urinary tract infection and fever of unknown origin in the immediate postoperative period. One woman developed radiation colitis after radiotherapy.

In the laparoscopic hysterectomy group, two women died because of a recurrent endometrial carcinoma. Of these two women, one was a 57-year-old woman with Figo stage 1c grade 2 disease, and no postoperative radiotherapy had a locoregional recurrence 12 months after surgery and died 2 months later. A stent was inserted for bowel obstruction, but the extensiveness of the metastases and her general condition did not allow for any adjuvant therapy. The other was a 64-year-old woman with the mixed cell-type tumour stage 3a grade 2 underwent pelvic radiotherapy and had a recurrence 11 months after surgery. Her general condition did not allow for

adjuvant chemotherapy, and she died 18 months after surgery. Other complications in the laparoscopic hysterectomy group were a urinary tract infection, deterioration of pre-operative micturition problems with long-term catheterization, back pain for which a neurologist was consulted but found no abnormalities. One woman developed radiation colitis after radiotherapy. No other complications (such as blood transfusions, visceral damage or port-site metastasis) occurred in either group.

Quality of life and recovery

Overall, only four questionnaires were missing, and thus, the return rate of the questionnaires was 97%. Table 4 and Fig. 2a, b and c show the differences in total scores on the three questionnaires between laparoscopic and abdominal hysterectomy. No scale or subscale was in favour of abdominal hysterectomy. The difference between groups in

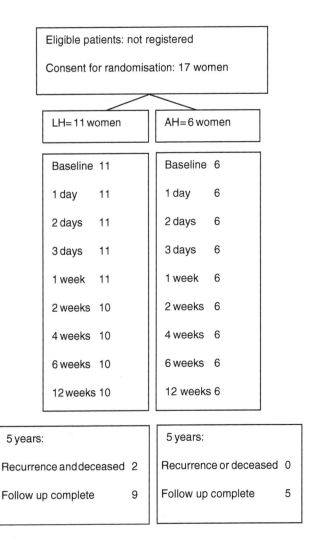

Fig. 1 Flowchart of the study

Table 2 Data on surgical procedures and oncological outcome by treatment group

	LH (n=11)	AH (n=6)	P value
Intra-operative laparoconversion	1 (9%)	n.a.	n.a.
Operation time (min)	122 [96–168]	80 [70–192]	0.03
Blood loss (mL)	200 [0–550]	350 [300–1450]	0.01
Hospitalization (days)	5 [4–16]	8 [5–11]	0.03
Clinical follow-up (months)	54 [18–80]	64 [50–81]	0.09
Diseased after recurrence	2 (18%)	0	0.40
Postoperative histology			
Normal	1 (9%)	0	
Atypical hyperplasia	0	1 (17%)	
Endometrial carcinoma[a]	10 (91%)	5 (83%)	0.60
Postoperative radiotherapy	3 (27%)	3 (50%)	0.34

Data shown as absolute numbers (percentage) or median [range]. $p = p$ value for differences between groups using Fisher's exact test in cases of 2-by-2 tables, and Mann–Whitney test in cases of non-normal distributed numerical variables

AH abdominal hysterectomy, *LH* laparoscopic hysterectomy, *n.a.* not applicable

[a] Endometrial carcinomas were stage 1b grade 1 (2 patients), 1c grade 1, 2a grade 1, and 3a grade 1 in the AH group, and 1a grade 1, 1b grade 1 (3 patients), 1b grade 2, 1c grade 1, 1c grade 2 (2 patients), 2b grade 1 and 3a grade 2 in the LH group. All histologies showed endometroid type adenocarcinoma, except one woman in the LH group with stage 3a grade 2 mixed cell-type tumour (endometroid and serous adenocarcinoma)

the RAND-36 total score was 142 units (95% confidence interval (CI) 46; 236) in favour of laparoscopic hysterectomy. Furthermore, in three RAND-36 subscales relating to physical well-being, statistically significant treatment effects in favour of laparoscopic hysterectomy were found (data not shown). One QoR-40 subscale and the total RI-10 showed borderline significant differences. Note that the difference between the treatment groups are presented after correction for differences in baseline values between the groups. The estimated increase per 10 units higher level in the total RAND-36 score at baseline between two patients was 7 (95%CI 4; 11) units. This was independent of both timepoint and treatment group. Furthermore, the estimated increase in the total RAND-36 score at 12 weeks after surgery compared with

1 week after surgery was 122 (95% CI 67; 178) units in both groups.

Conclusions

In this RCT, the difference in recovery was assessed between total laparoscopic hysterectomy and total abdominal hysterectomy, both with bilateral salpingo-oophorectomy, in patients scheduled for hysterectomy for reason of atypical endometrial hyperplasia or endometrial carcinoma. After baseline correction, we report a statistically significant difference in postoperative quality of life as measured by RAND-36, favouring laparoscopic hysterectomy. This difference between the treatment groups was present all along the

Table 3 Complications by treatment group

AH abdominal hysterectomy, *LH* laparoscopic hysterectomy, *n.a.* not applicable

Data shown as absolute numbers (percentage). $p = p$ value for difference between groups using Fisher's exact test

[a] Deterioration stress urinary incontinence

[b] TVT increased residual urine with self-catheterization

[c] Note that three women in each group received radiotherapy

	LH (n=11)	AH (n=6)	P value
Blood loss >1,000 cm³	0	1 (17%)	0.35
Fever (unknown origin)	0	1 (17%)	0.35
Urinary tract infection	1 (9%)	1 (17%)	1.0
Cervical stump problems	0	1 (17%)	0.35
Urinary symptoms	1 (9%) [a]	1 (17%) [b]	1.0
Temporary low saturation	0	1 (17%)	0.35
Atrial flutter	0	1 (17%)	0.35
Back pain	1 (9%)	0	1.0
Radiation colitis	1 (33%) [c]	1 (33%) [c]	1.0
Total complications	4	8	n.a.
No of patients with complications	3 (27%)	5 (83%)	0.05

Table 4 Estimated increase in questionnaire score level (95% confidence interval) by treatment group, by unit increase in baseline score and point of measurement using a linear mixed model

	RAND-36	QoR-40	RI-10
Treatment group[a]			
LH	142 (46; 236)	9 (−3; 21)	7 (0; 14)
AH	0 (reference)	0 (reference)	0 (reference)
Baseline effect			
per 10 units[b]	7 (4; 11)	5 (1; 9)	n.a.
Time after surgery			
1 day	n.a.	0 (reference)	n.a.
2 days	n.a.	4 (−3; 12)	n.a.
3 days	n.a.	4 (−4; 11)	n.a.
1 week	0 (reference)	13 (6; 20)	0 (reference)
2 weeks	−8 (−64; 47)	26 (18; 33)	0 (−3; 2)
4 weeks	49 (−6; 105)	n.a.	4 (1; 6)
6 weeks	130 (74; 185)	n.a.	6 (4; 9)
12 weeks	122 (67; 178)	n.a.	8 (5; 11)

Example: On average, the estimated level of the total RAND-36 score in the LH group was 142 units higher as compared with the AH group, at each timepoint from 2 to 12 weeks after surgery. The estimated increase per 10 units higher level in the total RAND-36 score at baseline between two patients was 7 units. This was independent of both timepoint and treatment group. Furthermore, the estimated increase in the total RAND-36 score at 12 weeks after surgery, compared to 1 week after surgery, was 122 units in both groups

Because the data fit very well to the parallel-line model the differences over time after surgery is estimated to be identical in both groups (see also Fig. 2a, b and c)

LH laparoscopic hysterectomy, *AH* abdominal hysterectomy, *RAND-36* RAND 36-Item Short Form Health Survey, *QoR-40* Quality of Recovery-40, *RI-10* Recovery Index-10, *n.a.* not applicable

[a] Difference between groups after correction for baseline differences

[b] The baseline effect is the increase in postoperative score per 10 units increase at baseline

recovery period until 12 weeks after surgery. All subscales of RAND-36 and QoR-40, as well as the RI-10, showed a favourable outcome after laparoscopic hysterectomy compared with abdominal hysterectomy. This is in agreement with other studies on quality of life after surgery in (potential) endometrial carcinoma patients [5, 9–11] and our previous findings in a larger benign population [2]. We found that the laparoscopic procedure took longer to perform, but with regard to other surgical and oncological outcomes, the present study is limited by its small sample size. These data may however be useful in future meta-analysis on the topic.

Lymphadenectomy has not been performed in this study amongst women with clinical stage I disease with expected low-grade endometrial carcinoma based on endometrial biopsy. Recently, two RCTs have failed to

demonstrate any advantage over routine lymphadenectomy in endometrial carcinoma patients [18]. Nonetheless, routine lymphadenectomy in endometrial carcinoma is still under debate [19]. It is common practice throughout the Netherlands to perform hysterectomy and bilateral salpingo-oophorectomy in these women and advice postoperative radiotherapy as based on the PORTEC studies [16, 20]. Thus, the results from our trial are limited to the population undergoing this type of treatment. Furthermore, note that PORTEC-2 data were not yet available at the time of the study [21], and no vaginal brachytherapy has been applied in the study.

In hysterectomies performed for potential malignant indications, recurrence and survival rates are of utmost importance. Although, there are no indications that laparoscopy is less safe [5, 12], this has not definitively been proven until now. In the present study, two women in the laparoscopic arm had a recurrence and died due to their malignancy. One woman had a bad prognosis due to a high-stage mixed cell tumour. In line with the PORTEC study, the other woman had not received postoperative radiotherapy to minimize her risk of locoregional recurrence. With a FIGO stage 1c grade 2 and aged 57 years, she was, however, rather close to the range of less favourable prognostic factors with indication for radiotherapy.

Not only the route of hysterectomy, e.g. abdominal or laparoscopic hysterectomy, may influence recurrence rates and all other potential factors should thus be reported in according studies. In the present study, for example, an intra-uterine manipulator has been used. The impact on outcomes as compared with, e.g. vaginal manipulation with a tube only is not known until now. In two previous studies on peritoneal washings before and after manipulation with an intra-uterine device, spread of malignant cells could be demonstrated in 2 out of 82 women with negative peritoneal washings prior to manipulation [22, 23]. Only one of these two women has sufficiently long follow-up (28 months) to report that no recurrence of malignancy has occurred [23]. Another histological phenomenon, "vascular pseudo invasion" of tumour into the blood vessels, has been described after manipulation with an intra-uterine balloon causing high intra-uterine pressures. Since this may have consequences for the staging and further therapy, this phenomenon may be regarded as undesirable and awareness among pathologists is needed [24].

The finding that quality of life was better after laparoscopic hysterectomy goes hand in hand with a different spectrum of complications as compared with other types of hysterectomy. A meta-analysis on benign indications reported a significant 2.6-fold increased risk of urinary tract injury [1]. Whether this also applies to endometrial

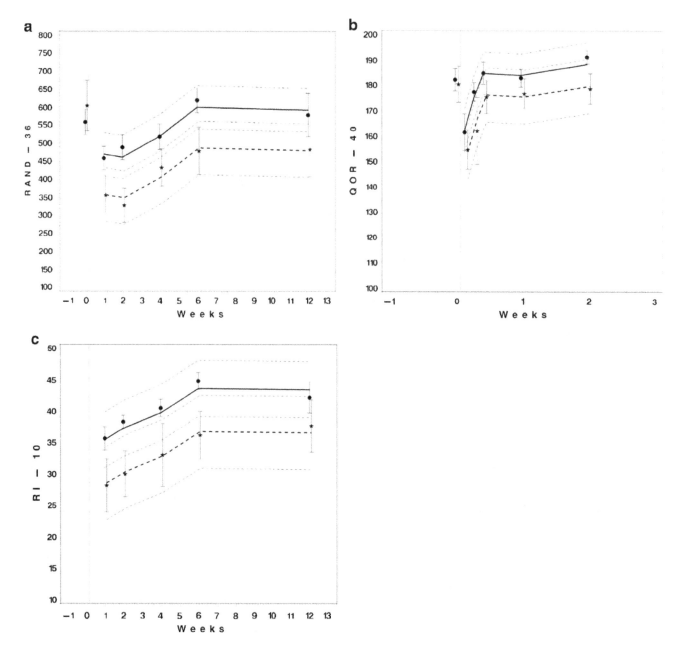

Fig. 2 a, b and **c**. The mean levels of the questionnaire scores after surgery by treatment group. The *symbols* indicate the observed mean and the *vertical bars* indicate ±one standard deviation. The *thick lines* indicate the estimated mean profiles and the *thin, short dashed lines* indicate the appropriate 95% confidence bands using a linear mixed model that accounts for the baseline value. Women in the laparoscopic hysterectomy group: *dot, solid line*. Women in the abdominal hysterectomy group: *star, thick dashed line*. *RAND-36* RAND 36-Item Short Form Health Survey, *QoR-40* Quality of Recovery-40, *RI-10* Recovery Index-10. Note that the data fit very well to the *parallel-line* model

carcinoma patients has not yet been unravelled, and cannot be concluded from the present study. The incidence of major complications in laparoscopic hysterectomy may, however, be highly reduced with experience of the surgeon. In Finland, the incidence of urinary tract injury in laparoscopic hysterectomy decreased from 1.4% to 0.7% in recent years [25]. Ureteral damage now happens in only 0.3% of cases, which seems comparable to abdominal

hysterectomy. Dependent on patient preference, the potential risks should be weighed against the improved quality of life after surgery in individual cases.

The conclusion from this small RCT was that laparoscopic hysterectomy was associated with better quality of life in the recovery period as compared to abdominal hysterectomy in women with atypical endometrial hyperplasia and endometrial carcinoma.

Acknowledgements   We thank J.M. (Hanny) Pijnenborg, MD, PhD for her careful review of the gynaecologic oncology aspects of the paper.

Conflicts of interest   The authors report no conflicts of interest.

References

1. Nieboer TE, Johnson N, Lethaby A et al (2009) Surgical approach to hysterectomy for benign gynaecological disease. Cochrane Database Syst Rev. 8:CD003677
2. Kluivers KB, Hendriks JC, Mol BW, Bongers MY, Bremer GL, de Vet HC, Vierhout ME, Brolmann HAM (2007) Quality of life and surgical outcome after total laparoscopic hysterectomy versus total abdominal hysterectomy for benign disease: a randomized, controlled trial. J Minim Invasive Gynecol 14:145–152
3. Kluivers KB, Johnson NP, Chien P, Vierhout ME, Bongers M, Mol BW (2008) Comparison of laparoscopic and abdominal hysterectomy in terms of quality of life: a systematic review. Eur J Obstet Gynecol Reprod Biol 136:3–8
4. Tozzi R, Malur S, Koehler C, Schneider A (2005) Analysis of morbidity in patients with endometrial cancer: is there a commitment to offer laparoscopy? Gynecol Oncol 97:4–9
5. Zullo F, Palomba S, Russo T et al (2005) A prospective randomized comparison between laparoscopic and laparotomic approaches in women with early stage endometrial cancer: a focus on the quality of life. Am J Obstet Gynecol 193:1344–1352
6. Fram KM (2002) Laparoscopically assisted vaginal hysterectomy versus abdominal hysterectomy in stage I endometrial cancer. Int J Gynecol Cancer 12:57–61
7. Zorlu CG, Simsek T, Seker Ari E (2005) Laparoscopy or laparotomy for the management of endometrial cancer. JSLS 9:442–446
8. Malzoni M, Tinelli R, Cosentino F, Perone C, Rasile M, Iuzzolino D, Malzoni C, Reich H (2009) Total laparoscopic hysterectomy versus abdominal hysterectomy with lymphadenectomy for early-stage endometrial cancer: a prospective randomized study. Gynecol Oncol 112:126–133
9. Kornblith AB, Huang HQ, Walker JL, Spirtos NM, Rotmensch J, Cella D (2009) Quality of life of patients with endometrial cancer undergoing laparoscopic international federation of gynecology and obstetrics staging compared with laparotomy: a Gynecologic Oncology Group study. J Clin Oncol 27(32):5337–5342
10. Mourits MJ, Bijen CB, Arts HJ, ter Brugge HG, van der Sijde R, Paulsen L, Wijma J, Bongers MY, Post WJ, van der Zee AG, de Bock GH (2010) Safety of laparoscopy versus laparotomy in early-stage endometrial cancer: a randomised trial. Lancet Oncol 11(8):763–771
11. Janda M, Gebski V, Brand A, Hogg R, Jobling TW, Land R, Manolitsas T, McCartney A, Nascimento M, Neesham D, Nicklin JL, Oehler MK, Otton G, Perrin L, Salfinger S, Hammond I, Leung Y, Walsh T, Sykes P, Ngan H, Garrett A, Laney M, Ng TY, Tam K, Chan K, Wrede CD, Pather S, Simcock B, Farrell R, Obermair A (2010) Quality of life after total laparoscopic hysterectomy versus total abdominal hysterectomy for stage I endometrial cancer (LACE): a randomised trial. Lancet Oncol 11 (8):772–780
12. Zullo F, Palomba S, Falbo A, Russo T, Mocciaro R, Tartaglia E, Tagliaferri P, Mastrantonio P (2009) Laparoscopic surgery vs laparotomy for early stage endometrial cancer: long-term data of a randomized controlled trial. Am J Obstet Gynecol 200(3):296.e1–296.e9
13. de la Orden SG, Reza MM, Blasco JA, Andradas E, Callejo D, Pérez T (2008) Laparoscopic hysterectomy in the treatment of endometrial cancer: a systematic review. J Minim Invasive Gynecol 15:395–401
14. van der Zee KI, Sanderman R (1993) Het meten van de gezondheidstoestand met de Rand – 36, een handleiding. Noordelijk Centrum voor gezondheidsvraagstukken, Groningen
15. Kluivers KB, Hendriks JC, Mol BW, Bongers MY, Vierhout ME, Brölmann HA, de Vet HC (2008) Clinimetric properties of 3 instruments measuring postoperative recovery in a gynecologic surgical population. Surgery 144:12–21
16. Creutzberg CL, van Putten WL, Koper PC, Lybeert ML, Jobsen JJ, Wárlám-Rodenhuis CC, De Winter KA, Lutgens LC, van den Bergh AC, van de Steen-Banasik E, Beerman H, van Lent M (2000) Surgery and postoperative radiotherapy versus surgery alone for patients with stage-1 endometrial carcinoma: multicentre randomised trial. Lancet 355:1404–1411
17. Verbeke G, Molenberghs G (1997) Linear mixed models in practice: a SAS-oriented approach. Springer, New York
18. ASTEC study group, Kitchener H, Swart AM, Qian Q, Amos C, Parmar MK (2009) Efficacy of systematic pelvic lymphadenectomy in endometrial cancer (MRC ASTEC trial): a randomised study. Lancet 373:125–136
19. Benedetti PP, Basile S, Maneschi F (2008) Systematic pelvic lymphadenectomy vs. no lymphadenectomy in early-stage endometrial carcinoma: randomized clinical trial. J Natl Cancer Inst 100:1707–1716
20. Mourits MJ, Bijen CB, de Bock GH (2009) Lymphadenectomy in endometrial cancer. Lancet 373:1169
21. Nout RA, Smit VT, Putter H, Jürgenliemk-Schulz IM, Jobsen JJ, Lutgens LC, van der Steen-Banasik EM, Mens JW, Slot A, Kroese MC, van Bunningen BN, Ansink AC, van Putten WL (2010) PORTEC Study Group. Vaginal brachytherapy versus pelvic external beam radiotherapy for patients with endometrial cancer of high-intermediate risk (PORTEC-2): an open-label, non-inferiority, randomised trial. Lancet 375:816–823
22. Eltabbakh GH, Mount SL (2006) Laparoscopic surgery does not increase the positive peritoneal cytology among women with endometrial carcinoma. Gynecol Oncol 100:361–364
23. Lim S, Kim HS, Lee KB, Yoo CW, Park SY, Seo SS (2008) Does the use of a uterine manipulator with an intrauterine balloon in total laparoscopic hysterectomy facilitate tumor cell spillage into the peritoneal cavity in patients with endometrial cancer? Int J Gynecol Cancer 18:1145–1149
24. Logani S, Herdman AV, Little JV, Moller KA (2008) Vascular "pseudo invasion" in laparoscopic hysterectomy specimens: a diagnostic pitfall. Am J Surg Pathol 32:560–565
25. Brummer TH, Seppälä TT, Härkki PS (2008) National learning curve for laparoscopic hysterectomy and trends in hysterectomy in Finland 2000–2005. Hum Reprod 23:840–845

3

Robot-assisted radical hysterectomy—perioperative and survival outcomes in patients with cervical cancer compared to laparoscopic and open radical surgery

Grigor Gortchev · Slavcho Tomov ·
Latchesar Tantchev · Angelika Velkova ·
Zdravka Radionova

Abstract In this study, perioperative outcomes and survival data in patients with early cervical cancer operated with three surgical methods: robot-assisted, laparoscopic and open, are to be analyzed. From January 2006 to May 2010, 294 patients with T1B1 cervical cancer were studied retrospectively. Robot-assisted radical hysterectomy (RARH) was performed in 73 (24.8%) of them, laparoscopic-assisted radical vaginal hysterectomy (LARVH) in 46 (15.6%) and, in 175, (59.5%), abdominal radical hysterectomy (ARH). Mean hospital stay of patients with RARH and LARVH was 4.1 ± 0.7 and 4.8 ± 0.5, respectively, and of those with ARH, 9.6 ± 1.0 days ($p=0.001$). Mean operative time was 152.2 ± 26.5 min for the robotic group as it was significantly shorter in comparison with the laparoscopic group (232.1 ± 61.7 min) and laparotomy group (168.2 ± 31.1 min) ($p=0.001$). The application of Cox regression analysis found that the regional lymph node metastases were of significant value for disease-free survival (DSF), and the nodal status and recurrence presence—for overall survival (OS). Type of surgical procedure did not influence DSF, as well as OS. RARH has been established to be a safe procedure with proven advantages in regard to operative time and hospital stay. The absence of significant differences in DSF and OS is a substantial reason to continue, from an oncologic point of view, the application of this method on patients with T1B1 cervical cancer.

G. Gortchev (✉) · S. Tomov · L. Tantchev · A. Velkova ·
Z. Radionova
Gynecologic Oncology Clinic, Medical University,
8A, Georgi Kochev Blvd,
Pleven 5800, Bulgaria
e-mail: oncogynec@yahoo.com

Keywords Robot-assisted radical hysterectomy · Cervical cancer · Perioperative outcomes · Survival outcomes

Background

After the first attempts of Nezhat et al. and Canis et al. in the radical laparoscopic hysterectomy, the beginning of the minimally invasive surgery for treatment of cervical carcinoma had been initiated [1, 2].

Conventional laparoscopy has some shortcomings, which premise that the method is mastered with difficulty for a longer period of time, and requires the development of specific coordination skills. The nature of the laparoscopic instruments proposes decreased tactile sensation and paradoxical movements. Hand tremor increases toward the distal end. The effector end of the instruments is with limited motions. The monitor reproduces the operative field in two dimensions, which is connected with a change in the coordination of the "eye–hand" feedback. In most cases, the surgeon works in insufficiently ergonomic position and environment. All these circumstances shape a barrier difficult to be surmounted by a beginning laparoscopist, especially in the cases when a radical laparoscopic surgery is needed [3].

Robotic surgical systems overcome a great part of the disadvantages of the classic laparoscopy. Robotic instruments have seven degrees of freedom, similar to those of the human arm, as the computer interphase eliminates the natural tremor. Sitting behind the console, the surgeon works comfortably in an ergonomic environment, and the image is three-dimensional. In 2006, Sert and Abeler describe the technique of the first robot-assisted laparoscopic radical hysterectomy (Piver type III) [4]. Data about more than 300 radical robotic hysterectomies for cervical cancer have been published from 2006 to 2009 [4–12]. Literature data concern basically the perioperative results because of the short period of incorporation of the robotic technology in the gynecologic oncology practice [6, 7, 13]. There are a few publications, which assess the survival outcomes of patients with cervical cancer and compare the three radical surgical methods—robotic, laparoscopic, and open [9, 14].

The goal of this study was to analyze our experience in the robotic radical hysterectomy and to compare the perioperative outcomes and preliminary results of survival of patients with early cervical cancer with those of the laparoscopic and open radical surgery.

Material and methods

From January 2006 to May 2010 in the Gynecologic Oncology Clinic, Medical University Pleven, Bulgaria, 294 patients with T1b1 cervical cancer were operated. Robot-assisted radical hysterectomy (RARH) was accomplished in 73 (24.8%) of them, laparoscopic-assisted radical vaginal hysterectomy (LARVH) in 46 (15.6%), and abdominal radical hysterectomy (ARH) in 175 (59.5%). From January 2006 to December 2007, the LARVH cohort of patients was treated. The program in robot-assisted gynecologic surgery and telemedicine, which major task was the implementation and development of the robotic technology in the gynecologic oncology practice, started in January 2008 at our institution. The operating team, consisting of console surgeon, bed-side assistant and bed-side nurse, was trained on porcine model to work with the robotic system at the European training center in Strasbourg. The console surgeon was trained additionally at the Division of Gynecology Oncology, Department of Obstetrics and Gynecology, University of North Carolina at Chapel Hill, USA. The application of the LARVH was gradually reduced after the installation of the robotic system da Vinci S and the beginning of the robotic program. RARHs included in the analysis were accomplished from May 2008 to May 2010, and the radical abdominal hysterectomies from January 2006 to May 2010. All robotic and laparoscopic procedures were accomplished by one surgeon, and the open procedures by two surgeons using one and the same operative methods.

Patients' data were collected retrospectively from the hospital record (history of present illness) and the Bulgarian National Cancer Registry. The da Vinci S system (Intuitive Surgical, Sunnyvale, CA, USA), located in the operating room for laparoscopic and telesurgery (OR1, Karl Storz, Germany) was used for the robotic surgery. The location of the da Vinci S system components is adapted to the specific conditions in OR1. The surgeon's console is located on the left side of the patient, the patient cart—facing the patient's feet, and the vision cart, bed-side assistant and scrub nurse—on the right side of the patient. Patient is placed on the operating table in dorsal lithotomy and in steep Trendelenburg position. Insufflation of CO_2 is accomplished in the upper left abdominal quadrant with Optical Veress (Karl Storz). RARH, which we perform, corresponds to class III radical hysterectomy according to Piver et al. [15]. A detailed description of the positioning and placement of trocars and the operative technique was presented by us in a publication in *Gynecological Surgery* journal [16].

The laparoscopic-assisted radical vaginal hysterectomy technique applied by us is similar to LARVH type III, described by Koehler et al. [17].

Data were processed with the statistical package SPSS 13.1., as the following methods were applied: descriptive analysis, variation analysis, cross tabulation, ANOVA, and χ^2 tests. Log rank, Breslow, and Tarone–Ware methods were used for the assessment of influence availability of the investigated parameters on survival, and the Cox regression model was applied for quantitative assessment of the influence of these factors on survival.

Findings

The mean age of the patients with RARH was 46.0± 11.2 years, and of those with LARVH and ARH, 42.5± 9.9 years and 49.0±11.0 years, respectively, as it was significantly lowest in the group with LARVH ($p=0.001$). In the abdominal radical surgery group, the cases between 50 and 59 years of age (49/28.0%) were predominating, and in the minimally invasive surgery, between 40 and 49 years of age (RARH, 24/32.9%; LARVH, 17/37.0%) ($p=0.003$). The preoperative stage, according to FIGO for the whole group of 294 patients, was assessed as Ib1. Metastases in the regional pelvic lymph nodes were diagnosed after the performance of the operative intervention in 59 (20.1%) patients (pT1b1 pN1 pM0). The distribution of the cases with metastatic lymph nodes according to the operation type was as follows: RARH, 12/16.4%; LARVH, 5/10.9%; and ARH, 42/24.0%, as the differences were insignificant ($p=0.095$). The average number of the removed lymph nodes was 11.4±7.0 (range 2–56) for RARH, 11.3±5.2 (range 3–24) for LARVH, and 15.9±7.7 (range 2–46) for ARH. The differences between RARH and ARH, and between LARVH and ARH are significant ($p=0.001$). The histological study determined that in the robotic cohort 65 (89.0%) of the patients were with squamous cell carcinoma (SCC) and 8 (11.0%) with adenocarcinoma; in the laparoscopic cohort, 41 (89.1%) were with SCC and 5 (10.9%) with adenocarcinoma, and in the laparotomy cohort, they were respectively 167 (95.4%) and 8 (4.6%) ($p=0.116$).

The values of the preoperative hematocrit, postoperative hematocrit on the first day after the operation, and the difference between the pre- and postoperative hematocrit, were investigated. The average preoperative hematocrit values distinguished significantly (RARH, 0.369±0.039; LARVH, 0.375±0.037; ARH, 0.359±0.042) (p=0.035), and those of the postoperative hematocrit insignificantly (RARH, 0.317± 0.035; LARVH, 0.330±0.031; ARH, 0.318±0.045) (p= 0.153). The difference between the pre- and postoperative hematocrit was insignificant (RARH, 0.052±0.039; LARVH, 0.045±0.036; ARH, 0.041±0.035) (p=0.253). The main patient and tumor characteristics are summarized in Table 1.

The operative time was determined as the time between the beginning of the skin incision and the last skin stitch placement (incision time—skin closed time). Mean operative time was 152.2±26.5 min for the robotic group and significantly shorter in comparison with the laparoscopic group (232.1±61.7 min) and laparotomy group (168.2± 31.1 min) (p=0.001). The RARH and LARVH learning

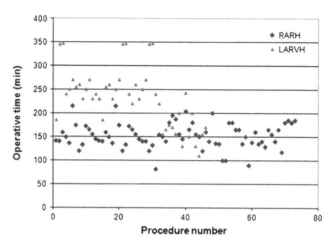

Fig. 1 Learning curve of the robot-assisted radical hysterectomy and laparoscopic-assisted radical vaginal hysterectomy

curve is presented in Fig. 1. The robotic radical hysterectomy learning curve was without considerable variations. The mean operative time of the first ten patients in the

Table 1 Main patient and tumor characteristics

	RARH (n=73)	LARVH (n=46)	ARH (n=175)	p values
Age (years)				
Mean	46.0	42.5	49.0	0.001
SD	±11.2	±9.9	±11.0	
Range	(24–75)	(20–69)	(20–78)	
Predominating age group	40–49 years	40–49 years	50–59 years	
	24 (32.9%)	17 (30.0%)	49 (28.0%)	0.003
Preoperative Htc				
Mean	0.369	0.375	0.359	0.035
SD	±0.039	±0.037	±0.042	
Range	(0.260–0.460)	(0.280–0.460)	(0.230–0.470)	
Postoperative Htc				
Mean	0.317	0.330	0.318	0.153
SD	±0.035	±0.031	±0.045	
Range	(0.230–0.390)	(0.270–0.390)	(0.230–0.490)	
Htc difference				
Mean	0.052	0.045	0.041	0.253
SD	±0.039	±0.036	±0.035	
Range	(0.043–0.061)	(0.034–0.055)	(0.033–0.049)	
Cancer type				
SCC	65 (89.0%)	41 (89.1%)	167 (95.4%)	0.116
Adenocarcinoma	8 (11.0%)	5 (10.9%)	8 (4.6%)	
Total number of nodes				
Mean	11.4	11.3	15.9	0.001
SD	±7.0	±5.2	±7.7	
Range	(2–56)	(3–24)	(2–46)	
N0	61 (83.6%)	41 (89.1%)	133 (76.0%)	
N1	12 (16.4%)	5 (10.9%)	42 (24.0%)	0.095

robotic cohort was insignificantly higher in comparison with that one of the remaining 63 patients, respectively, 153.9±27.4 and 151.0±26.6 min ($p=0.832$). Learning curve of the radical laparoscopic hysterectomies shows comparatively high and stable level for the first 20 patients (mean operative time 263.2±49.4) and insignificant tendency toward a reduction for the remaining 26 (mean operative time 223.4±62.5) ($p=0.071$) (Fig. 1). The frequency of the complications in both groups with different mean operative time appeared statistically insignificant in the robotic ($p=0.688$), as well as in the laparoscopic cohort ($p=0.345$). We did not study the learning curve of the abdominal radical hysterectomies as this operative technique is applied according to a standardized method by all surgeons at our institution before 2006.

The average length of hospital stay for the patients with RARH and LARVH was 4.1±0.7 and 4.8±0.5 days, respectively and 9.6±1.0 days for those with ARH as the differences were with high significance in favor of the minimally invasive procedures ($p=0.001$).

The complications rate for the whole group of 294 patients was 4.4% ($n=13$). Only in one of them (7.7%) from the laparotomy cohort, an intraoperative ureteral lesion was found. The remaining 12 (92.3%) complications were established in the postoperative period. The complications in the different types of surgical interventions are presented in Table 2. There were no conversions in the robotic and laparoscopy groups.

Adjuvant therapy was conformed to a standard for the treatment of cervical carcinoma, approved by the Guild of the Bulgarian Radiotherapists. The postoperative external beam radiotherapy was carried out on 235 (79.9%) patients at a dose of 50 Gy to the whole pelvis. Chemoradiation was applied to all patients with metastases in the regional lymph nodes (20.1%/59) as the external beam radiotherapy dose was 50 Gy, combined with cisplatin at a dose of 40 mg/m^2.

The mean follow-up period was 316.3±192.0 days in the robotic group, 1,531.6±612.2 days in the laparoscopic group and 808.3±385.3 days in the laparotomy group ($p=0.001$).

Using the univariate and Cox regression analysis, the disease-free survival (DSF) and overall survival (OS) of the patients, operated with the three types of radical procedures— robotic, laparoscopic and open, were studied. Because of the different time of inclusion in the study and the different follow-up time, the univariate analysis was carried out by the method of Kaplan–Meier; as for determination of DFS, the investigated event was recurrence appearance, and for OS, death, caused by oncologic disease. In 29 (9.9%) of the patients, a recurrence was found, as the mean recurrence time was 2,161.8±57.6 days (95% CI, 2,048.8–2,274.7), and cumulative DFS, 81.8%. Frequency of recurrences, distributed according to the particular types of operative interventions, was as follows: RARH, 1 (1.4%); LARVH, 3 (6.5%); ARH, 25 (14.3%) ($p=0.001$). With the univariate analysis were analyzed the probable factors, influencing the time for recurrence appearance as follows: metastases in the regional lymph nodes, histological type of tumor, type of operation, complication presence. Significant dependence was established between DFS and the metastases in the lymph nodes (Table 3). DFS was highest in patients with robotic surgery (95.8%±4.1%), lower in the laparoscopic group (91.5%± 4.8%), and lowest in the laparotomy group (77.4%± 6.5%) as the differences were significant ($p=0.019$) (Fig. 2). Histological type of tumor and complications appearance did not influence the DFS ($p>0.05$). After application of the multivariate analysis with Cox regression model, only the regional lymph nodes status from the significant factors preserved its statistical significance, as the presence of metastases in them increased 4.1 times the probability for recurrence appearance (95% CI, 1.35–12.34).

Univariate analysis of the OS established that from the whole group of 294 patients, 23 (7.8%) have died, as 2 (4.3%) of them were with LARVH, 21 (12.0%) were with ARH, and all that have undergone RARH are alive ($p=0.004$). Cumulative OS was 88.2% at mean survival time of 2,242.5±45.6 days (95% CI, 2,153.0–2,331.9). The following factors with probable influence over the OS were examined: status of the regional lymph nodes, type of operation, histological tumor type, complication presence, and recur-

Table 2 Intra- and postoperative complications in robotic, laparoscopic, and open radical hysterectomy	Complications	RARH ($n=73$)	LARVH ($n=46$)	ARH ($n=175$)	p value
	Intraoperative				
	Ureteral lesion	–	–	1	
	Postoperative				
	Ureterovaginal fistula	1	–	1	
	Lymphocele	2	–	–	
	Pelveocellulitis	–	1	4	
	Lung thromboembolia	–	–	1	
	Hydronephrosis (unilateral, moderate)	–	–	2	
	Total n (%)	3 (4.1)	1 (2.2)	9 (5.1)	0.676

Table 3 Influence of the metastases in the regional lymph nodes on disease-free survival, mean recurrence time, overall survival, and survival mean time

	N1	N0	*p* value		
			Log rank	Breslow	Tarone–Ware
DFS (%)	65.1±10.0	85.3±4.6			
MRT (days)	1,794.5±174.8	2,233.3±57.3	0.001	0.007	0.003
	(95% CI, 1,451.9–2,137.0)	(95% CI, 2,120.9–2,345.7)			
OS (%)	62.3±10.3	93.3±1.9			
SMT (days)	1,769.1±175.7	2,333.1±38.5	0.0001	0.001	0.0001
	(95% CI, 1,427.8–2,113.4)	(95% CI, 2,257.7–2,408.5)			

MRT mean recurrence time, *CI* confidence interval, *SMT* survival mean time

rence appearance. Only the nodal status, the type of operation and recurrence appearance out of all parameters displayed significant dependence with the OS. The influence of the regional lymph node metastases on OS is presented in Table 3. OS in ARH was 84.9%, in LARVH 94.9%, and in RARH 100% (p=0.037) (Fig. 3). Patients with recurrence had 52.5%OS at mean survival time of 1,171.4 ±170.5 days (95% CI, 837.3–1,505.5), and those without recurrence 90.4% and 2,278.7±42.5 days, respectively (95% CI, 2,195.4–2,362.0)(p=0.001). Histological type of tumor and comp-lication appearance did not influence OS (p>0.05).

The nodal status and recurrence presence preserved their significance in the Cox regression analysis. The risk for death of cervical cancer is 6.6 times higher in the presence of metastases in the regional lymph nodes, and 6.3 times higher of recurrences.

Discussion

The predominant part of the literature studies, which investigate the minimally invasive methods (robotic and/or laparoscopic) for treatment of early cervical carcinoma, are retrospective and case matched [6, 7, 9, 14]. Estape et al. have analyzed 32 patients who underwent robotic radical hysterectomy from August 2006 to April 2008. These cases were matched to a historical cohort of patients with total laparoscopic radical hysterectomy (July 2004–July 2006) and radical abdominal hysterectomy (May 2002–July 2006) [9]. Maggioni et al. have collected prospectively data for 40 patients with robotic radical hysterectomy, and compared them with a retrospective group of patients with abdominal radical hysterectomy [12].

Only a few authors compare the three operative approaches– robotic, laparoscopic, and open [6, 9]. Normally, the comparative analyses include either robotic and laparoscopic surgery or robotic and open surgery [4, 7, 11–13, 18, 19].

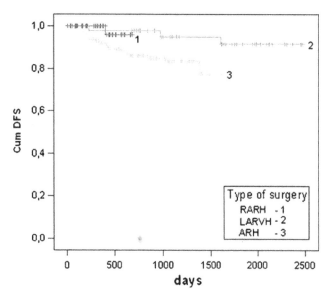

Fig. 2 Disease-free survival and type of surgery

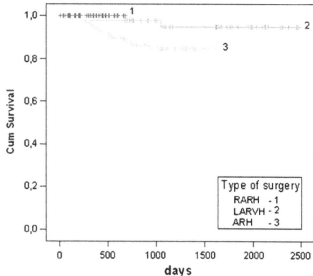

Fig. 3 Influence of type of surgery on the overall survival

Obermair et al. published in 2008 the design of a multicenter prospective randomized controlled trial, which compared laparoscopic or robotic radical hysterectomy with abdominal radical hysterectomy [20].

Our study, like the one of Cantrell et al., is entirely retrospective [14]. We analyze 294 patients with T1b1 cervical cancer, operated by three radical approaches: robotic, laparoscopic, and open. The operative interventions have been accomplished by one and the same team, at one institution, for a period of 4 years and 5 months (January 2006–May 2010). In contrast with Obermair's article, we compare the three methods separately. Although the laparoscopic and robotic surgeries are minimally invasive methods, they require mastering of different surgical skills in order to be applied. For example, LARVH, in contrast to the total laparoscopic radical hysterectomy, has a specific vaginal stage.

The weakness of our study is in its retrospective nature, as well as in the fact that it is not randomized and multicenter. The strength of the study is the comparison of outcome in patients, operated with three different types of radical procedures—robotic, laparoscopic, and open.

In the perioperative parameters, significant differences in favor of the robotic radical surgery were determined in the analysis of the mean age, mean operative time, and mean hospital stay ($p=0.001$).

Statistically significant lower mean age of the robotic group of patients in comparison with the open approach group was indicated in the studies of Boggess et al., Estape et al., and Maggioni et al. [7, 9, 12]. We attribute the lower mean age of the patients with LARVH and RARH in our series to two fundamental causes: a tendency toward a reduction in the age limit of the diagnosed cases with cervical cancer among the female population on one side, and the preferences of younger women to be operated with minimally invasive methods on the other [21].

Operative time is one of the main parameters, which corresponds with the severity of the operative trauma. Articles with a small number of patients present a longer operative time, because of less initial experience (Ko et al., $n=16$; mean operative time MOT=0450 hours; Lowe et al., $n=7$; MOT=260 min; Nezhat et al., $n=13$; MOT=323 min) [11, 13, 19]. The duration of the first robotic radical hysterectomy performed by us was approximately 4 h (215 min), and of the tenth—3 h (180 min). No significant difference was found in the mean operative time between the group of the first 10 patients and the group of the rest 63 patients. No difference was established in the complication rate between both groups as well. That is why we decided to analyze the operative time of all patients, operated by us, without excluding the first cases.

Our data for the mean operative time for RARH are similar to those of Estape et al. (2.4±0.8 h/144 min), and for LARVH and ARH correspond to the data of Magrina et al. (220.4±

37.5 and 166.8±33.2, respectively, $p=0.001$) [6, 9]. In the multicenter study, presented by Lowe et al., five console surgeons participated, as nobody of them has had any preceding experience in the laparoscopic surgery. This fact and relatively the small number of cases operated by the particular surgeons, explain the longer mean operative time (215 min) in comparison with our data (152.2 min) [22].

The length of hospital stay reflects the differences in the postoperative outcomes of the patients subjected to different operative procedures. Factors that determine the time of discharge from hospital are the possibility of the patient to ambulate independently, recovery of the functions of the gastrointestinal tract, permitting oral ingestion of food, normalization of clinical parameters, as well as adequate pain control with oral drugs. Recovery of urinary bladder function (residual urine <50 ml) is not a determinant. Patients with residual urine >50 ml can be discharged from the hospital with a Foley catheter. Recovery of urinary bladder function is followed up ambulatory.

The differences in the mean hospital stay in our study are with high significance in favor of the minimally invasive procedures (RARH and LARVH, respectively 4.1±0.7 and 4.8±0.5 days) in comparison with the open radical approach (9.6±1.0 days) ($p=0.001$). Our data about the radical robotic hysterectomy are similar to those of Maggioni et al. (3.7± 1.2 days) and Sert et al. (4 days) [4, 12]. However, there are a lot of studies that present shorter hospital stay, ranging from 1 to 2.6 days [6, 7, 9, 11, 22]. The requirement of the National Health Insurance System for a minimum postoperative hospital stay of 2 days for the minimally invasive procedures was one of the basic reasons for the longer hospital stay of our patients with robotic surgery.

Average number of the removed lymph nodes in radical hysterectomy for cervical carcinoma range widely from 9.2 to 33.8 [7, 18]; as according to the type of the operative approach, the variations are in the following limits: robotic, from 11.5 to 33.8; laparoscopic, from 15 to 31; open, from 9.2 to 27.7 [4, 6, 7, 13, 18]. Our data are close to the lower range for the robotic radical hysterectomies and, in the data of Maggioni et al., are significantly lower in comparison with those of the abdominal radical surgery ($p<0.05$) [12]. Admitting the fact that in all cases, the zone of dissection visually is without residual lymph tissue, we think that the differences are determined mainly by the individual anatomy of the pelvic lymphatic system and the criteria differences for counting out the lymph nodes by the particular pathologists. Moreover, the size of the lymphatic dissection is not identical with the different authors. Feuer et al. perform dissection from the common iliac artery to the circumflex iliac vein, Persson et al. begin the lymphadenectomy from the common iliac lymph nodes, continue with the external iliac and finish with the obturator lymph nodes, and Magrina et al., in cases with indications, include the paraaortal lymph nodes in the dissection [6, 10, 18]. The distal margin of our lymph node dissection is determined by the circumflex iliac vessels, and the proximal, by the bifurcation of the common iliac artery. On suspicion of lymph node metastases, we carry out frozen section examination. If metastases are proven, the dissection zone is extended along the common iliac artery.

Hematocrit is a laboratory parameter, which is used for acute and chronic blood loss assessment, as well as for changes in the water–electrolyte balance. In mammals, hematocrit is independent of body size. We used this parameter for indirect assessment of the intraoperative blood loss. No significant differences in the values of the postoperative hematocrit ($p=0.153$), and the difference between the pre- and postoperative hematocrit in the three operative methods ($p=0.253$) were established.

Literature data about the complications rate in radical robotic surgery vary in a wide range —from 7.8% to 59% [7, 10]. Different criteria for defining the minor complications and the different patients' follow-up period are the main reasons for that variety. Moreover, differences in the criterion for early and late postoperative complications exist. Magrina accepts, for early complications, those that have occurred to 6 weeks after the operation, while Maggioni, those that have occurred to 1 month after the operation [6, 12]. No significant differences in the frequency of the complications were established in all publications that compare the robotic with the open and/or laparoscopic surgery [9, 12, 13, 18, 19]. The rate of our complications for RARH was 4.1% ($n=3$) and did not differ significantly from that one of LARVH (2.2%/$n=1$) and ARH (5.1%/$n=9$) ($p=0.676$). Readmission for treatment of complications arising in five patients was necessary—two with ureterovaginal fistulas (RARH and ARH), one with symptomatic lymphocele (RARH), one with severe pelveo-cellulitis (LARVH), and one with pulmonary thrombembolia, terminated fatally (ARH). Correction of the ureterovaginal fistulas was performed via open surgery, while the patient with the symptomatic lymphocele was subjected to laparoscopy. The remaining cases were treated conservatively.

Data for the follow-up period, recurrences and mortality rate in patients with cervical cancer who have undergone radical robotic hysterectomy are reported in few articles [5, 6, 9, 10, 14]. In a case-matched analysis of robotic radical hysterectomy compared with laparoscopy and laparotomy, Estape et al. present mean patient's follow-up period of 284.2 ± 152.1 days (robotic group), 941.6 ± 273.9 days (laparoscopy group), and $1,382.4\pm592.7$ days (laparotomy group), respectively [9]. In our study, significantly shortest was the mean follow-up period for the robotic group (316.3 ± 192.0 days), followed by the laparotomy group (808.3 ± 385.3 days) and laparoscopic group ($1,531.6\pm612.2$ days), respectively ($p=0.001$). Significant differences in favor of

the minimally invasive approaches (RARH and LARVH) in comparison with the open surgery, with regard to the frequency of recurrences ($p=0.001$) and mortality rate ($p=0.004$), are observed.

The outlined by the univariate analysis trends in our study for better DFS and OS of patients with robotic surgery in comparison with those with laparoscopic and open radical surgery, were not confirmed by the Cox regression model. The metastases in the regional lymph nodes (for DFS and OS) and the recurrence appearance (for OS) were the only parameters, which preserved their significance. Our results are close to those of Cantrell et al. The authors have studied retrospectively the progression-free survival (PFS) and OS in 71 patients with cervical carcinoma, who have undergone type III robotic radical hysterectomy and compared them with a group of open radical hysterectomies. No significant differences were found in PFS ($p=0.27$) and OS ($p=0.47$) between both groups [14].

Conclusion

In conclusion, analysis of the perioperative parameters shows that RARH is a reliable procedure with proven advantages with regard to the mean operative time and hospital stay in patients with early cervical cancer. Data on the survival are preliminary. We recognize that the follow-up period for the patients with robotic hysterectomy is short. After accumulation of sufficient number of cases and sufficient follow-up period from a statistical reliability point of view, it will be clarified in what direction the results will be altered. The absence of significant differences in the DFS and the OS currently, however, is a substantial reason to continue from an oncologic point of view, the application of this method on patients with T1b1 cervical cancer.

Declaration of interest The authors report no conflicts of interest. The authors alone are responsible for the content and writing of the paper.

References

1. Nezhat CR, Burrell MO, Nezhat FR, Benigno BB, Welander CE (1992) Laparoscopic radical hysterectomy with paraaortic and pelvic node dissection. Am J Obstet Gynecol 166(3):864–865
2. Canis M, Mage G, Wattiez A, Pouly JL, Manhes H, Bruhat MA (1990) Does endoscopic surgery have a role in radical surgery of cancer of the cervix uteri? J Gynecol Obstet Biol Reprod (Paris) 19:921
3. Ballantyne G, Marescaux J, Giulianotti P (2004) Primer of robotic and telerobotic surgery. Lippincott Williams & Wilkins, Philadelphia
4. Sert B, Abeler V (2007) Robotic radical hysterectomy in early-stage cervical carcinoma patients, comparing results with total

laparoscopic radical hysterectomy cases. The future is now? Int J Med Robot 3(3):224–228

5. Kim YT, Kim SW, Hyung WJ, Lee SJ, Nam EJ, Lee WJ (2008) Robotic radical hysterectomy with pelvic lymphadenectomy for cervical carcinoma: a pilot study. Gynecol Oncol 108(2):312–316

6. Magrina JF, Kho RM, Weaver AL, Montero RP, Magtibay PM (2008) Robotic radical hysterectomy: comparison with laparoscopy and laparotomy. Gynecol Oncol 109(1):86–91

7. Boggess JF, Gehrig PA, Cantrell L, Shafer A, Ridgway M, Skinner EN et al (2008) A case–control study of robot-assisted type III radical hysterectomy with pelvic lymph node dissection compared with open radical hysterectomy. Am J Obstet Gynecol 199(4):357.e1–357.e7

8. Fanning J, Fenton B, Purohit M (2008) Robotic radical hysterectomy. Am J Obstet Gynecol 198:649.e1–649.e4

9. Estape R, Lambrou N, Diaz R, Estape E, Dunkin N, Rivera A (2009) A case matched analysis of robotic radical hysterectomy with lymphadenectomy compared with laparoscopy and laparotomy. Gynecol Oncol 113(3):357–361

10. Persson J, Reynisson P, Borgfeldt C, Kannisto P, Lindahl B, Bossmar T (2009) Robot assisted laparoscopic radical hysterectomy and pelvic lymphadenectomy with short and long term morbidity data. Gynecol Oncol 113(2):185–190

11. Lowe MP, Hoekstra AV, Jairam-Thodla A, Singh DK, Buttin BM, Lurain JR et al (2009) A comparison of robot-assisted and traditional radical hysterectomy for early-stage cervical cancer. J Robot Surg 3(1):19–23

12. Maggioni A, Minig L, Zanagnolo V, Peiretti M, Sanguineti F, Bocciolone L et al (2009) Robotic approach for cervical cancer: comparison with laparotomy: a case control study. Gynecol Oncol 115(1):60–64

13. Nezhat F (2008) Minimally invasive surgery in gynecologic oncology: laparoscopy versus robotics. Gynecol Oncol 111(2 Suppl):S29–S32

14. Cantrell LA, Mendivil A, Gehring PA, Boggess JF (2010) Survival outcomes for women undergoing type III robotic radical hysterectomy for cervical cancer: a 3-year experience. Gynecol Oncol 117(2):260–265

15. Piver MS, Rutledge F, Smith JP (1974) Five classes of extended hysterectomy for women with cervical cancer. Obstet Gynecol 44:265–272

16. Gortchev G, Tomov S, Tanchev L, Velkova A, Radionova Z (2010) Da Vinci S robotic surgery in the treatment of benign and malignant gynecologic tumors. Gynecol Surg 7:153–157

17. Koehler C, Possover M, Klemm P, Tozzi R, Schneider A (2002) Renaissance der Operation nach Schauta. Gynaekologe 35:132–145

18. Feuer G, Benigno B, Krige L, Alvarez P (2009) Comparison of a novel surgical approach for radical hysterectomy: robotic assistance versus open surgery. J Robot Surg 3:179–186

19. Ko EM, Muto MG, Berkowitz RS, Feltmate CM (2008) Robotic versus open radical hysterectomy: a comparative study at a single institution. Gynecol Oncol 111(3):425–430

20. Obermair A, Gebski V, Frumovitz M, Soliman PT, Schmeler KM, Levenback C (2008) A phase III randomized clinical trial comparing laparoscopic or robotic radical hysterectomy with abdominal radical hysterectomy in patients with early stage cervical cancer. J Minim Invasive Gynecol 15(5):584–588

21. Valerianova Z, Vukov M, Dimitrova N (2009) Cancer incidence rates per 100,000 by primary sites and age at diagnosis in Bulgaria 2007 – females. Bulgarian National Cancer Registry 18:48–58

22. Lowe MP, Chamberlain DH, Kamelle SA, Johnson PR, Tillmanns TD (2009) A multi-institutional experience with robotic-assisted radical hysterectomy for early stage cervical cancer. Gynecol Oncol 113(2):191–194

4

Single-port hysterectomy with pelvic lymph node dissection in the porcine model: feasibility and validation of a novel robotic lightweight endoscope positioner

Pedro F. Escobar · Jason Knight · Matthew Kroh ·
Sricharan Chalikonda · Jihad Kaouk · Robert Stein

Abstract The purpose of this study was to evaluate the feasibility and validity of a modified single-port robotic lightweight endoscope in the performance of single-port hysterectomy with pelvic lymph node dissection in the porcine model. Task completion times were recorded for each component of the procedure: port placement, docking of the surgical robot, operative time for the procedures. For each task, linear regression modeling was performed using SPSS to determine whether a correlation existed between task completion time and increasing surgeon experience. All robotic-assisted LESS procedures were performed successfully without the addition of laparoscopic ports or open conversion. Regression analysis demonstrated a strong correlation between the number of procedures and task completion time for robot docking and pelvic lymph node dissection, correlation coefficients 0.74 and 0.77, $p=0.001$, respectively.

This study demonstrated the feasibility and effectiveness of a new, compact single-port robotic voice-activated endoscope at improving laparoscope guidance during the performance of single-port hysterectomy with pelvic lymph node dissection in the porcine model. Further work is needed to better define the ideal operative procedure

for single-site surgery in oncology and integration of new single-port robotic platforms into clinical practice.

Keywords Robotic surgery · Single-port surgery · LESS · Single-port laparoscopy

Background

Innovations in minimally invasive surgical technology have allowed laparoscopic surgeons to perform increasingly complex surgeries through smaller incisions. An emerging area in minimally invasive surgery is single-port laparoscopy (SPL), or laparoendoscopic single-site surgery (LESS). SPL entails performing laparoscopic surgery utilizing a multi-channel port system, typically placed through a single umbilical skin incision. New technologies have improved the success and reproducibility of these single-access approaches, including the use of flexible laparoscopes, flexible instruments, and internal retractors. However, significant obstacles still exist mainly due to physical impediments of instrumentation.

Working within a confined space, typically the umbilicus, results in several shortcomings. These disadvantages include conflict of instruments sharing a common port, different or inferior retraction in the operative field, unstable flexible endoscopes, and surgeon fatigue and discomfort secondary to poor ergonomics. Recently, there has been interest in the application of robotic technology to these procedures [1–4]. Fusion of these concepts, single-site surgery and robotic technology is an area of active research and innovation in minimally invasive surgery. The purpose of this study was to evaluate the feasibility and validity of a modified single-port

P. F. Escobar (✉) · J. Knight · M. Kroh · S. Chalikonda ·
J. Kaouk · R. Stein
Department of OB/GYN and Women's Health Institute,
Cleveland Clinic,
Desk A-81, 9500 Euclid Avenue,
Cleveland, OH 44195, USA
e-mail: escobap@ccf.org

robotic lightweight endoscope (ViKY-XL) in the performance of single-port hysterectomy with pelvic lymph node dissection in the porcine model.

Material and methods

This pilot training study was performed at the Cleveland Clinic, c-SITE, Cleveland, OH, USA. All procedures performed in this training protocol have been approved by the Institutional Animal Care and Use Committee (IACUC) at the Cleveland Clinic, Protocol no. (2009–0086). Task completion times were recorded for each component of the procedure: port placement, docking of the surgical robot, operative time for the hysterectomy with BSO, and operative time for pelvic lymph node dissection. For each task linear regression modeling was performed using SPSS (version 19.0.0) to determine whether a correlation existed between task completion time and increasing surgeon experience.

Robotic lightweight endoscope positioner

The ViKY® System "Vision Control for endoscopY" (Endocontrol Medical, La Tronche, France) is a compact motorized endoscope driver designed to improve surgeon ergonomics (Fig. 1). The original model followed foot pedal commands, which moved the endoscope in the x, y, and z axes. Keeping the same architecture, but with a larger platform, the modified ViKY® XL system includes a compact motorized voice-activated (Bluetooth) endoscope manipulator specially designed for single-access surgery. The platform has a diameter of 182 mm and weighs 2.2 kg. The main ring of the system is fastened on one of the lateral operating room table rails through a height adjustment mechanism. Three degrees of freedom are integrated into the main ring of the system. Media File 1

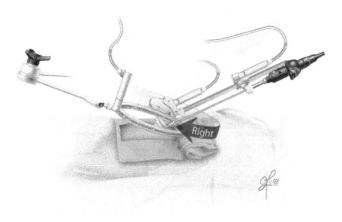

Fig. 1 Robotic endoscope driver moving camera toward field right

The study was performed on 12 healthy female pigs. Normal health status was determined preoperatively by physical examination, blood chemistry, and quarantine (according to the IACUC protocol). Food was withheld from the pigs for 24 h before surgery. All animals were provided water ad libitum. Pre-operative care, anesthesia, and euthanasia were overseen by a staff veterinarian. After induction, all pigs were positioned in dorsal lithotomy position for the surgical procedures. At the conclusion of the lab, the pigs remained under general anesthesia and were humanely euthanized.

Access was obtained using the Hasson technique through a 1.5–2.0 cm umbilical incision allowing insertion of the SILS™(Covidien, Mansfield, CT, USA) single-port robotic trocar system. The abdominal cavity was insufflated to an intra-abdominal pressure of 12 mmHg. The surgical table was tilted to a 35° Trendelenburg position to displace the abdominal viscera cranially. The urinary bladder was then drained directly to ease visualization of the pelvis.

The ViKY® System was docked into one of the lateral surgical table rails through a height/pivot adjustment mechanism. An Olympus 5-mm LTF-VH deflectable tip video laparoscope (Olympus Surgical and Industrial America Inc, Center Valley, PA, USA) was then coupled with the system. A Bluetooth ear-piece was utilized to aurally control the platform's 3 degrees of freedom (in/out, left/right, up/down) (Media File 1). Articulated Maryland graspers, curved scissors, and 5-mm Ligasure blunt tip vessel sealer were then used for lymph node dissections and hysterectomies/oophorectomies. The iliac artery and vein were first identified, the retroperitoneal space entered and developed in a caudal–cranial fashion. The lymphatic tissue was removed using the Maryland grasper and 5-mm Ligasure (Covidien, Mansfield, CT, USA).

Findings

All robotic-assisted LESS procedures were performed successfully without the addition of laparoscopic ports or open conversion. The lightweight/compact system allowed the surgeon to stand next to the surgical table in an ergonomic fashion without restricting the freedom of motion and limiting endoscope-instrument clashing.

Mean animal weight was 26.14 kg (23–29 kg). Mean task completion times are noted in Table 1. Figure 2 illustrates the trend in task completion times with increasing number of procedures, $p=0.001$. Regression analysis demonstrated a strong correlation between increasing surgeon experience and decreasing task completion time for robot docking and pelvic lymph node dissection, correlation coefficients 0.74 and 0.77, respectively (Figs. 3 and 4). No statistically significant improvement in task completion time was noted for port placement or hysterectomy with oophorectomy. No intraoperative complications were observed.

Table 1 Task completion time

Task	Mean completion time (range)
Port placement	4.75 min (3–7 min); SD, 1.22
Docking	7.25 min (4–13 min); SD, 2.93
Hysterectomy, oophorectomy	20.92 min (15–25 min); SD, 2.94
Pelvic node dissection	64.25 min (48–85 min); SD, 11.89

Discussion

This study demonstrated the feasibility and effectiveness of a new, compact single-port robotic voice-activated endoscope at improving laparoscope guidance during the performance of single-port hysterectomy with pelvic lymph node dissection in the porcine model. This robotic voice-activated endoscope driver contributed to a stable endoscopic image, and allowed significant improvement in operating times.

Ergonomics has a major influence on the acceptance and dissemination of new surgical technology. There are several inherent limitations of LESS when compared to laparoscopy and robotic techniques. These disadvantages include conflict between instruments, diminished triangulation, different or inferior retraction in the operative field, unstable flexible endoscopes, and surgeon fatigue and discomfort secondary to poor ergonomics. To alleviate inherent problems attributable to the single-site approach, several ad hoc novel flexible instruments and optics have been developed in the last few years.

Perhaps the most significant advantage of this robotic system when coupled with an articulated endoscope is improved visualization and stability of the surgical field as well as improved ergonomics, minimizing instrument conflict thereby potentiating greater precision and accuracy. Our results are consistent with a previous study by Crouzet et al. for reconstructive and extirpative urological surgery using the porcine model [5]. The authors concluded that with single-port access, the robotic endoscope allows more room for the surgeon compared to an assistant. This is also consistent with data published regarding the da Vinci SI for single-site surgery in urology. Using the current da Vinci SI via a single-site approach for radical prostatectomies in a preclinical setting, Desai et al. concluded that conflict of the robotic arms was worse compared to multiport cadaveric procedures, but closure/suturing was easier [6]. Consequently, White et al. reported early surgical outcomes on 20 patients who underwent robotic laparoendoscopic single-site radical prostatectomy (R-LESS RP) [7]. The authors concluded that R-LESS RP was technically feasible and reduces some of the difficulties encountered with conventional LESS.

The robotic platform as we know it today (da Vinci S and da VinciSI) is not ideal for robotic single-site surgery due to spatial constraints and a significant amount of exterior instrument collisions, but future versions of the device will surely provide integral elements to further the development of single-port gynecologic surgery [8]. Current research within our group has focused on the evaluation of novel single-port robotic platforms for procedures in gynecologic oncology [9, 10]. Preliminary data demonstrates that the performance of various oncology procedures using novel single-site robotic platforms is feasible, and more importantly, overcomes inherent limitations of LESS.

Fig. 2 Trends in task completion time

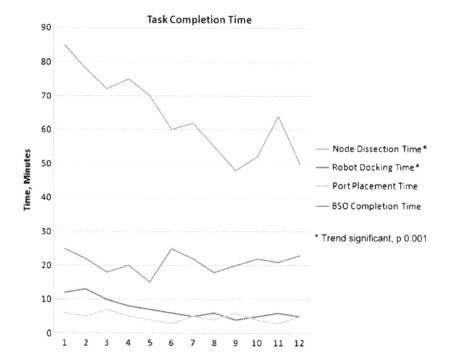

Fig. 3 Learning curve for robot setup

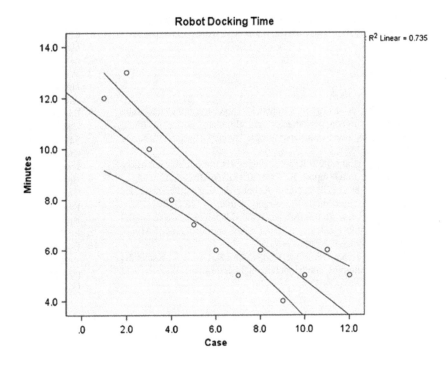

Conclusion

In conclusion, we report here the feasibility of a surgical robot with master–slave function for visual field control for single-port surgery. The novel advantage of the system when coupled with a flexible 5-mm endoscope is the control, and stability of the vision field for LESS. This is an advantage when performing ergonomically complex procedures such as node dissections during via a single-port approach. Further work is needed to better define the ideal operative procedure for single-site surgery in oncology and integration of new single-port robotic platforms into clinical practice.

Fig. 4 Learning curve for lymph node dissection with ViKY

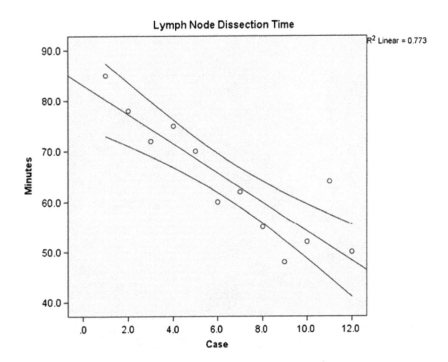

Declaration of interest   The authors report no conflicts of interest. The authors alone are responsible for the content and writing of the paper.

References

1. Joseph RA et al (2010) "Chopstick" surgery: a novel technique improves surgeon performance and eliminates arm collision in robotic single-incision laparoscopic surgery. Surg Endosc 24 (6):1331–1335
2. Kaouk JH et al (2009) Robotic single-port transumbilical surgery in humans: initial report. BJU Int 103(3):366–369
3. Haber GP et al (2010) Novel Robotic da Vinci instruments for laparoendoscopic single-site surgery. Urology 76(6):1279–1282
4. Escobar PF et al (2009) Robotic-assisted laparoendoscopic single-site surgery in gynecology: initial report and technique. J Minim Invasive Gynecol 16(5):589–591
5. Crouzet S, Haber GP, White WM, Kamoi K, Goel RK, Kaouk JH (2010) Single-port, single-operator-light endoscopic robot-assisted laparoscopic urology: pilot study in a pig model. BJU Int 105:682–685 [PubMed]
6. Desai MM, Aron M, Berger A et al (2008) Transvesical robotic radical prostatectomy. BJU Int 102(11):1666–1669
7. White MA, Haber GP, Autorino R et al (2010) Robotic laparoendoscopic single-site radical prostatectomy: technique and early outcomes. Eur Urol 58(4):544–550
8. Barret E, Sanchez-Salas R, Ercolani MC, Rozet F, Galiano M, Cathelineau X, Tanoue K, Yasunaga T, Kobayashi E, Miyamoto S, Sakuma I, Dohi T (2011) Natural orifice transendoluminal surgery and laparoendoscopic single-site surgery: the future of laparoscopic radical prostatectomy. Future Oncol 7(3):427–434
9. Haber GP, White MA, Autorino R, Escobar PF, Kroh MD, Chalikonda S, Khanna R, Forest S, Yang B, Altunrende F, Stein RJ, Kaouk JH (2010) Novel robotic da Vinci instruments for laparoendoscopic single-site surgery. Urology 76(6):1279–1282, Epub 2010 Oct 27
10. Escobar PF, Kebria M, Falcone T (2011) Evaluation of a novel single-port robotic platform in the cadaver model for the performance of various procedures in gynecologic oncology. Gynecol Oncol 120(3):380–384, Epub 2011 Jan 8

5

Medical debulking with gonadotrophin-releasing hormone agonists to facilitate vaginal hysterectomy

Joan Melendez · Ravi Bhatia · Abiodun Fakokunde · Wai Yoong

Abstract Although the superiority of vaginal compared to abdominal hysterectomy is well established, most gynaecologists still prefer the abdominal route for removal of benign large uteri >14 weeks. Gonadotrophin-releasing hormone agonists such as goserelin can reduce uterine bulk by up to 60% and was initially used to convert a midline to Pfannenstiel incision in abdominal hysterectomy. The conversion of an abdominal to a potential vaginal hysterectomy by uterine size reduction would prove advantageous, and the authors present data from a case control study of 12 women with uteri >14 weeks who successfully underwent vaginal hysterectomy following preoperative treatment with goserelin. Women scheduled for hysterectomy for menorrhagia with non-prolapsing clinical uterine size of >14 weeks were offered an attempt at vaginal hysterectomy after pre-treatment with goserelin. A group of women with comparable uterine size who underwent abdominal hysterectomy for similar indication served as control. Pre- and postoperative data such as haemoglobin, myoma size, uterine weight, duration of procedure and complications were collected prospectively. Both groups had comparable preoperative haemoglobin, subjective preoperative uterine bulk (median 16 weeks) and body mass index. The vaginal hysterectomy group received a median of two goserelin injections prior to surgery, and the uterine weight at histology was similar in both groups (median 580 vs 609 g, $p<0.05$). The duration of surgery was twice as long in vaginal compared to abdominal hysterectomy (153.7 vs 85 min, $p<0.05$), but analgesia use and the length of inpatient stay were lower in the study group (2.62 vs 3.5 days, $p<0.05$). In women with >14 week-size uteri, treatment with gonadotrophin agonists reduces uterine size sufficiently to allow safe vaginal hysterectomy. Although duration of surgery was longer, women who underwent vaginal hysterectomy required less analgesia and had shorter inpatient stay.

Keywords Vaginal hysterectomy · Medical debulking · Gonadotrophin-releasing hormone agonist

Background

Laparotomy is still the preferred route of surgical access in women requiring a hysterectomy for menorrhagia or fibroid, although it is well documented that intraoperative and postoperative morbidity, analgesia use and hospital stay are significantly lower with the vaginal route [1–4]. The abdominal route could be attributed to personal preference as well as lack of training and experience, and should vaginal hysterectomy (VH) become more widespread, the potential for cost saving and improved patient experience is significant: one study already demonstrated that the cost of abdominal and laparoscopic hysterectomy were 34.5% and 72% respectively higher than for vaginal hysterectomy [5].

The most common reason cited by gynaecologists for favouring abdominal over the vaginal approach is large uterine bulk, and many would be reluctant to attempt VH in patients with an estimated uterine size of 12–14 weeks [6, 7]. Observational and comparative studies by Magos et al. [8], Harmanli et al. [5] and Sahin [9], however, all demonstrate that uteri of up to 20 weeks could be removed vaginally. Interestingly, contrary to accumulating evidence supporting the vaginal approach particularly for this group,

J. Melendez · R. Bhatia · A. Fakokunde · W. Yoong (✉)
Department of Obstetrics and Gynaecology,
North Middlesex University Hospital,
London N18 1QX, UK
e-mail: wai.yoong@nmh.nhs.uk

the American College of Obstetrics and Gynecology recommends against vaginal hysterectomy for women with uterine size of >12 weeks.

That the "average practicing gynaecologist, through deliberate effort, could increase his/her VH rate to 95% within 5 years" [10] was a great motivation for us as was the challenge of developing the confidence to progressively increase the size of the uteri that could be removed through the vaginal route (only 3.9% of hysterectomies for fibroid uteri were performed vaginally [11]).

Stoval and colleagues have used gonadotrophin-releasing hormone (GnRH) agonists as a preoperative adjunct to medically debulk uteri, thus enabling hysterectomy, which otherwise would have been approached abdominally, to be performed vaginally [12].

In this study, we present data from a prospective case control study of 12 women with enlarged uteri without prolapse who were treated with a GnRH agonist in order to facilitate vaginal hysterectomy; the control group comprised patients with enlarged uteri who underwent total abdominal hysterectomy (TAH) for a similar indication (i.e. menorrhagia).

Materials and methods

This was a prospective case control study undertaken in a teaching hospital in London over a 2-year period. Between 2006 and 2008, women scheduled for hysterectomy for menorrhagia with clinical uterine size of >14 weeks were offered an attempt at VH after pre-treatment with goserelin acetate. Women in the study group received either one or two intramuscular doses of 3.6 mg of goserelin (Zoladex, Astra Zeneca, Ltd.) while a group of women with comparable uterine size who underwent TAH for menorrhagia served as control; this study therefore achieves Oxford level II evidence. Oophorectomies were not routinely performed in either group.

VHs were performed by two consultant gynaecologists (WY and AF) who were experienced at doing the procedure for prolapse (as part of the repertoire of most trained gynecologists) but were attempting to gain more experience at removing larger non-prolapsing uteri >14 weeks through

the vaginal route. TAH in the control groups was performed by consultant gynaecologist colleagues of the two senior authors or senior trainees under their direct supervision. All patients received an intravenous bolus dose of 1.2 g Augmentin intraoperatively and wore antiembolic stockings and/or sequential compression stockings. VH patients had a vaginal pack and indwelling urinary catheter in situ until the following morning. Postoperative pain management included oral narcotics, non-steroidal anti-inflammatory medications and, in addition, patient-controlled analgesia for the first day in the TAH group.

Patient characteristics such as age, ethnicity, parity, body mass index (BMI), uterine size on scan and clinical size at surgery, preoperative administration of GnRH analogues, histological uterine weight and histopathology report were recorded. Peri-and postoperative complications (including surgical, blood transfusion and pyrexia) and other important outcome measures such as change in haemoglobin concentration, operative time and length of postoperative hospital stay were also compared.

Findings

Prospective data from 12 patients were collected from the study and control groups, respectively. The two groups had statistically comparable median age (49 vs 48 years), pre-treatment uterine length on ultrasound scan (12.1 vs 10.5 cm), preoperative haemoglobin (12.8 vs 12.6 g/dl) and BMI (31.72 vs 24.25 g/m^2) ($p>0.05$ in all cases). Women who had VH had higher parity than women who underwent TAH (3 vs 1.5, $p<0.05$) (Table 1).

The median subjective uterine size of the VH group prior to goserelin injections was 18 weeks (range 15–20 weeks), while the subjective uterine bulk at the time of surgery (median 16 vs 16 weeks) and histological uterine weight (median 580 vs 609 g) were comparable in both groups ($p>0.05$) (Fig. 1). The subjective median decrease in clinical uterine bulk was thus 11.11%.

The median duration of surgery (137 vs 81.6 min) and estimated blood loss (629 vs 422 ml) (both $p>0.05$) were significantly higher in the vaginal compared to the abdominal hysterectomy group, but this was skewed by

Table 1 Patient characteristics

Patient characteristics	VH ($n=12$) Median (range)	TAH ($n=12$) Median (range)	p value[*]
Age (years)	49 (41–51)	48 (39–51)	NS
Parity	3 (1–4)	1.5 (0–4)	0.04
Uterine length on USS (cm)	12 (9–16)	10.65 (8–14)	NS
Clinical size at time of surgery (weeks)	16 (12–22)	16 (12–22)	NS
Previous abdominal surgery	1/12	2/12	NS

NS not significant

[*]$p<0.05$ is taken to infer statistical significance

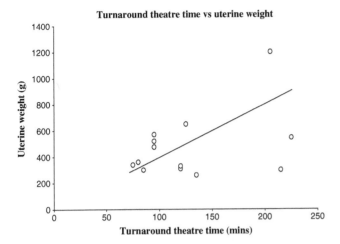

Fig. 1 Uterine weight vs duration of surgery

an outlier in the VH group whose specimen weighed 1,200 g. Analgesia requirements and length of inpatient stay were significantly lower in the VH group (2.41 vs 4.1 days, p<0.05) (Table 2). Nine of the 12 TAH patients required intramuscular opioids postoperatively compared to only one in the VH group.

Serious postoperative morbidity was minimal in both groups: in the VH group, two women had pyrexia (>38°C) postoperatively which resolved within 24 h with antibiotics, and the patient who had the 1,200-g uterus removed required two units of blood for blood transfusion.

Conclusion

Hysterectomy remains one of the commonest gynaecological operations, and the Cochrane review on the subject [13] concluded (on the basis of safety, reduced postoperative pain, shortened length of stay and higher patient satisfaction) that VH should be performed in preference to TAH, and if not possible, then a laparoscopically assisted approach may then be used. Furthermore, both Harry Reich and Ray Garry, pioneers of laparoscopic hysterectomy, agreed that "evidence based studies support the use of vaginal hysterectomy if possible over laparoscopic and abdominal hysterectomy" [14, 15]. Despite this, there is

still reluctance for gynaecologists to perform VH, particularly in the absence of prolapse and when the uterine size exceeds 12 weeks. In fact, only 15% of hysterectomies for fibroids in the USA [16] were performed vaginally, although many authors have now reported successful vaginal removal of enlarged uteri of up to 20 weeks [8, 9] using techniques such as bisection, Lash intramyometrial coring, vaginal myomectomy and wedge resection.

Stovall and colleagues were the first to describe the concept of medically debulking the enlarged uterus to facilitate VH and were able to show a success rate of 70% for uteri between 14 and 18 weeks. When translated in to cost analyses, significant potential savings could be made, which would easily compensate for the cost of preoperative GnRH analogues expenditure [17]. Previous costing by Johns and colleagues from the USA [18] indicated that the average hospital charge for VH was US $700 less than TAH (US $5,869 vs $6,552) while more contemporaneous data from the UK suggest similar reimbursement tariffs for both VH and TAH but more net profit with the former because of the shorter duration of inpatient stay.

While laparoscopy is a useful adjunct to VH when extensive adhesiolysis is contemplated or when there is suspected adnexal pathology, we concur with previous authors [2, 8, 10] that laparoscopic assistance is not otherwise necessary for the vaginal removal of a moderately enlarged uterus.

Our study corroborates the previous findings that the neoadjuvant use of GnRH analogues can help facilitate vaginal hysterectomies in moderately large uteri and further demonstrates positive advantages compared to a cohort of patients with similar uterine size at surgery who underwent TAH. We admit that our case control series is neither large (12 women in each group) nor randomised and thus can be subject to type II bias. We are also aware that many exceptional vaginal surgeons are able to remove large uteri even without the use of GnRH analogues. Our study simply seeks to suggest that medical debulking using GnRH analogues can convert an abdominal to a potentially safe VH and is a simple and cost-effective way through which an "average" gynaecologist can improve skill and confidence in attempting the vaginal route. We feel that in the

Table 2 Peri- and postoperative outcome measures

Outcome measure	VH (n=12) Median (range)	TAH (n=12) Median (range)	p value*
Theatre turnover time (min)	153.7 (80–225)	85 (50–170)	0.01
Estimated blood loss (ml)	629 (200–1,600)	422 (100–700)	NS
Histological uterine weight (g)	580 (475–1,200)	609 (450–1,218)	NS
Length of stay (days)	2 (1–5)	3.5 (3–9)	0.02
Postoperative pyrexia >38°C	2	0	NS
Transfusion	1	0	NS

NS not significant

*p<0.05 is taken to infer statistical significance

first year of our study, size regression achieved with goserelin gave us the confidence that VH for the "bulky" uteri is possible and motivated us to attempt removal by the vaginal route unless otherwise contraindicated. Through deliberate effort and building on experience as a result of this study, both senior authors have been able to remove progressively larger uteri so much so that analogues are currently used only for trial of VH >20 weeks or to effect amenorrhoea in order to maximise preoperative haemoglobin.

There is therefore little doubt that with sufficient impetus, motivation and training, units can increase their vaginal hysterectomy rates for non-prolapsing uteri from under 40% to nearly 100% over a period of a few years [10].

Acknowledgements The authors are indebted to the medical writings of Mr. A. Magos, Mr. R. Varma and Professor S. Sheth in stimulating their interest in vaginal hysterectomy for the larger non-descending uteri.

Declaration of interest The authors report no conflicts of interest. The authors alone are responsible for the content and writing of the paper.

References

1. Harmanli OH, Byun S, Dandolu V, Gaughan JP, Grody MHT (2006) Vaginal hysterectomy for the enlarged uterus. Gynecol Obstet Invest 6:4–8
2. Unger JB (1999) Vaginal hysterectomy for the woman with a moderately enlarged uterus weighing 200 to 700 grams. Am J Obstet Gynecol 180(6 Pt 1):1337–1344
3. Harmanli OH, Gentzler CK, Byun S, Dandolu MH, Grody T (2004) A comparison of abdominal and vaginal hysterectomy for the large uterus. Int J Gynaecol Obstet 87(1):19–23
4. Switala I, Cosson M, Lanvin D, Querleu D, Crepin G (1998) Is vaginal hysterectomy important for large uterus of more than 500 g? Comparison with laparotomy. J Gynecol Obstet Biol Reprod (Paris) 27(6):585–592
5. Kovac SR (2000) Hysterectomy outcomes in patients with similar indications. Obstet Gynecol 95:787–793
6. Doucette RC, Sharp HT, Alder SC (2001) Challenging generally accepted contraindications to vaginal hysterectomy. Am J Obstet Gynecol 184(7):1386–1389, discussion 1390–1
7. Synder TE, Stovall TG (2002) Use of gonadotrophin releasing hormone agonist before hysterectomy. In: Sheth S, Studd J (eds) Vaginal hysterectomy. Martin Dunitz, London, pp 111–127, Chapter 10
8. Magos A, Bournas N, Sinha R, Richardson RE, O'Connor H (1996) Vaginal hysterectomy for the large uterus. BJOG 103 (3):246–251
9. Sahin Y (2007) Vaginal hysterectomy and oophorectomy in women with 12–20 weeks' size uterus. Acta Obstet Gynecol Scand 86(11):1359–1369
10. Varma R, Tahseen S, Loukugamage AU, Kunde D (2001) Vaginal route as the norm when planning hysterectomy for benign conditions: change in practice. Obstet Gynecol 97:613–616
11. Vessey MP, Villard-Mackintosh L, McPherson K, Coulter A, Yeates D (1992) The epidemiology of hysterectomy: findings in a large cohort study. BJOG 99:402–407
12. Stovall TG, Summit RL Jr, Washburn SA, Ling FW (1994) Gonadotropin-releasing hormone agonist use before hysterectomy. Am J Obstet Gynecol 170(6):1744–1748, discussion 1748–51
13. Nieboer TE, Johnson N, Lethaby A, Tavender E, Curr E, Garry R, van Voorst S, Mol BW, Kluivers KB (2009) Surgical approach to hysterectomy for benign gynaecological disease. Cochrane Database Syst Rev 8(3):CD003677
14. Reich H (2007) Total laparoscopic hysterectomy: indications, techniques and outcomes. Curr Opin Obstet Gynecol 19:337–344
15. Garry R (2009) The best way to determine the best way to undertake a hysterectomy (commentary). BJOG 116:473–477
16. Lepine LA, Hillis SD, Marchbanks PA, Koonin LM, Morrow B, Kieke BA et al (1997) Hysterectomy surveillance-United States 1980–93. CDC Surveillance summaries, August 8, 1997. MMWR Morb Mortal Wkly Rep 1997, 46(SS4):1–15
17. Bradham DD, Stovall TG, Thompson CD (1995) Use of GnRH agonist before hysterectomy: a cost simulation. Obstet Gynecol 85 (3):401–406
18. Johns DA, Carrera B, Jones J, DeLeon F, Vincent R, Safely C (1995) The medical and economic impact of laparoscopically assisted vaginal hysterectomy in a large metropolitan not for profit hospital. Am J Obstet Gynecol 172:1709–1719

6

Laparoscopic supracervical hysterectomy: impact of body mass index and uterine weight

Munawar Hussain · Funlayo Odejinmi

Abstract Obesity is a risk factor for the development of uterine fibroids and dysfunctional uterine bleeding which may require hysterectomy. Vaginal hystectomy for enlarged uteri due to fibroids can be difficult and challenging while abdominal hysterectomy increases the risk of infection and bleeding. This prospective study was conducted to compare the operative outcome of laparoscopic supracervical hysterectomy in women with high body mass index (BMI) with enlarged or normal sized uteri. Patients were divided in to four groups according to body mass index and uterine weight. Group 1 included patients with BMI$\geq$25 kg/m^2 and uterine weight of $\geq$280 g, group 2 included patients with BMI$\geq$25 kg/m^2 and uterine weight of <280 g, group 3 (BMI $\leq$25 kg/m^2 and uterine weight $\geq$280 g) and group 4 (BMI$\leq$25 kg/m^2 and uterine weight of $\leq$280 g) were not included in the final analysis. There was no conversion to laparotomy, any intraoperative complications or difference in the mean duration of hospital stay in both groups. However, the operative time and blood loss in group 1 was more as compared to group 2. Laparoscopic supracervical hysterectomy is feasible and can be safely performed regardless of BMI or uterine weight.

Keywords Obesity · Large uterus · Fibroid uterus · Menorrhagia · Laparoscopic supracervical hysterectomy

M. Hussain
St. Michael's Hospital and Bristol Centre
for Reproductive Medicine,
Bristol, UK

M. Hussain (✉)
St. Michael's Hospital, University Hospitals Bristol NHS Trust,
Bristol BS2 8EG, UK
e-mail: dr_72hussain@yahoo.com

F. Odejinmi
Whipps Cross University Hospital NHS Trust,
London E11 1NR, UK
e-mail: jimi@doctors.org.uk

Background

Despite the introduction of various alternative therapies for menorrhagia, hysterectomy still remains one of the most commonly performed procedures worldwide [1]. Vaginal hysterectomy should be the preferred choice but when it is not feasible or possible, laparoscopic hysterectomy is the next preferred procedure as this is associated with less postoperative pain and quick recovery. Enlarged uteri due to fibroids pose difficulty in choosing the route of hysterectomy; although vaginal hystectomy is possible, it can be technically difficult and challenging. Laparoscopic hysterectomy, on the other hand, is considered hazardous in majority of these cases due to lack of expertise. Consequently, most hysterectomies for enlarged uteri are still being performed abdominally and often with midline incision with all its associated complications [2].

Obesity is an increasing problem and is a risk factor for the development of uterine fibroids and dysfunctional uterine bleeding which may require hysterectomy [3]. Obesity increases the risks of bleeding and infection after abdominal as well as vaginal hysterectomy [4]. Laparoscopic supracervical hysterectomies (LSH) are gaining popularity because of their safety and faster postoperative recovery [5, 6]. To reduce the complications of abdominal hysterectomies, LSH may be an alternative for large uteri in women with high body mass index (BMI). As there is very limited literature on this specific subject, we conducted this prospective observational study to analyze the operative outcome of LSH performed in women with high body mass index with enlarged and normal sized uteri.

Material and methods

This prospective comparative study was conducted in advanced laparoscopic surgery unit of Whipps Cross University Hospital London from June 2007 till June 2011. This was conducted as a continuous prospective audit of clinical practice after obtaining approval from the hospital research and development committee.

Body mass index (BMI) was calculated by measuring the weight in kilograms divided by height in meters squared. Patient's BMI was graded as overweight (BMI 25–30 kg/m^2), obese (BMI 30–40 kg/m^2) or morbidly obese (BMI>40 kg/m^2) as proposed by the World health Organization classification system of obesity. The uterine weight was measured in grams and stratified into two groups, weight≤280 g and ≥280 g. Patients were divided into four groups according to their BMI and uterine weight. Group 1 included patients with BMI≥25 kg/m^2 and uterine weight of ≥280 g, group 2 included patients with BMI≥25 kg/m^2 and uterine weight of <280 g, group 3 included patients with BMI≤25 kg/m^2 and uterine weight ≥280 g and group 4 included patients with BMI≤25 kg/m^2 and uterine weight of ≤280 g.

Preoperative clinical evaluation included assessment of uterine size and mobility, pelvic ultrasonography or MRI if required, and endometrial sampling was performed with or without hysteroscopy if clinically indicated. Patients were fully counseled regarding the proposed procedure and available alternatives, written information was provided and an informed consent was taken. Patients were included in the study if menorrhagia was resistant to medical treatment or had failed endometrial ablation therapy, history of at least three normal cervical smears and were happy to have cervical screening in the future. Previous pelvic surgery or endometriosis was not a contraindication to LSH. Exclusion criteria were a history of abnormal cervical smears, endometrial hyperplasia or carcinoma, suspicious adnexal mass, uterine prolapse or patients not willing to retain the cervix. No upper limit of the uterine size was set as exclusion criteria. All procedures were performed by one surgeon.

Surgical procedure

A modified five-port technique to perform LSH in women with enlarged uteri where the uterus extended beyond the true pelvis is explained in a previous article [7]. Briefly, all patients underwent the procedure under general anesthesia with endotracheal intubation and in modified lithotomy position. Their bladders were catheterized and a Clearview™ (Clinical Innovations) uterine manipulator was inserted through the cervix for manipulation of the uterus. Pneumoperitoneum was created by Veress needle at the left subcostal region 2 cm below the costal margin in the midclavicular line, i.e., Palmers point, and

a 5-mm port was then inserted at this point. A 0° 5-mm laparoscope was used to inspect the abdomen for the duration of the operation. A second 5-mm port was placed on the contralateral side, in the right hypochondrium, and two other ancillary (5 mm) ports were inserted laterally at the level of the umbilicus depending upon the size of the uterus, above the level of the ovarian ligaments lateral to the epigastric vessels and a 10-mm suprapubic port 4 cm above the pubic symphysis in the midline (Fig. 1). The right side of the procedure was carried out with the laparoscope in the right subcostal port and likewise the left side was carried out with the laparoscope in the left subcostal port. Bipolar diathermy forceps were used for coagulation and harmonic scalpel was used for coagulation and cutting the pedicles. On both sides, the infundibulopelvic or ovarian ligament with the tube and round ligaments were coagulated and divided, the uterovesical fold was then opened and bladder resected downwards (this was important especially where there is a large fibroid at the level of isthmus of the uterus). On both sides, the uterine arteries were skeletonized, coagulated and divided. Then, the uterus was transected from the cervix using the Lap Loop™ (Roberts Surgical). Endocervical canal was cored out to destroy any remnant endometrial tissue. A tissue morcellator was then used to remove the uterine specimen from the abdominal cavity.

Data collection, power calculation and statistical analysis

Data was prospectively collected on a standardized proforma and entered onto a computerized database. The

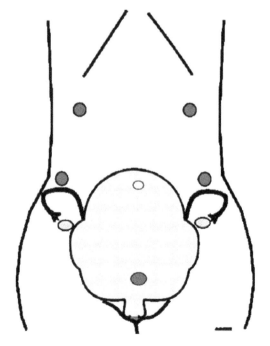

Fig. 1 Port sites in the modified five-port technique of LSH for large uteri [7].

database included patient demographics, examination findings, operative indications, operative time, blood loss, operative complications, uterine weight and duration of hospital stay and details of histology of the uterine specimens. Operative blood loss was calculated by measuring the volume of fluid in the suction system and subtracting the amount of irrigation used during the procedure. The operating time was calculated from the insertion of the Veress needle to skin closure of the last port site.

The study was powered as a two-group study to detect medium to large effects which would be of clinical relevance and powered on the basis that the Mann–Whitney test would be used to investigate the significance of differences. On this basis, for a medium to large effect size, a minimum sample size of at least $n=40$ per group would have at least 80% power for standard level of significance (alpha=0.05) in a two-sided test.

Continuous data were reported as mean±1SD with 95% confidence intervals and were compared by unpaired Student's t-test, while noncontinuous data were reported as median and interquartile range and compared by Mann–Whitney U test. Categorical variables were presented as percentages and 95% CI and compared by Fisher's exact test. Deviation of variables from Gaussian distribution was assessed by Shapiro–Wilk test. A probability value of <0.05 was considered to be statistically significant. Statistical analysis was performed using intercooled Stata, ver.8.0 (Stata Corporation, College Station, TX).

Results

Table 1 shows the patients' demographic characteristics and operative parameters. There were 44, 41, 14 and 12 patients in groups 1, 2, 3 and 4, respectively. Due to the small number of patients in groups 3 and 4, they were not included in the final analysis.

Patients in groups 1and 2 were comparable with respect to age, parity, BMI, operative indications and operative procedure performed. The mean BMI in groups 1 and 2 were 33 and 34 kg/m^2, respectively; however, 18% (8/44) patients in group 1 and 17% (7/41) patients in group 2 were morbidly obese (BMI>40 kg/m^2). The uterine size and the weight of the uterine specimens were substantially bigger (P< 0.0001) in group 1. In group 1, the mean uterine size was 20 weeks; however, 50% (22/44) of the uteri were more than 20 weeks in size; likewise, the mean uterine weight was 574 g, but 52% (23/44) of the uteri weighed were more than 500 g and 17% (4/23) out of these uteri weighed more than 1 kg. The operative time and blood loss was statistically more in group 1 as compared to group 2.

There was no conversion to open procedure, no intra-operative complications, no blood transfusion and no difference in the mean duration of hospital stay in both groups. Histopathology confirmed leiomyoma in 97% and 94% cases and adenomyosis in the remaining 3% and 6% cases in groups 1 and 2, respectively, and there were no malignancies.

Table 1 Patient characteristics and operative parameters

Parameter observed	Group I ($n=44$)	Group II ($n=41$)	P value
Age (years)[a]	45.8±4.3 (44.5–47.1)	47.0±4.9(45.3–48.4)	0.28
Parity[a]	1.8±1.3 (1.4–2.2)	1.8±1.2 (1.4–2.0)	0.96
BMI (kg/m^2)[a]	33.5±5.7 (31.8–35.2)	34±6.1 (32.1–35.9)	0.69
Indications of Hysterectomy[b]			
Menorrhagia and fibroids	41 (93%, 95% CI 81–99)	39 (95%, 95% CI 83–99)	>0.999
Menorrhagia and D.U.B	1 (2%, 95% CI 0–1.2)	1 (2.4%, 95% CI 0–1.3)	
Chronic pelvic pain	2 (5%, 95% CI 0–1.5)	0	
Pressure symptoms	0	1 (2.4%, 95% CI 0–1.3)	
Uterine size (weeks)[c]	20 (10–30)	10 (8–16)	<0.0001
Operative procedure[b]			
LSH	36 (82%, 95% CI67–92)	33(80%, 95% CI65–91)	>0.999
LSH+BSO	8 (18%, 95% CI8–32)	8 (20%, 95% CI8–35)	>0.999
Operative time (minutes)[a]	97.3±38.9 (85.5–108.2)	56.5±20.5 (50.0–63.0)	<0.0001
Intraoperative blood loss (ml)[a]	273±171 (221–324)	180±103 (147–212)	0.003
Uterine weight (g)[a]	574±246 (499–649)	147±47(132–162)	<0.0001
Hospital stay (days)[a]	2.1±0.52 (1.9–2.2)	2.0±0.53 (1.7–2.0)	0.04

DUB dysfunctional uterine bleeding, *BSO* bilateral salpingoophrectomy

[a] Data are mean±1SD (95% CI) and analyzed by unpaired Student's t-test

[b] Data are percentage and 95% confidence interval, analyzed by Fisher's exact test

[c] Data are median (range), analyzed by Mann–Whitney U test

Discussion

In this study, majority (>90%) of the hysterectomies in both groups were performed due to menorrhagia and fibroids in the uterus. The uterine size and the weight of the uterine specimens were substantially higher in group 1 resulting in long operative time and more blood loss as compared to group 2. The median operative times and blood loss was more in our study as compared to other studies on this subject [7–9]. Considering the larger uterine size in our study, it is not surprising to observe that it took us more time to operate, and there was more blood loss. It has been shown that uterine weight is an independent factor to increase the operative time, blood loss and complications during abdominal and laparoscopic hysterectomy especially when the uterine weight is more than 500 g [10, 11]. Although the median blood loss was more in group 1, it was in such a limited amount that none of the patients required blood transfusion in either group. Moreover, most of the actual operative time in group 1 was spent in morcellation of the enlarged uteri due to fibroids, adding to the total length of the procedure. Additional factor of high BMI might also have contributed towards more operative time as the laparoscopic entry and actual procedure is difficult in this group of women. Although laparoscopic hysterectomy in obese women is safe and feasible, it can be associated with more operative time, more blood loss and conversion to laparotomy [12]. We did not encounter any operative complications and there was no conversion to open procedure. Thus, despite the longer operative time and relatively more blood loss, LSH was completed with low morbidity while maintaining the benefits of minimally invasive surgery in a high risk group of women with high BMI and enlarged uteri.

Despite the increasing prevalence of obesity with associated menstrual problems and proven benefits of LSH, there is still limited literature on the specific subject of LSH for obese women with large uteri. Although few studies have addressed LSH for large uteri [7, 9], while others [13–15] have shown the safety and feasibility of total laparoscopic and supracervical hysterectomy for large uteri, none have specifically addressed LSH for large uteri in obese women.

The increasing prevalence of obesity with associated fibroids uterus and menstrual problems the world over is such that the practicing gynecologist would expect more patients from this group attending for hysterectomy [16]. Originally, obesity was considered as a relative contraindication for laparoscopic surgery, but with improved technology and skills, the current evidence suggests that laparoscopic hysterectomy is feasible and safe in obese women; however, it is associated with relatively more operative time and risk of bleeding [12, 17–19]. Although our data is specifically for laparoscopic supracervical hysterectomy, it is consistent with the results of the above-mentioned studies with regard to operative time, blood loss, complication rate and duration of hospital stay and has highlighted the limited role of BMI in the surgical outcome of LSH.

LSH is gaining popularity not only among gynecologists but also among the patients. Traditionally, gynecologists have been trained for either abdominal or vaginal hysterectomy, and the choice of route of hysterectomy depends on the uterine size and mobility as well as the preference and experience of the surgeon. [2]. In our opinion, LSH can be successfully performed in obese women with enlarged uteri by modifying the operative technique. We suggest a modified five-port technique for LSH in enlarged uteri as explained in "Material and methods". It is our particular placement of the ports that enabled us to remove large uteri satisfactorily. Despite the large uterus, this operative technique provides good exposure of both pelvic side walls because the laparoscope can be placed on the left side for left-sided pedicles and likewise on the right side for the right-sided pedicles.

The limitations of this study include observational nature and the relatively small number of patients; however, it has sufficient power to detect medium to large effect size of clinical relevance. We believe this study is an important contribution to the very limited literature available on the subject of laparoscopic supracervical hysterectomy for women with high BMI and enlarged uteri. This study will encourage other surgeons to consider this procedure in this group of women to prevent the complications associated with abdominal hysterectomy. However, more gynecologists will have to master their skills to operate upon obese women with enlarged uteri.

Conclusions

This study suggests that laparoscopic supracervical hysterectomy is feasible and can be safely performed in large women with large uteri rather than the traditional approach of laparotomy by midline incision. However, relatively longer operative times and more blood loss can be expected in this group of women. Larger prospective studies are needed to complement our results.

Conflict of interest   The authors report no conflicts of interest. The authors alone are responsible for the content and writing of the paper.

References

1. Garry R (2009) The future of hysterectomy. BJOG 112:133–139
2. Davies A, Hart R, Magos A, Hadad E, Moris R (2002) Hysterectomy: surgical route and complications. Eur J Obstet Gynecol Reprod Biol 104:148–151

3. Osler M, Daugbjerg S, Frederiksen BL, Ottesen B (2011) Body mass and risk of complications after hysterectomy on benign indications. Hum Reprod 26:1512–1518

4. Löfgren M, Poromaa IS, Stjerndahl JH et al (2004) Operative infections and antibiotic prophylaxis for hysterectomy in Sweden: a study by the Swedish National Register for Gynecologic Surgery. Acta Obstet Gynecol Scand 83:1202–1207

5. Esdaile BA, Chalian RA, Del Priore G et al (2006) The role of supracervical hysterectomy in benign disease of the uterus. J Obstet Gynaecol 26:52–58

6. Bojahr B, Raatz D, Schonleber G et al (2006) Perioperative complication rate in 1,706 patients after a standardized laparoscopic supracervical hysterectomy technique. J Minim Invasive Gynecol 13:183–189

7. Shahid A, Sankaran S, Odejinmi F (2011) Laparoscopic subtotal hysterectomy for large uteri using modified five port technique. Arch Gynecol Obstet 283:79–81

8. Erian J, El-Shawarby SA, Hassan M et al (2008) Laparoscopic subtotal hysterectomy using the plasma kinetic and lap loop systems: an alternative approach in the surgical management of women with uterine fibroids. Eur J Obstet Gynecol Reprod Biol 137:84–87

9. Lyons TL, Adolph AJ, Winer WK (2004) Laparoscopic supracervical hysterectomy for the large uterus. J Am Assoc Gynecol Laparosc 11:170–174

10. Bonilla DJ, Mains L, Whitaker R et al (2007) Uterine weight as a predictor of morbidity after a benign abdominal and total laparoscopic hysterectomy. J Reprod Med 52:490–498

11. O'Hanlan KA, McCutcheon SP, McCutcheon JG (2011) Laparoscopic hysterectomy: impact of uterine size. J Minim Invasive Gynecol 18:85–91

12. Heinberg EM, Crawford BL 3rd, Weitzen SH et al (2004) Total laparoscopic hysterectomy in obese versus non obese patients. Obstet Gynecol 103:674–680

13. Fiaccavento A, Landi S, Barbieri F et al (2007) Total laparoscopic hysterectomy in cases of very large uteri: a retrospective comparative study. J Minim Invasive Gynecol 14:559–563

14. Kondo W, Bourdel N, Marengo F et al (2011) Surgical outcomes of laparoscopic hysterectomy for enlarged uteri. J Minim Invasive Gynecol 18:310–313

15. Mueller A, Renner SP, Haeberle L et al (2009) Comparison of total laparoscopic hysterectomy (TLH) and laparoscopy-assisted supracervical hysterectomy (LASH) in women with uterine leiomyoma. Eur J Obstet Gynecol Reprod Biol 144:76–79

16. Osler M, Daugbjerg S, Frederiksen BL et al (2011) Body mass and risk of complications after hysterectomy on benign indications. Hum Reprod 26:1512–1518

17. O'Hanlan KA, Dibble SL, Fisher DT (2006) Total laparoscopic hysterectomy for uterine pathology: impact of body mass index on outcomes. Gynecol Oncol 103:938–941

18. Mueller A, Thiel F, Lermann J et al (2010) Feasibility and safety of total laparoscopic hysterectomy (TLH) using the Hohl instrument in non obese and obese women. J Obstet Gynaecol Res 36:159–164

19. Holub Z, Jabor A, Kliment L et al (2001) Laparoscopic hysterectomy in obese women: a clinical prospective study. Eur J Obstet Gynecol Reprod Biol 98:77–82

7

The well-being of women following total laparoscopic hysterectomy versus total abdominal hysterectomy for endometrial cancer

Sivakami Rajamanoharan · Tim Duncan · Jafaru Abu

Abstract Total laparoscopic hysterectomies (TLH) are increasingly being used in the management of endometrial carcinoma. There is insufficient research on patient satisfaction and well-being after TLH for malignant endometrial disease. The objective of this questionnaire-based retrospective study was to compare post-operative well-being after total abdominal hysterectomy (TAH) versus TLH for endometrial carcinoma. Eighty-one women who underwent a TLH or TAH for endometrial carcinoma and atypical endometrial hyperplasia in a tertiary UK hospital were the sample of this study. Data regarding well-being and post-operative satisfaction were obtained via a self-administered questionnaire. Results were analysed. The primary outcome was health-related well-being. The length of post-operative hospital stay, satisfaction with scar, return to normal activities, severity of post-operative pain and sexual activity were secondary outcome measures. Seventy women responded (TAH $n=41$; TLH $n=29$). There was no difference between overall well-being between both groups. TLH group reported a shorter hospital stay (TAH=4 days; TLH=2 days; $p=0.000$), a quicker return to normal activities

with 24.4% of the TAH group taking 12 weeks or more, compared to 3.4% of the TLH group ($p=0.019$) and increased satisfaction with their scars than the TAH group ('very' or 'fairly satisfied' with scar TAH 92.7%; TLH 100%; $p=0.039$). This study has found that patients' well-being after endometrial carcinoma is not significantly affected by surgical technique. This is in line with previous studies using patients with benign disease. However, laparoscopic techniques do have a reduced impact on a patient's life through shorter hospital stays and quicker return to normal activities

Keywords Total laparoscopic hysterectomy · Total abdominal hysterectomy · Endometrial carcinoma · Patient well-being

Introduction

In the UK in 2007, there were 7,536 cases of endometrial carcinoma diagnosed [1]. Hysterectomy via the abdominal route, with bilateral salpingo-oophorectomy and peritoneal washings, has been the mainstay of treatment. Advances in minimally invasive surgery led to the introduction of laparoscopically assisted vaginal hysterectomy (LAVH), laparoscopic hysterectomy (LH) and total laparoscopic hysterectomy (TLH) [2]. In LAVH, the round ligaments and the infundibulopelvic ligaments are secured laparoscopically and the rest of the procedure is completed via the vaginal route; whereas in LH the uterine vessels are secured laparoscopically before completing the rest of the procedure vaginally. With TLH, the entire hysterectomy is performed laparoscopically and the only vaginal component is removal of the uterus. Currently, TLH is used alongside total abdominal hysterectomy (TAH) in the management of endometrial cancer. Some studies have showed that TLH compared to TAH is associated with a reduction in the amount of total blood loss at operation,

S. Rajamanoharan
Chelsea and Westminster Hospital, NHS Foundation Trust,
369 Fulham Road,
London SW10 9NH, UK
e-mail: Sivakami1986@hotmail.com

T. Duncan
Department of Gynaecological Oncology,
Norfolk and Norwich University Hospitals,
Colney Lane,
Norwich NR4 7UY, UK
e-mail: tim.duncan@nnuh.nhs.uk

J. Abu (✉)
Department of Obstetrics and Gynaecology,
Nottingham University Hospitals,
City Campus,
Nottingham NG1 5PB, UK
e-mail: jafaru.abu@nuh.nhs.uk

reduced requirement for post-operative analgesia and reduced hospital stay [3–6]. Whilst major complications such as urinary tract injury have been shown to be slightly higher in patients having TLH compared to TAH, there was no statistically significant difference in such complication rates between the two procedures [3, 4]. Many surgeons are now opting for TLH in patients who present with stage 1a endometrial carcinoma, as the disease-free interval and overall survival rates after TLH have proved similar to that after TAH [6].

The majority of studies that have compared the two techniques have focussed on surgical outcomes such as blood loss and operative time. Many argue that such measures are indirect indicators of patient satisfaction with a procedure. However, a patient's well-being, frequently expanded to a holistic notion of a patient's physical, social, emotional and spiritual well-being or 'quality of life', is considered a more direct measure of an intervention's impact on a patient [7]. One of the largest studies which examined quality of life as a secondary outcome after TAH versus laparoscopic hysterectomy procedures (i.e. grouping TLH, LH and LAVH together) reported that laparoscopic hysterectomy procedures were associated with a better quality of life [8]. A systematic review into quality of life after LH versus TAH which studied 30 previous trials also found similar results. The authors stated that in the seven studies which focused on quality of life as an outcome measure, patients who had laparoscopic hysterectomies reported a quality of life that was equal to or better than those who had received a TAH [9].

Only two studies have looked exclusively at TLH with quality of life or patient well-being as the primary outcome [10, 11]. One found that TLH patients had more 'post-operative vitality' than TAH patients [10], whereas the other reported that there was no significant difference in 'psychological well-being' or 'sexuality' after both procedures [11]. Notably, both studies only recruited patients with benign disease, therefore the impact of surgery when already dealing with the diagnosis of malignancy has yet to be established. Most studies comparing laparoscopic and abdominal approaches to hysterectomy have concentrated on benign disease, these patients cohorts are likely to be differ significantly to those undergoing surgery for endometrial cancer. Recently, there have been Australian [12] and Dutch [13] randomised controlled trails addressing quality of life for patients in this important group. Our study aims to compare patient well-being after TLH versus TAH for endometrial cancer in a UK population.

Materials and methods

Participants

This questionnaire-based, retrospective study was conducted in a large UK teaching hospital. Women who had undergone a TLH or TAH for an initial presentation of endometrial malignancy or atypical hyperplasia at one tertiary centre over a period of 23 months (January 2007 through to November 2008) were identified. Women who had presented with endometrial malignancy were staged pre-operatively with magnetic resonance imaging (MRI). Those with a uterine size of <12 weeks gestation were considered eligible (total $n=81$; TAH $n=49$; TLH n=32). Patients who had presented pre-operatively with benign pathology were excluded.

Baseline patient characteristics of pre-operative use of hormone replacement therapy (HRT), parity, menopausal status, body mass index (BMI), age and American Society of Anesthesiologists (ASA) score were obtained from hospital records. Patient well-being post-operatively was assessed via a self-administered questionnaire (Appendix I) that was distributed by mail, together with a covering letter. Completed questionnaires were also returned in a prepaid stamped envelope.

Questionnaire

The questionnaire was derived from the validated SF-36 health questionnaire [14]. It included participants' details (name, age and date on which they completed the questionnaire) and questions under seven broad themes. (1) Health in general—a visual analogue scale to express opinion of general health (0='poor' to 100='excellent') and a structured question inquiring about opinion of health now compared to 1 year ago. (2) Limitations on activities of daily living (vigorous activities, moderate activities, using the stairs, bathing and dressing). (3) Recovery after hospital (post-operative hospital stay, time taken to return to normal activities and satisfaction with scar). (4) Severity of post-operative pain. All questions referring to pain consisted of a visual analogue scale due to its documented validity in measuring pain intensity [15]. (5) Post-operative sexual activity. The women were asked to comment on their sexual activity now compared to before the operation. A visual analogue scale was used to assess pain on resumption of sexual activity post-operatively. (6) Ideas concerning their general health. (7) General comments. This comprised of a free text box asking participants to comment on anything they felt was not covered by the preceding questions.

Surgical procedure

Antibiotics and thrombo-prophylaxis were administered to all women prior to surgery according to the hospital protocol. The abdominal hysterectomies were performed or supervised by consultant gynaecological oncologists. Total abdominal hysterectomies were performed via a lower abdominal transverse incision and involved complete removal of the uterus including the corpus and the cervix as well as bilateral salpingo-oophorectomy with or without pelvic lymph node dissection or sampling. The laparoscopic hysterectomies were also performed by consultant gynaecological oncologists. Four small incisions are made: three 5-mm trocar ports in the lower abdomen and one 10-mm intra-umbilical camera port. TLH procedure involved securing the round ligament and infundibulopelvic ligaments with a blood vessel sealing device such as the Ligasure 5. The bladder was then reflected with monopolar diathermy scissors and the uterine vessels secured at the edge of a trans-vaginal tube (McCartney tube). The cervix is then excised from the vaginal vault at the edge of the trans-vaginal tube and the whole specimen removed vaginally. If required, lymph nodes were dissected laparoscopically and retrieved via the McCartney tube. Laparoscopic vaginal vault closure was with O-monocryl suture.

Outcome measures

The primary outcome of this retrospective study was health-related well-being after TAH versus TLH for early-stage endometrial carcinoma. The length of post-operative hospital stay, satisfaction with scar, return to normal activities, severity of post-operative pain and sexual activity were secondary outcome measures.

Statistical analysis

Differences in women's baseline characteristics (age, parity, menopausal status, BMI, HRT use and SA score) and the duration of time from operation to questionnaire completion were compared between the two groups. The mean and standard deviation were calculated for parametric data; median and inter-quartile range for non-parametric data. Data from visual analogue scales was measured in millimetres, the measurement corresponding to a number from 0 (no pain) to 100 (worst pain). Qualitative data from theme VII was grouped into categories and analysed separately. Differences between the two groups were tested for statistical significance using chi^2 test for categorical data; independent t test for parametric continuous data and Mann–Whitney U test for non-parametric continuous data. A p value of <0.05 was considered significant. All data was analysed using SPSS 14.0 software (SPSS USA 2005).

Results

Eighty-one questionnaires were sent out in total. Seventy (87.5%) were completed and returned (TAH n=41; TLH n=29). Of the 11 women that did not respond, one had undergone a TAH for stage 1A endometrial carcinoma, but sadly

died 5 months after the operation due to the development of an unrelated primary carcinoma of the colon with associated liver metastasis.

The study groups were balanced for age, menopausal status, BMI, pre-operative parity and ASA score. There were however differences in the levels of pre-operative HRT use and the median duration of time from the operation to questionnaire completion (Table 1). Whilst endometrial carcinoma was the main indication for surgery in both groups, there was a substantial number of TLH carried out for atypical hyperplasia (8, 25%) than TAH (3, 6.1%). Detailed analysis of the histological type, stage and grade of disease is given in Table 2.

Analysis of the primary outcome (Table 3) revealed no statistically significant difference between the two groups, with both groups expressing a good sense of health-related well-being. Upon analysis of secondary outcomes, a number of differences were evident between the two groups (Table 4). The number of days spent in hospital post-operatively differed significantly along with the duration of time taken to return to normal activities with 24.4% of the TAH group taking 12 weeks or more, compared to 3.4% of the TLH group. Two women were able to return home within 2 days of a TLH procedure, whilst the minimum stay after a TAH was 2 to 4 days. Satisfaction with the surgical scar was significantly higher in the TLH group, 92.7% of the TAH group said they were 'very' or 'fairly satisfied' compared to 100% of the TLH group; $p=0.039$. No difference in the severity of post-operative pain was reported.

Of those who answered the questionnaire, 60% (TAH= 21, 51.2%; TLH=21, 72.4%) wrote a comment in question

Table 1 Patients' pre-operative baseline characteristics, current age and time duration from operation to questionnaire completion by treatment group

		TAH ($n=49$)	TLH ($n=32$)	p value
ASA score[a]		2 (1–2)	2 (1–3)	0.568
HRT use	Yes	1 (2)	5 (16)	0.017*
	No	48 (98)	25 (78)	
Pre-menopausal		6 (12)	6 (19)	0.351
Post-menopausal		43 (88)	24 (75)	
BMI (kg/m²)[a]		32 (21–60)	33 (26–40)	0.856
Parity[a]		2 (1–3)	2 (2–2.5)	0.881
Current age (years)[a]		65 (58–73)	60 (50–70)	0.083
Time from operation to questionnaire completion (months)[a]		10 (5–18)	6 (4–9)	0.007*

Data expressed as absolute numbers (percentage)

TAH total abdominal hysterectomy, *TLH* total laparoscopic hysterectomy, *HRT* hormone replacement therapy, *BMI* body mass index, *ASA* American Society Anesthesiologists

[a] Median (inter-quartile range)

Table 2 Patients' pre-operative diagnosis, MRI staging, post-operative histological type, histological stage and histological grade of endometrial carcinoma

		TAH (*n*=49)	TLH (*n*=32)	*p* value
Pre-operative diagnosis [*n* (%)]	Endometrial carcinoma	42 (85.7)	20 (62.5)	0.038*
	Atypical hyperplasia	3 (6.1)	8 (25.0)	
	Complex hyperplasia	1 (2.0)	1 (3.1)	
	Other	2 (4.1)	2 (6.3)	
MRI Stage [*n* (%)]	IA	5 (10.2)	9 (28.1)	0.076
	IB	10 (20.4)	6 (18.8)	
	IC	7 (14.3)	0	
	IIA	2 (4.1)	0	
	IIB	2 (4.1)	1 (3.1)	
	IIIA	2 (4.1)	0	
	IIIB	0	0	
	IIIC	3 (6.1)	0	
	IV	1 (2.0)	0	
	Primary tumour not identified	2 (4.1)	4 (12.5)	
	No MRI	15 (30.6)	12 (37.5)	
Post-operative histological type [*n* (%)]	Endometroid Adenocarcinoma	40 (81.6)	27 (84.4)	0.018*
	Carcinosarcoma	6 (12.2)	0	
	Serous papillary carcinoma	2 (4.1)	0	
	Benign disease	1 (2.0)	5 (15.5)	
Post-operative histological stage [*n* (%)]	IA	4 (8.2)	10 (31.3)	0.011*
	IB	21 (42.9)	12 (37.5)	
	IC	8 (16.3)	1 (3.1)	
	IIA	1 (2.0)	0	
	IIB	5 (10.2)	1 (3.1)	
	IIIA	7 (14.3)	3 (9.4)	
	IIIB	0	1 (3.1)	
	IIIC	2 (4.1)	0	
	IV	1 (2.0)	0	
	No histological stage reported	0	4 (12.5)	
Post-operative histological grade [*n* (%)]	I	16 (32.7)	15 (46.9)	0.187
	II	23 (46.9)	9 (28.1)	
	III	8 (16.3)	4 (12.5)	
	No histological grade reported	2 (4.1)	4 (12.5)	

Data expressed as absolute numbers (percentage of group)

TAH total abdominal hysterectomy, *TLH* total laparoscopic hysterectomy, *MRI* magnetic resonance imaging

7.1, the general comments free text section. Six women (TAH=4, TLH=2) commented on the negative impact of radiotherapy and chemotherapy on their health-related well-being. Four women said their recovery had been affected by post-operative wound infections (TAH=3, TLH=1). Nine women (TAH=8, TLH=1) stated that they experienced negative symptoms or problems since their operation. Comments from the TAH group included 'tire more easily' (four women), 'backache', 'sensitive bowels', 'feel that hysterectomy has aged me', 'sex has become very painful' and having 'bouts of depression'. One woman from the TLH group remarked on having 'trapped wind' and 'difficult sleeping'. Four women from the TAH group stated that the negative aspects of their health-related well-being were not due to the operation but due to other health conditions, such as asthma and musculoskeletal pain from a previous road traffic accident.

Eleven women commented on the 'excellent' quality of care received whilst in hospital (TAH=6, TLH=5); however, two women (TAH=1, TLH=1) felt the care they received post-operatively was 'less than expected' and they 'felt left on my own a little to cope with the emotional feelings experienced'. Thirteen women (TAH=4, TLH=9) expressed their satisfaction with the surgical procedure they had experienced, whilst 8 out of the 21 in the TLH group who answered question 7.1 expressed particular contentment in laparoscopic

Table 3 Primary outcome: scores on well-being between the two groups

Question—responses		TAH (n=41)	TLH (n=29)	p value[a]
1.1 Opinion of health at present (visual analogue scores)		70 (55.5–81.0)	76 (61.0–84.0)	0.375
1.2 Health now compared to one year ago	Much better	12 (29.3)	10 (34.5)	0.253
	Somewhat better	3 (7.3)	7 (24.9)	
	About the same	21 (51.2)	9 (31.0)	
	Somewhat worse	4 (9.8)	2 (6.9)	
	Much worse	1 (2.4)	1 (3.4)	
2.1 No. whose activities of daily living were limited by health		30 (75.0)	21 (72.4)	0.809
6.1 'Get sick a little easier' than other people	True	3 (7.3)	0 (0.0)	0.108
	False	29 (70.7)	28 (96.6)	
	Don't know	9 (22.0)	1 (3.4)	
6.2 No. who felt they were 'as healthy as anybody' they know		33 (56.1)	20 (69.0)	0.338
6.3 No. who expected their health to 'get worse'		5 (12.2)	2 (6.9)	0.511
6.4 No. who felt their health was 'excellent'		27 (65.9)	22 (75.8)	0.920

Data expressed as absolute number (percentage of total group)

TAH total abdominal hysterectomy, *TLH* total laparoscopic hysterectomy

[a] p value for difference between the two groups using chi^2 test for categorical data, independent *t* test for parametric continuous data and Mann–Whitney *U* test for non-parametric continuous data

surgery, e.g. 'I feel grateful that I was lucky to have keyhole procedure and feel that it should become the rule rather than the exception'. Three women (TAH=1, TLH=2) stated that they would recommend laparoscopic surgery to others, or 'given the choice I would have gone for keyhole' (one woman from TAH group).

Table 4 Secondary outcome measures between the two groups

Question		TAH (n=41)	TLH (n=29)	p value[a]
3.1 No. of days of post-operative hospital stay[a]		4 (4–5)	2 (2–3)	0.000*
3.2 Duration of time taken to return to normal activities after operation (weeks)	0–2	0 (0)	2 (6.9)	0.019*
	2–4	2 (4.9)	4 (13.8)	
	4–6	5 (12.2)	10 (34.5)	
	6–8	12 (29.3)	8 (27.6)	
	8–10	8 (19.5)	2 (6.9)	
	10–12	4 (9.8)	2 (6.9)	
	12 or more	10 (24.4)	1 (3.4)	
3.3 Satisfaction with appearance of scar	Very satisfied	26 (63.4)	27 (93.1)	0.039*
	Fairly satisfied	12 (29.3)	2 (6.9)	
	A little unhappy	2 (4.9)	0 (0)	
	Very unhappy	1 (2.4)	0 (0)	
4.1 VAS score for severity of post-operative pain (mm)[b]	0–24 h	28 (8–75)	25 (8–54)	0.582
	24–48 h	26 (8.25–63.0)	25.3 (2–47)	0.252
	2 days–1 week	22.5 (5.3–53.0)	6 (1–41)	0.085
	1–4 weeks	9 (1–33.5)	5 (1–21)	0.404
	>4 weeks	3 (1–12)	2 (1–5)	0.646

Data expressed as absolute number (percentage of total group)

TAH total abdominal hysterectomy; *TLH* total laparoscopic hysterectomy; *VAS* visual analogue scale

[a] p value for difference between the two groups using chi^2 test for categorical data, independent *t* test for parametric continuous data and Mann–Whitney *U* test for non-parametric continuous data

[b] Median (inter-quartile range)

Discussion

We conducted a retrospective study looking at health-related well-being after total abdominal hysterectomy versus total laparoscopic hysterectomy for endometrial cancer patients. Our study concluded there was no difference in sense of well-being after either procedure. Two studies on post-operative well-being after TLH versus TAH, on patients with benign disease reported increased 'post-operative vitality' in the TLH group [10] whilst the other shared our study's conclusion that surgical approach did not affect patient's post-operative well-being [11].

Previous studies which included a similar cohort to the current study, with early stage endometrial cancer, suggest some measures of quality of life are improved but not all [12, 13]. Obermair et al. demonstrated that physical well-being and body image were improved after TLH, but emotional and social well-being were not [12]. This suggests that parameters of quality of life are not globally improved with TLH, which may explain overall well-being similar in the two arms of our study. Our positive findings include a significant difference in the number of post-operative days spent in hospital, the time taken by women to return to normal activities and overall satisfaction with their scar - all favouring the TLH group. The short length of hospital stay and reduced time taken to return to normal activities associated with TLH is in line with previous studies looking at the same parameters [3–6, 12, 13]. In addition to economic benefits, both findings illustrate a substantial effect on a patient's life through minimising the impact of surgery on work and family life. This in turn positively affects the lives of a patient's family and loved ones. The importance of this was evident in a study that focussed on the health-related concerns of patients undergoing major surgery from the perspective of patients, surgeons and health care professionals. It found that concerns about family support, the impact of major surgery on family or their spouse and spiritual support were themes frequently raised by the patients, but often overlooked by surgeons and health care professionals [16].

We also found a significantly increased level of satisfaction with scars following total laparoscopic hysterectomy when compared to total abdominal hysterectomy, this correlates with the improved body image seen in the LACE trial [12]. Although such a finding may appear mundane, research into the effect of scars, including surgical scars, on patients' emotional and psychological well-being has concluded that it can have a considerable influence over quality of life [17].

Despite previous reports of reduced pain after laparoscopic procedures, we found that there was no difference in reported pain intensity between the two groups. We asked women to rate pain intensity using a visual analogue scale in order to maintain our focus on quality of life as opposed to clinical or surgical outcomes. However, this does not take into account differences in the quantity of analgesia used between the two groups to achieve good pain control. Indeed decreased levels of analgesia use in TLH than TAH have previously been reported [4].

The free text box of our questionnaire was to give women the freedom to express their opinions without the constraints of a semi-structured or structured interview. Whilst this does not give data that can be compared easily, it helps us acknowledge themes that we have overlooked but patients have reported as important such as the impact of radiotherapy and chemotherapy on well-being, and the quality of hospital care they received during their admission.

A disadvantage of our study is that it was carried out retrospectively. Therefore we were unable to establish each group's pretest well-being and eliminate differences in baseline characteristics such as the time duration between surgery and questionnaire completion. This has a particular impact on memory of post-operative pain and the healing of scars. Notably however, the TLH group reported increased satisfaction with their scars, despite having newer and therefore less well-healed scars.

Conclusion

As the popularity of TLH increases over the traditional abdominal approach in the management of endometrial carcinoma, it is important to assess the impact not only in terms of surgical outcomes but also in terms of patient well-being and satisfaction. Our study has shown that there is no difference in reported overall well-being, although other studies suggest that only particular aspects of quality life are improved. Therefore, future studies in this area should be employing more specific questionnaires addressing individual aspects of well-being, to accurately determine the true impact of the route of surgery on patients' recovery. TLH is associated with increased satisfaction with scars, decreased hospital stay and notably a significantly faster return to normal activities which not only impacts on a woman's psychological well-being but also their ability to return to employment or role within the family.

Acknowledgements We would like to thank Dr. Sasikala Rajamanoharan for her invaluable statistical advice and critique of the final manuscript and Susan Carter for her tireless clerical assistance throughout the study.

Funding No funding was solicited or required for this study.

References

1. Office of National Statistics (2007) Cancer statistics registrations: registrations of cancer diagnosed in 2007, England, Scotland, Wales and Northern Ireland

2. Reich H, DeCaprio J, Glynn MF (1989) Laparoscopic hysterectomy. J Gynecol Surg 5:213–216

3. O'Hanlan KA, Huang GS, Garnier AC, Dibble SL, Reuland ML, Lopez L, Pinto RL (2005) Total laparoscopic hysterectomy versus total abdominal hysterectomy; cohort review of patients with uterine neoplasia. JSLS 9(3):277–286

4. Schindlebeck C, Klauser K, Dian D, Janni W, Friese K (2008) Comparison of total laparoscopic, vaginal and abdominal hysterectomy. Arch Gynecol Obstet 277:331–337

5. Müller A, Thiel FC, Renner SP, Winkler M, Häberle L, Beckmann MW (2010) Hysterectomy—a comparison of approaches. Dtsch Arztebl Int 107(20):353–359

6. Obermair A, Manolitsas TP, Leung Y, Hammond IG, McCartney AJ (2004) Total laparoscopic hysterectomy for endometrial cancer patterns of recurrence and survival. Gynecol Oncol 92:789–793

7. Fitzpatrick R, Fletcher A, Gore S, Jones D, Spiegelhalter D, Cox D (1992) Quality of life measure in health care. I: application and issues in assessment. BMJ 305:1074–1077

8. Garry R, Fountain J, Mason S, Napp V, Brown J, Hawe J, Clayton R, Abbott J, Philips G, Whittaker M, Lilford R, Bridgman S (2004) The evaluate study: two parallel randomised trials, one comparing laparoscopic with abdominal hysterectomy, the other comparing laparoscopic with vaginal hysterectomy. BMJ 328:129–136

9. Kluivers KB, Johnson NP, Chien P, Vierhout ME, Bongers MY, Mol BWJ (2008) Comparison of laparoscopic and abdominal hysterectomy in terms of quality of life: a systematic review. Eur J Obstet Gynecol 136:3–8

10. Kluivers KB, Hendriks JC, Mol BW, Bongers MY, Bremers GL, de Vet HC, Vierhout ME, Broimann HA (2007) Quality of life and surgical outcome after total laparoscopic hysterectomy versus total abdominal hysterectomy for benign disease: a randomized, controlled trial. J Minim Invasive Gynecol 14(2):142–152

11. Ellstrom MA, Astrom M, Moller A, Olsson JH, Hahlin M (2003) A randomized trial comparing changes in psychological well-being and sexuality after laparoscopic and abdominal hysterectomy. Acta Obstet Gynecol Scand 82(9):871–875

12. Janda M, Gebski V, Brand A, Hogg R, Jobling TW, Land R, Manolitsas T, McCartney A, Nascimento M, Neesham D, Nicklin JL, Oehler MK, Otton G, Perrin L, Salfinger S, Hammond I, Leung Y, Walsh T, Sykes P, Ngan H, Garrett A, Laney M, Ng TY, Tam K, Chan K, Wrede CD, Pather S, Simcock B, Farrell R, Obermair A (2010) Quality of life after total laparoscopic hysterectomy versus total abdominal hysterectomy for stage I endometrial cancer (LACE): a randomised trial. Lancet Oncol 11(8):772–780

13. Kluivers KB, Ten Cate FA, Bongers MY, Brölmann HA, Hendriks JC (2011) Total laparoscopic hysterectomy versus total abdominal hysterectomy with bilateral salpingo-oophorectomy for endometrial carcinoma: a randomised controlled trial with 5-year follow-up. Gynecol Surg 8(4):427–434

14. Brazier JE, Harper R, Jones NMB, O'Cathain A, Thomas KJ, Usherwood T, Westlake L (1992) Validating the SF-36 health survey questionnaire: new outcome measure for primary care. BMJ 305:160–164

15. Katz J, Melzack R (1999) Measurement of pain. Surg Clin North Am 79:231–252

16. Ammerman DJ, Watters J, Clinch JJ, Hébert PC, Wilson KG, Morris DB, Fergusson D (2007) Exploring quality of life for patients undergoing major surgery: The perspectives of surgeons, other healthcare professionals, and patients. Surgery 141(1):100–109

17. Brown BC, McKenna SP, Siddhi K, McGrouther DA, Bayat A (2008) The hidden cost of skin scars: quality of life after skin scarring. J Plast Reconstr Aesthetic Surg 61:1049–1058

8

Vaginal cuff dehiscence in laparoscopic hysterectomy: influence of various suturing methods of the vaginal vault

M. D. Blikkendaal · A. R. H. Twijnstra ·
S. C. L. Pacquee · J. P. T. Rhemrev ·
M. J. G. H. Smeets · C. D. de Kroon · F. W. Jansen

Abstract Vaginal cuff dehiscence (VCD) is a severe adverse event and occurs more frequently after total laparoscopic hysterectomy (TLH) compared with abdominal and vaginal hysterectomy. The aim of this study is to compare the incidence of VCD after various suturing methods to close the vaginal vault. We conducted a retrospective cohort study. Patients who underwent TLH between January 2004 and May 2011 were enrolled. We compared the incidence of VCD after closure with transvaginal interrupted sutures versus laparoscopic interrupted sutures versus a laparoscopic single-layer running suture. The latter was either bidirectional barbed or a running vicryl suture with clips placed at each end commonly used in transanal endoscopic microsurgery. Three hundred thirty-one TLHs were included. In 75 (22.7 %), the vaginal vault was closed by transvaginal approach; in 90 (27.2 %), by laparoscopic interrupted sutures; and in 166 (50.2 %), by a laparoscopic running suture. Eight VCDs occurred: one (1.3 %) after transvaginal interrupted closure, three (3.3 %) after laparoscopic interrupted suturing and four (2.4 %) after a laparoscopic running suture was used ($p=.707$). With regard to the incidence of VCD, based on our data, neither a superiority of single-layer laparoscopic closure of the vaginal cuff with an unknotted running suture nor of the transvaginal and the laparoscopic interrupted suturing techniques could be demonstrated. We hypothesise that besides the suturing technique, other causes, such as the type and amount of coagulation used for colpotomy, may play a role in the increased risk of VCD after TLH.

Keywords Vaginal cuff dehiscence · Laparoscopic hysterectomy · Barbed suture · Laparoscopic suturing

M. D. Blikkendaal · A. R. H. Twijnstra · C. D. de Kroon ·
F. W. Jansen (✉)
Department of Gynaecology, Leiden University Medical Centre,
PO Box 9600, 2300 RC Leiden, the Netherlands
e-mail: f.w.jansen@lumc.nl

S. C. L. Pacquee · J. P. T. Rhemrev · M. J. G. H. Smeets
Department of Gynaecology, Bronovo Hospital,
PO Box 96900, 2509 JH The Hague, the Netherlands

Background

Vaginal cuff dehiscence (VCD) after hysterectomy is an adverse event with potential severe morbidity. The incidence of VCD after total laparoscopic hysterectomy (TLH) varies between 0.3 and 3.1 % [1–7]. This is higher compared with the abdominal (AH) and vaginal (VH) approach [1, 8]. Since the continuous increment in the number of hysterectomies performed laparoscopically, the aetiology of VCD and explanations for its association with TLH have been subjected to research. Patient characteristics, such as smoking, diabetes, advanced age, radiation therapy and chronic steroid administration, next to precipitating factors such as sexual intercourse, postoperative cuff infection and/or hematoma and increased abdominal pressure (e.g. coughing, vomiting and straining at toilet) have been addressed with regard to their association with VCD [1, 9, 10]. Nevertheless, none of these factors are unique for TLH. Therefore, an explanation could very well be found in some specific procedural steps used to achieve a hysterectomy by laparoscopic approach. Some authors state that electrosurgical colpotomy, often used in TLH, is responsible for suboptimal vaginal cuff healing, due to tissue necrosis and prolonged devascularisation [11]. Recently, several studies compared the influence of various vaginal vault closure techniques on the incidence of VCD after TLH. Jeung et al. conducted the only prospective study on this topic and found no difference between laparoscopically sutured interrupted figures-of-eight versus knotted double-layer running sutures (1.6 and 0.8 %, respectively) [5]. On the other hand, Uccella et al. reported a threefold increased incidence associated with laparoscopic single-layer interrupted suturing compared with transvaginal closure with interrupted sutures (0.18 and 0.64 %, respectively) [7]. However, Siedhoff et al. compared a barbed running suture with other laparoscopic suturing techniques and found no VCDs in the barbed suture group versus a VCD rate of 3.1 % for other methods of closure [6]. Similarly, Einarsson et al. described a non-comparative cohort in which the vaginal cuff was closed with a barbed suture. An incidence of 0.6 % of the patients requiring vaginal cuff re-suturing was found [3].

Internationally, the aetiology of VCD is still a matter of concern. Either in its technique (TLH) as in the used technology (electrosurgical colpotomy and/or suturing method), an explanation could be found for the higher incidence of VCD. In our quest to further improve vaginal vault closure, we have been using various suturing methods. At first, we switched from transvaginal closure of the vaginal vault to laparoscopic closure with interrupted sutures. Thereafter, we started using running sutures: both barbed suturing and an unknotted running suturing technique with clips. To compare these methods, a power analysis indicated that we would have needed 1,349 cases in each arm to detect a desired reduction of 50 % in the VCD rate of 3.4 % [11] (80 % power, type I error 0.05). Since we regarded an adequately powered prospective study to be impossible to perform and given the need for more information, we conducted a retrospective cohort study based on prospectively collected data on this subject. This study aims to compare the incidence of vaginal cuff dehiscence with transvaginal closure of the vaginal vault versus laparoscopic closure with knotted interrupted sutures versus laparoscopic closure with two different unknotted single-layer running suturing methods.

Methods

A university hospital (Leiden University Medical Centre, Leiden) and an affiliated teaching hospital (Bronovo Hospital, The Hague) participated in this study. All patients who underwent a TLH for benign and (pre)malignant indications between January 2004 and May 2011 were enrolled. Three gynaecologists (JPTR, MJGHS and FWJ) performed all procedures and used similar techniques and instruments over time. According to the surgeon's preference and availability, the procedures were performed by one or two surgeons. At the start of the study, all surgeons were already experienced in advanced laparoscopic surgery.

TLH was carried out similar to a recently described technique [12]. Briefly, all classic surgical steps are carried

out laparoscopically, using bipolar energy for dissection of the ligaments and coagulation of the vascular pedicles. The bladder peritoneum is dissected with ultrasonic energy and the cervico-vaginal fascia is identified anteriorly. Hereafter, the sacro-uterine ligament is dissected posteriorly and the vaginal fornix is opened circularly using ultrasonic energy, while cranial traction with the uterine manipulator is provided. To the surgeon's preference, during this step (additional), bipolar energy is used as well. The vaginal cuff is sutured transvaginally (interrupted sutures with Vicryl no. 0, Ethicon, Johnson & Johnson Medical GmbH, Norderstedt, Germany) or laparoscopically (interrupted sutures or a running suture, both single-layer). In every stitch, a full thickness bite of approximately 1 cm is obtained, containing recto-vaginal fascia and vaginal mucosa posteriorly and vaginal mucosa and pubo-cervical fascia anteriorly. In laparoscopic closure of the vaginal vault, Vicryl no. 0 is used for the interrupted sutures, which are secured with intracorporeal tied knots. In case of a running suture, two different suturing methods are used according to the surgeon's preference. In one method, a double-armed barbed suture (Quill™ Self-Retaining System; Angiotech Pharmaceuticals Inc., Vancouver, British Columbia, Canada) is used, in which the barbs change direction at mid-point. This suture is bidirectionally sutured from the midline to both lateral angles of the vaginal cuff [13]. In the other, we adopted (off label) a suturing technique commonly used in transanal endoscopic microsurgery (TEM). In this technique a regular Vicryl no. 0 with a suture staple placed at the distal end of the wire is sutured from the right to the left angle of the vaginal cuff, after which another suture staple is placed at the proximal end to secure the suture (suture clip forceps for TEM, Richard Wolf GmbH, Knittlingen, Germany). In all suturing methods, both utero-sacral ligaments are incorporated in the repair and the peritoneum is unclosed.

Patients were evaluated by anamnesis and physical examination 6 weeks postoperatively. Sexually active patients were instructed not to restart sexual intercourse until after this evaluation. All data were derived from a database supplemented by a chart review. For all patients, the type of suture (transvaginal interrupted, laparoscopic interrupted or laparoscopic running) was registered. Furthermore, patient characteristics (age, body mass index (BMI, in kilograms per square metre) and ASA classification) and procedure characteristics (operating time (in minutes, skin-to-skin), blood loss (in milliltre), uterus weight (in grams) and adverse outcomes) were obtained. Adverse events were registered for type of complication, severity (i.e. requiring re-intervention or not) and moment of onset, up to 6 weeks after discharge (i.e. marking the legitimate adverse event reporting period), according to the definitions and regulations as determined by the

Guideline Adverse Events of the Dutch Society of Obstetricians and Gynaecologists [14].

The primary outcome was the incidence of VCD by type of suture (transvaginal interrupted (group 1) versus laparoscopic interrupted (group 2) versus laparoscopic running (group 3)). According to literature, we defined VCD as a partial or complete separation of the vaginal cuff that required surgical intervention, regardless of the presence of an open peritoneum and/or evisceration [1]. As a secondary assessment, we collected additional data of all these patients to identify possible characteristics associated with this complication. This included the trigger event to onset of dehiscence, presenting symptoms at the time of dehiscence, presence of an open peritoneum, presence of evisceration, type of repair, the interval time (in days) between TLH and dehiscence, relevant comorbidities (i.e. smoking, diabetes, use of immune suppressing drugs and radiotherapy), relevant accompanying complications (i.e. vaginal cuff cellulitis, infection or hematoma), indication for surgery, menopausal status, type of energy used for colpotomy (bipolar, ultrasonic or a combination) and use of prophylactic antibiotics at the time of hysterectomy. All procedures in which the vaginal cuff was sutured by conventional open approach (i.e. after conversion to laparotomy or after a minilaparotomy for specimen retrieval) were excluded.

To calculate differences between the groups, SPSS 17.0 statistical software (Chicago, IL, USA) was used. A Pearson chi-square test was used to compare proportions, and a one-way analysis of variance (ANOVA) was used for continuous variables. Pairwise t tests with Bonferroni's correction were used for post hoc multiple comparison. If the condition of a normal distribution (kurtosis between -1 and $+2$) was not met, additionally a Kruskal–Wallis test was performed to confirm the p value calculated by the ANOVA. p values <0.05 were considered statistically significant.

Findings

During the study period, a total of 333 TLHs were performed. Of these, two procedures were converted to laparotomy. These two procedures were excluded from further analysis (no VCD reported). Finally, 331 TLHs were included in the analysis. In 75 patients (22.7 %), the vaginal vault was closed by transvaginal approach. Laparoscopic interrupted sutures were used for closure in 90 procedures (27.2 %), and a laparoscopic running suture was used in 166 procedures (50.2 %, 81 barbed sutures and 85 TEM sutures). The baseline characteristics of these three groups are detailed in Table 1. Compared with group 2, patients in group 1 had a lower ASA classification ($p=.014$), while blood loss was higher ($p=.003$). Compared with group 3, patients in group 1 had a lower BMI ($p=.014$), while blood

loss was higher ($p\leq.001$). This difference in blood loss is partly caused by two procedures in group 1 with an estimated blood loss of 2,300 and 950 mL, respectively (uterus weight 880 and 650 g, respectively; length of surgery 335 and 160 min, respectively). Nevertheless, after exclusion of these two statistical outliers, the differences in blood loss remained significant (mean blood loss in group 1, 188 mL; SD ±178 mL; $p=.028$ compared with group 2 and $p=.002$ compared with group 3). All other baseline characteristics were comparable between each group.

Overall, eight vaginal cuff dehiscences occurred: one (1.3 %) after transvaginal interrupted closure, three (3.3 %) after interrupted laparoscopic suturing and four (2.4 %) after a laparoscopic running suture was used (Table 2). There was no statistical difference with regard to VCD between these three groups ($p=.707$). In addition, we plotted all procedures in a consecutive order—separately for each surgeon—and marked the cases complicated by a VCD. These graphs showed that the VCDs did not tend to occur more frequently within the beginning period of each suturing method (not shown). Furthermore, the overall complication rate (regarding all severities) (20.0 versus 17.8 versus 13.3 %, $p=.373$) and the rate of complications requiring re-intervention (2.7 versus 3.3 versus 3.0 %, $p=.773$) were similar between the groups as well. In all but three patient records (99.1 %), both anamnesis and physical examination during the postoperative clinical evaluation after 6 weeks were clearly registered. Table 3 represents the characteristics of all patients that presented with a vaginal cuff dehiscence. Within the patient and procedure characteristics, no obvious predisposing factors could be identified. All patients received prophylactic antibiotics at time of hysterectomy. During all the procedures, ultrasonic energy and bipolar coagulation were alternately used for colpotomy and haemostasis. All eight patients presented with (heavy) vaginal blood loss. Two cases were (most likely) accompanied by another complication. In the first, an old vaginal vault haematoma appeared to be present during exploration in the operating room. In the last case, based on anamnesis and physical examination, sexual intercourse most likely caused an abscess to 'spontaneously' drain. In at least half of the cases, the patient had marked intercourse as the trigger event for the complaint; all presented with abdominal pain. In two cases a small dehiscence of the peritoneum was present. However, no evisceration occurred. In three patients, a vaginal cuff dehiscence occurred after the 6 weeks follow-up examination, on the 57th, 71st and 75th day, respectively, all after sexual intercourse. Except for one of these patients in which some granulation tissue was treated with silver nitrate, anamnesis and physical examination during the regular follow-up examination did not reveal other abnormalities in the postoperative course. One case was complicated by a fallopian tube prolapse. In this case, both the prolapse

Table 1 Baseline characteristics of all procedures by suture method of the vaginal vault (transvaginal interrupted versus laparoscopic interrupted versus laparoscopic running) (n=331)

	Group 1, transvaginal interrupted sutures (n=75)		Group 2, laparoscopic interrupted sutures (n=90)		Group 3, laparoscopic running sutures (n=166)		ANOVA: Overall	Bonferroni: group 1 versus 2	Bonferroni: group 1 versus 3	Bonferroni: group 2 versus 3
	Mean±SD	Range	Mean±SD	Range	Mean±SD	Range	p value	p value	p value	p value
Age (years)	47.2±7.3	(32.5–66.1)	47.5±8.5	(32.8–79.3)	49.0±9.1	(29.0–78.3)	.230	–	–	–
BMI (kg/m^2)	25.3±3.6	(18.1–35.0)	26.3±5.2	(16.2–44.1)	27.5±6.1	(17.5–48.0)	.013	NS	.014	NS
ASA classification[a]	1[b]±0.4	(1–2)	1[b]±0.5	(1–3)	1[b]±0.6	(1–3)	.018	.014	NS	NS
Length of surgery (min)[a]	141±49	(60–335)	128±32	(70–240)	129±40.0	(50–260)	.082	–	–	–
Blood loss (mL)[a]	226±312	(25–2300)	129±148	(25–1,000)	120±122	(25–800)	<.001	.003	<.001	NS
Uterus weight (g)	283±181	(35–822)	228±163	(35–700)	249±197	(31–950)	.202	–	–	–

SD standard deviation, *NS* not significant

[a] *p* value was confirmed by Kruskal–Wallis test because of a non-normal distribution

[b] Median

and the vaginal cuff dehiscence could be managed laparoscopically. In all other cases, vaginal (re)suturing of the dehiscence was sufficient. After repair, further recovery was uneventful in all eight patients.

Discussion

VCD is a potentially severe adverse event. Internationally, the reason for the increased incidence of VCD after TLH is still a matter of concern. The used suturing method of the vaginal vault is mentioned as an aetiological factor. In our comparison of laparoscopic suturing of the vaginal cuff with a single-layer unknotted running suture and both laparoscopic and transvaginal closure with knotted interrupted sutures, we found the lowest incidence of VCD after transvaginal suturing (1.3 %). This was followed by both the barbed suture and the running vicryl suture with TEM clips (2.4 %), which proved to be an easy to adopt alternative. However, based on our data, no statistical superiority of either of these suturing methods could be proven. Regardless of these suturing techniques, the incidence of VCD after TLH remains high compared with abdominal and vaginal hysterectomy. Therefore, other steps of the procedure unique to TLH, such as the amount and type of coagulation used for colpotomy, should be assessed in future research as possible determinants for the onset of VCD.

To our knowledge, the present study is the first to compare single-layer running suturing techniques with interrupted sutures for closure of the vaginal cuff. Additionally, cuff closure using a running vicryl suture with TEM clips is a newly introduced alternative to other suturing techniques currently in use. The safety and effectiveness of barbed sutures already has been demonstrated in two other studies [3, 6]. However, one was non-comparative and in the other a more time-consuming double-layer suturing method was used. Furthermore, the barbed suture proved to be relatively easy to learn [6]. In our experience as well, both the single-layer barbed suture and the single-layer running vicryl suture with TEM clips proved to be easy to adopt and as safe—regarding incidence of VCD—as transvaginal and laparoscopic closure of the vaginal cuff with interrupted sutures.

Both techniques allow laparoscopic closure of the vaginal vault to be less time-consuming, due to their unknotted fashion. However, some concern is expressed regarding adhesion formation of the intestine to the tail of the barbed suture, which in turn potentially could cause bowel obstruction [15–17].

As shown in Table 1, due to the retrospective design of our study, some differences in the baseline characteristics occurred. Especially with regard to the aetiology of VCD, the observed differences in mean BMI and mean intraoperative blood loss are, however, not clinically relevant.

Table 2 Incidence of vaginal cuff dehiscence and other complications by type of suture (n=331)

	Group 1, transvaginal interrupted sutures (n=75)	Group 2, laparoscopic interrupted sutures (n=90)	Group 3, laparoscopic running sutures (n=166)	p value
Vaginal cuff dehiscence (%)	1 (1.3)	3 (3.3)	4 (2.4)	.707
Overall complications (%)	15 (20.0)	16 (17.8)	22 (13.3)	.373
Requiring (re)intervention (%)	2 (2.7)	3 (3.3)	5 (3.0)	.773

Furthermore, the same counts for the difference in ASA classification between group 1 and group 2, since none of the patients presenting with a VCD suffered from a systemic disease which potentially could induce this complication (e.g. diabetes or chronic cough due to chronic obstructive pulmonary disease). Finally, given the relatively long study period (in which the same surgical techniques and instruments were used), we had to rule out a possible influence of surgical experience to explain these differences. However, near the end of the study period, VCD tended to occur as (in)frequent as at the beginning.

VCD is still a matter of concern to those who perform TLH. Although techniques for suturing of the vaginal cuff have changed rapidly over the past years, only one prospective study on this subject has been published [5]. It compared laparoscopic closure with interrupted and running sutures, however, with a double-layer suturing method and with an extracorporeal knotting technique. Recently, Uccella et al. advocated a superiority of transvaginal closure based on data of their own retrospective cohort and a review of literature in which they found a threefold increase in the incidence of VCD associated with laparoscopic closure [7]. Our study suggests a similar difference between transvaginal closure and laparoscopic closure with knotted interrupted sutures. However, they did not compare the use of laparoscopic running suturing methods. Given the fact that transvaginal closure cannot always be accomplished in all women, alternatives to this suturing method should be studied. Unfortunately, a prospective intention-to-treat study to test this superiority will be hard to perform. Based on a pooled incidence of 0.18 % [7] (transvaginal closure) versus 2.4 % (laparoscopic running unknotted suture, present study), we measured that at least 405 patients should be included in each arm to obtain adequate power (two-sided test for independent samples with 80 % power and 5 % type I error). To ensure that the same surgical technique is applied in all procedures, ideally, a single-centre study needs to be conducted. As a result, the conclusions drawn from the present study have to be strengthened by pooling of data with future publications on this topic.

Several explanations why hysterectomy by laparoscopic approach is prone to have a higher rate of VCD have been put forward. Firstly, regarding initial sexual intercourse as a precipitating event, it has been suggested that the rapid recovery after the laparoscopic approach, compared with the abdominal approach, facilitates swift return to everyday activities and early resumption of (sexual) activities, which could predispose rupture of the vaginal vault [10, 18]. On the other hand, this assertion does not seem to hold, whereas also in our study most VCDs related to intercourse occurred after the regular 6 weeks postoperative follow-up examination, which is considered to be sufficient time for primary wound healing [9–11, 18–20].

Secondly, several studies suggested that the amount and type of energy used for colpotomy could be predisposing for VCD [5, 18, 21, 22]. Gruber et al. performed a histopathologic assessment to compare the thermal damage after the use of ultrasonic, monopolar and bipolar energy for colpotomy in swine. They concluded that ultrasonic energy causes the least and bipolar energy the greatest tissue damage [21]. In all our procedures, including those complicated by a VCD, ultrasonic energy was used for colpotomy and additional bipolar energy was used for haemostasis (Table 3). The amount of coagulation used in the cases in which a VCD occurred compared with the procedures after which no VCD occurred is, however, unclear. Nevertheless, in order to maintain sufficient vascularisation, minimising the use of bipolar energy for haemostasis seems advisable. Preferably, only arterial bleeders should be coagulated and one should rely on the sutures to control venous oozing. This recommendation is supported by the lower reported incidence of VCD after conventional abdominal approach to hysterectomy, in which the vaginal vault is clamped and sutured and no coagulation is used on a regular basis [23].

Furthermore, several studies did address the type and class of suture material as a possible cause for vaginal cuff dehiscence [11, 19, 22]. However, review of the literature yields neither evidence nor consensus on the preferred suture material, concerning monofilament versus multifilament and delayed absorbability of the thread.

Finally, surgical characteristics such as the technical difficulty of laparoscopic surgery, the high complexity of laparoscopic knot tying and insufficient amounts of tissue incorporated in the

Table 3 Characteristics of all patients with a vaginal cuff dehiscence

Case	Age (years)	BMI (kg/m²)	ASA	Length of surgery (min)	Blood loss (mL)	Uterus weight (g)	Indication for hysterectomy	Postmenopausal	Prophylactic antibiotics at hysterectomy	Suture type	Energy used for colpotomy	Trigger event	Presenting symptoms	Time after hysterectomy (days)	Peritoneum open	Evisceration	Type of repair	Relevant comorbidities	Relevant accompanying complications
1	55	35	2	135	100	Unknown	EC	Yes	Yes	Transvaginal interrupted	Bipolar and ultrasonic	Spontaneous	VBL	13	No	No	Transvaginal resuturing	None	Vaginal vault haematoma
2	41	30	1	115	150	Unknown	DUB and UM	No	Yes	Laparoscopic interrupted	Bipolar and ultrasonic	Spontaneous	VBL	15	No	No	Transvaginal suturing	Smoking	None
3	49	25	2	120	155	Unknown	DUB	No	Yes	Laparoscopic interrupted	Bipolar and ultrasonic	Spontaneous	VBL	20	No	No	Transvaginal suturing	None	None
4	56	24	1	105	25	100	EC	Yes	Yes	Laparoscopic interrupted	Bipolar and ultrasonic	Spontaneous	VBL	28	No	No	Transvaginal suturing	None	Granulation
5	46	23	1	110	50	315	UM	Yes	Yes	Laparoscopic running (Quill™)	Bipolar and ultrasonic	Intercourse	VBL and pain	75	No	No	Transvaginal suturing	None	Granulation
6	40	26	1	125	25	360	UM	No	Yes	Laparoscopic running (Quill™)	Bipolar and ultrasonic	Intercourse	VBL and pain	71	Yes	No	Laparoscopic resuturing	None	Fallopian tube prolapse
7	50	25	1	105	200	150	UM	No	Yes	Laparoscopic running (TEM)	Bipolar and ultrasonic	Intercourse	VBL and pain	57	Yes	No	Transvaginal suturing	None	None
8	34	22	1	95	75	140	UM	No	Yes	Laparoscopic running (TEM)	Bipolar and ultrasonic	Intercourse	VBL and pain	41	No	No	Transvaginal suturing	None	Abscess (most likely[a])

EC endometrial cancer, *DUB* dysfunctional uterine bleeding, *UM* uterine myomas, *TEM* suture method adopted from transanal endoscopic microsurgery (see 'Methods' section), *VBL* vaginal blood loss

[a] Based on anamnesis and physical examination, this VCD most likely occurred after drainage of an abscess during sexual intercourse

suture have been suggested as reasons for the increased incidence of VCD in LH [5–7, 13]. The placement of sutures in 'big bites' of viable tissue seems justified [5, 18].

It is more likely that a VCD occurs secondary to an underlying factor such as a haematoma or a primary healing defect as a result of excessive coagulation. Hypothetically, in these cases, the vaginal wall epithelium remains approximated only by the suture. Therefore, as soon as the suture loses most of its tensile strength, a (partial) separation of the vaginal cuff occurs. This hypothesis is supported by the difference in days between surgery and VCD, which we found in the present study (Table 3). With regard to the barbed suture ($n=2$), the mean time to VCD was 73 days. For the other suturing methods ($n=6$), in which regular Vicryl no. 0 was used, the mean time to VCD was 29 days. This difference can be explained by the fact that the tensile strength of Vicryl is 25 % after 4 weeks (http://www.ecatalog.ethicon.com/sutures-absorbable), whereas the tensile strength of the barbed suture is still 80 % [6]. Sexual intercourse might only trigger breakdown of a partially dissolved suture, which in case of such a primary healing defect, causes a (partial) separation of the vaginal wall epithelium that would have occurred sooner or later anyway. In our opinion, the advice to refrain from intercourse up to 3 months after TLH, as suggested by others, is neither based on the pathophysiological process of VCD nor based on evidence [2, 24]. Similarly, given the ambiguous relationship of intercourse and VCD, we thus tend to emphasise to our patients that from a clinical point of view they themselves are not to blame for this embarrassing event.

The VCD rate of 3.3 % that we found for laparoscopic interrupted sutures was relatively high but was similar to the rate published by others before they started to use the barbed suture [6]. However, more importantly, in these cases the peritoneum remained closed and in none (of all our cases) an evisceration occurred. Especially the latter is important, since immediate reoperation is needed and its association with bowel perforation and/or necrosis, peritonitis and general sepsis [7, 9, 25].

Conclusion

In conclusion, based on our data, no superiority of one of the suturing methods over the other was found and the exact aetiology of VCD still remains unclear. Regardless of the suturing method, we hypothesise that the surgical approach towards the colpotomy in TLH in comparison to the abdominal approach, with additional (extensive) application of coagulation, has inherent its specific side effects. To enable future scientific analysis of pooled data, we would like to challenge others to publish their data and opinion on this important subject.

Declaration of interest The authors report no conflicts of interest. The authors alone are responsible for the content and writing of the paper.

References

1. Hur HC, Donnellan N, Mansuria S et al (2011) Vaginal cuff dehiscence after different modes of hysterectomy. Obstet Gynecol 118:794–801
2. Ceccaroni M, Berretta R, Malzoni M et al (2011) Vaginal cuff dehiscence after hysterectomy: a multicenter retrospective study. Eur J Obstet Gynecol Reprod Biol 158:308–313
3. Einarsson JI, Vellinga TT, Twijnstra AR et al (2010) Bidirectional barbed suture: an evaluation of safety and clinical outcomes. JSLS 14:381–385
4. Hwang JH, Lee JK, Lee NW et al (2011) Vaginal cuff closure: a comparison between the vaginal route and laparoscopic suture in patients undergoing total laparoscopic hysterectomy. Gynecol Obstet Invest 71:163–169
5. Jeung IC, Baek JM, Park EK et al (2010) A prospective comparison of vaginal stump suturing techniques during total laparoscopic hysterectomy. Arch Gynecol Obstet 282:631–638
6. Siedhoff MT, Yunker AC, Steege JF (2011) Decreased incidence of vaginal cuff dehiscence after laparoscopic closure with bidirectional barbed suture. J Minim Invasive Gynecol 18:218–223
7. Uccella S, Ghezzi F, Mariani A et al (2011) Vaginal cuff closure after minimally invasive hysterectomy: our experience and systematic review of the literature. Am J Obstet Gynecol 205:119
8. Agdi M, Al-Ghafri W, Antolin R et al (2009) Vaginal vault dehiscence after hysterectomy. J Minim Invasive Gynecol 16:313–317
9. Iaco PD, Ceccaroni M, Alboni C et al (2006) Transvaginal evisceration after hysterectomy: is vaginal cuff closure associated with a reduced risk? Eur J Obstet Gynecol Reprod Biol 125:134–138
10. Croak AJ, Gebhart JB, Klingele CJ et al (2004) Characteristics of patients with vaginal rupture and evisceration. Obstet Gynecol 103:572–576
11. Hur HC, Guido RS, Mansuria SM et al (2007) Incidence and patient characteristics of vaginal cuff dehiscence after different modes of hysterectomies. J Minim Invasive Gynecol 14:311–317
12. Einarsson JI, Suzuki Y (2009) Total laparoscopic hysterectomy: 10 steps toward a successful procedure. Rev Obstet Gynecol 2:57–64
13. Greenberg JA, Einarsson JI (2008) The use of bidirectional barbed suture in laparoscopic myomectomy and total laparoscopic hysterectomy. J Minim Invasive Gynecol 15:621–623
14. Twijnstra AR, Zeeman GG, Jansen FW (2010) A novel approach to registration of adverse outcomes in obstetrics and gynaecology: a feasibility study. Qual Saf Health Care 19:132–137
15. Thubert T, Pourcher G, Deffieux X (2011) Small bowel volvulus following peritoneal closure using absorbable knotless device during laparoscopic sacral colpopexy. Int Urogynecol J 22:761–763
16. Donnellan NM, Mansuria SM (2011) Small bowel obstruction resulting from laparoscopic vaginal cuff closure with a barbed suture. J Minim Invasive Gynecol 18:528–530
17. Einarsson JI, Grazul-Bilska AT, Vonnahme KA (2011) Barbed vs standard suture: randomized single-blinded comparison of adhesion formation and ease of use in an animal model. J Minim Invasive Gynecol 18:716–719

18. Nezhat CH, Nezhat F, Seidman DS et al (1996) Vaginal vault evisceration after total laparoscopic hysterectomy. Obstet Gynecol 87:868–870
19. Yuce K, Dursun P, Gultekin M (2005) Posthysterectomy intestinal prolapse after coitus and vaginal repair. Arch Gynecol Obstet 272:80–81
20. Yaakovian MD, Hamad GG, Guido RS (2008) Laparoscopic management of vaginal evisceration: case report and review of the literature. J Minim Invasive Gynecol 15:119–121
21. Gruber DD, Warner WB, Lombardini ED et al (2011) Laparoscopic hysterectomy using various energy sources in swine: a histopathologic assessment. Am J Obstet Gynecol 205:494–496
22. Walsh CA, Sherwin JR, Slack M (2007) Vaginal evisceration following total laparoscopic hysterectomy: case report and review of the literature. Aust N Z J Obstet Gynaecol 47:516–519
23. Thompson JD, Warschaw J (1997) Hysterectomy. In: Rock JA, Thompson JD (eds) Te Linde's operative gynecology, 8th edn. Lippincott, Philadelphia, pp 771–854
24. Shen CC, Hsu TY, Huang FJ et al (2002) Comparison of one- and two-layer vaginal cuff closure and open vaginal cuff during laparoscopic-assisted vaginal hysterectomy. J Am Assoc Gynecol Laparosc 9:474–480
25. Sinha R, Kadam P, Sundaram M et al (2011) Vaginal vault dehiscence with evisceration after total laparoscopic hysterectomy. Gynecol Surg 8:175–176

9

Can total laparoscopic hysterectomy replace total abdominal hysterectomy? A 5-year prospective cohort study of a single surgeon's experience in an unselected population

D. Ghosh · P. Wipplinger · D. L. Byrne

Abstract Total laparoscopic hysterectomy (TLH) has well-established advantages over total abdominal hysterectomy in benign gynaecology. We evaluated the outcome of a single surgeon who offered TLH as the default surgical procedure for all non-vaginal hysterectomies in an unselected gynaecology clinic population. TLH was offered as the default method of hysterectomy for patients from September 1, 2006, and data were collected up to August 31, 2011. Data were collected on indication for surgery, previous surgery, pelvic pathology, intraoperative findings, uterine weight and/or size, complications and conversion to open hysterectomy. Primary outcomes were the proportion of hysterectomies performed laparoscopically, complications and conversion rates. A total of 173 hysterectomies were performed; 18 (10 %) were total abdominal hysterectomy (TAH), 17 (10 %) were vaginal hysterectomies (VH), and 138 (80 %) were TLH. TLH rates increased from 51 % in year 1 to 100 % in years 3, 4 and 5 for women that elected for laparoscopic approach. The median uterine weight for TLH increased each year from 110 g (range 58–209 g) in year 1 to 240 g (range 70–584 g) in year 5. All patients were deemed suitable for laparoscopic approach irrespective of the uterine size and comorbidities by year 3 with only a single conversion in year 4. There were 11 major surgical complications: VH 0 (0 %), TAH 1 (5.6 %) and TLH 10 (7.2 %) and three (2.2 %) conversions to laparotomy. Once a surgeon's laparoscopic expertise plateaus, TLH can be offered to patients as the default procedure for non-vaginal hysterectomy in an unselected UK population with benign disease.

Keywords Learning curve · Total laparoscopic hysterectomy

D. Ghosh · P. Wipplinger · D. L. Byrne (✉)
Department of Gynaecology, Royal Cornwall Hospital,
Truro TR1 3LJ Cornwall, UK
e-mail: dominic.byrne@rcht.cornwall.nhs.uk

Background

Since the first total laparoscopic hysterectomy (TLH) was described [1], there is increasing evidence that it provides advantages over vaginal hysterectomy (VH) [2] and total abdominal hysterectomy (TAH) in benign gynaecology [3]. The National Institute for Health and Clinical Excellence promotes the advantages of laparoscopic hysterectomy for early endometrial cancer [4] and supports its use as a choice for benign hysterectomy [5].

TLH has been shown in randomised trials to result in a reduction in postoperative pain and an enhanced recovery when compared to open hysterectomy [3, 6]. It has also been shown that patients have a shorter hospital stay when compared with abdominal and vaginal hysterectomy [7]. Despite this evidence, laparotomy is currently the most common surgical route for hysterectomy [8].

Whilst the benefits for patients are proven, the technical and financial challenges of TLH have delayed its adoption into standard practice. TLH takes longer to perform [3] and carries higher equipment costs when compared to open hysterectomy [9]. Where direct and indirect costs of abdominal and laparoscopic hysterectomy were evaluated using combined data from controlled trials, shorter hospital stay was shown to compensate for the higher procedural costs of laparoscopic hysterectomy [10]. A cost comparison using a societal perspective model analysed hospital inpatient costs, equipment costs, lost wages and caregiver costs of robotic, laparoscopic and abdominal hysterectomy for endometrial cancer and predicted laparoscopy as the least expensive approach [11]. Further research to evaluate hysterectomy costs in benign gynaecology, including mapping the complete patient journey, is required where societal factors and economic benefits are likely to balance the cost in favour of TLH.

Laparoscopic hysterectomy is considered more difficult than abdominal hysterectomy [12]. The technical challenges of laparoscopic surgery may be daunting for a surgeon who is very competent at open hysterectomy, as it returns the surgeon to a novice status once again. Some surgeons relish the new challenges whilst others find it difficult to relearn and do not wish to change. The support and infrastructure to learn complex laparoscopic surgery is also variable and the service pressures of current roles may frustrate such development. The technical challenges of a laparoscopic approach include limited instrument mobility and positioning, as instruments are fixed at the port site. Laparoscopic surgery is visualised in two dimensions, so depth cannot be seen, it must be learned. These factors, accompanied by the altered ergonomics, increase the difficulty of a laparoscopic approach [13]. The learning curve for TLH has previously been studied and defined according to the number of procedures performed by assessing complication rates and the length of operating time in a novice and experienced laparoscopic surgeon. In the experienced surgeon, the learning curve reached a plateau at the first 10 cases [14]. The average duration of laparoscopic hysterectomy has been shown to be comparable to abdominal hysterectomy as experience is gained [15]. It should be expected that with increasing experience, surgeons would undertake more complex laparoscopic hysterectomies, which whilst expanding the applicability of the procedure, will conversely add to the operative time.

Methods

This study examines the 5-year outcome of a single surgeon with 25 years surgical experience of abdominal and vaginal hysterectomy who, after 12 years of preparatory training (comprising surgical training courses, personal mentoring and performing laparoscopically assisted vaginal hysterectomy, then TLH on selected patients), introduced TLH as the default method of non-vaginal hysterectomy from September 1, 2006.

We collected data on all hysterectomies, irrespective of route, performed by one surgeon over a 5-year period to determine what proportion was successfully carried out laparoscopically. As these data include all patients offered hysterectomy in one consultant general gynaecology clinic, it is a complete dataset and not subject to selection bias. Consequently, it will determine the true outcome if TLH is offered as the primary route for surgery. The cohort will also demonstrate any changes in selection criteria and case complexity as the surgeon's experience increases.

Patients were informed that TLH was a new procedure and early cases were told specifically how many procedures the surgeon had performed. All were told that conversion to an open procedure was a possibility and that they could elect for an open procedure from the outset. This cohort is a complete data set of the named surgeon's practice as all patients remained under his care irrespective of route of hysterectomy or indication for procedure. There was only one patient (in year 5) referred to another consultant for hysterectomy. This patient was listed for a TLH but requested an alternative surgeon as the procedure could be carried out sooner; in doing so, she accepted a TAH. So with the exception of this single patient, there is no selection bias in the population studied.

Outcome data were retrieved by a search of the Royal Cornwall Hospitals Trust theatre database for all patients undergoing hysterectomy between September 1, 2006 and August 31, 2011 (5-year complete data) under the care of one of the authors (DLB). Cases were cross-referenced with the surgeon's personal records to ensure all patients were included. The notes of all patients were collected and a standardised data set was recorded on a prepared pro forma.

The indication for surgery, any previous abdominal surgery and known pelvic pathology were recorded, along with the name of the listing surgeon, the operating surgeon and the patients named consultant. Intraoperative findings were recorded including size of uterus, adhesions, endometriosis or congenital abnormalities. Intraoperative and postoperative complications and conversion to laparotomy were recorded. The uterine weight and (or) size was recorded from the histopathology report. The reason for hysterectomy not being performed laparoscopically was also recorded.

Total laparoscopic hysterectomy was performed using a 10-mm zero degree laparoscope through the umbilicus with one lateral 5-mm port on each side. An additional 10-mm port was placed suprapubically. The procedure was performed using a bipolar Maryland forceps (Olympus, Hamburg, Germany) and a Lotus ultrasonic scalpel (SRA Developments Ltd, Ashburton, UK). The pedicles were secured and divided in turn to include the adnexae as necessary. In complex endometriosis cases, the ureters were dissected as required. A colpotomy cup was used to prevent gas escaping when the vagina was opened. In the early procedures, this was a McCartney Tube (LiNA Medical UK Ltd, Cullompton, UK) and in later procedures, a Hohl uterine manipulator (Storz GmbH &Co, Tuttlingen, Germany) incorporating a colpotomy cup was used. The vaginal vault was sutured laparoscopically with a continuous suture and intracorporeal knots. The suprapubic port site was closed with a deep suture. All wounds were then closed with absorbable skin sutures. In procedures with a large fibroid uterus, the laparoscope port was placed high in the abdomen and the umbilical port was used for instrumentation. In addition, in very large fibroid uterus cases, bilateral uterine artery occlusion was carried out at source at the start of the procedure. Large fibroid uteri were morcellated using a Rotocut morcellator (Storz GmbH &Co, Tuttlingen, Germany) to facilitate removal. A urinary catheter was inserted at the onset of the procedures and removed the following morning. Patients were discharged home the following day unless unsuitable.

In cases of abdominal hysterectomy, the procedure was performed through a pfannenstiel incision. The bowel was packed off and then a three or four pedicle traditional clamp hysterectomy, completed. The vault was closed with a continuous absorbable suture and the abdomen, closed in layers. A urethral catheter was inserted at the onset of the procedure and removed the next day. Patients were discharged on the third or fourth postoperative day unless unsuitable.

Vaginal hysterectomy was performed by infiltration of the cervix with local anaesthetic and adrenaline, and then circumcised. The vaginal skin was retracted and ascending pedicles taken along the uterus until the tubo-ovarian pedicles were divided. The ovaries were always retained at vaginal hysterectomy. The vagina was closed with absorbable suture, and a vaginal pack and urethral catheter was inserted. Both were removed the following day and patients were discharged on the third or fourth postoperative day unless unsuitable.

In all types of hysterectomy, patients were discharged when pain-free (with or without oral analgesics), when urinary catheter had been removed and the woman was fully mobile and confident to self care at home.

Findings

In the 5-year period, a total of 202 hysterectomies were recorded on the hospital database under the care of one author. Detailed review of the notes confirmed that 12 were patients actually under the care of other consultants, 11 patients had not in fact had a hysterectomy performed and two sets of notes were untraceable. In three cases, patients under the care of the named consultant underwent TLH by a locum consultant and these cases have been excluded. One patient transferred care to another consultant to expedite surgery. Thus, 173 patients had undergone a hysterectomy under the care of the named consultant, and notes were available for review. Of the 173 cases, 18 TAHs, 17 VHs and 138 TLHs were undertaken (Table 1).

Total abdominal hysterectomy

Eighteen TAHs were performed. All occurred in the first 2 years, with nine in each year except for one TAH which was performed in year 5 by another consultant. The one patient who had a TAH performed in year 5 by another consultant had opted for TAH instead of TLH to shorten her waiting time; this was a waiting list management issue, not a clinical decision. Nine patients were operated on by a doctor not trained to perform TLH and in the absence of the

Table 1 Number and percentage of total abdominal, vaginal and total laparoscopic hysterectomies performed each consecutive year of the study

Year	TAH; n (%)	VH; n (%)	TLH; n (%)	Total Hysterectomies
1	9 (27.3)	7 (21.2)	17[a] (51.5)	33
2	9 (23.1)	8 (20.5)	22[a] (56.4)	39
3	0	2 (6.1)	31 (93.9)	33
4	0	0	39[a] (97.4)	39
5	0[b]	0	29 (96.7)	29
Total	18 (10.4)	17 (9.8)	138 (79.8)	173

[a] Single conversion occurred

[b] One patient transferred care to another consultant for TAH to expedite surgery

named consultant. Ten patients had a TAH by the named consultant, of whom eight had been listed for this procedure by the named consultant and two patients had been listed for TAH by junior doctors. The indication for TAH was a large fibroid uterus (larger than 16 weeks gestation equivalent) in nine cases and three previous Caesarean sections in one case. At histology, the uterine size of these 10 cases performed over the 2 years by the consultant varied from 135 to 2,793 g, median weight (no weight recorded in three of these specimens). See Fig. 1 for comparison of uterine size and hysterectomy type by consecutive years of experience.

Vaginal hysterectomy

Seventeen patients underwent vaginal hysterectomy. All operations occurred in the first 3 years; none in the last 2 years. Eight patients underwent vaginal hysterectomy by the named consultant, for uterine prolapse; three had procidentia and five had a cervix at, or below, the introitus. Four

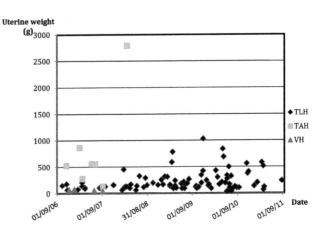

Fig. 1 For each route of hysterectomy, the weight of each individual uterus (where reported at histology) is plotted against the date surgery was performed

of these eight patients had additional vaginal wall surgery. Seven of these patients had been listed by the author and one listed by a junior doctor. The remaining nine patients were all listed, and operated on, by a specialty doctor in the absence of the consultant; seven of these also had a vaginal repair.

Total laparoscopic hysterectomy

TLH was undertaken in 138 patients; 99 patients had been listed for surgery by the named consultant and 39 by other doctors on behalf of the named consultant. In two cases, a subtotal hysterectomy was performed as the patients had requested that their cervix be retained. There were three conversions to laparotomy for the following reasons:

1. Case 13 (year 1) had a completed TLH, but the abdomen was opened by a colorectal surgeon to repair injury to adherent bowel, which had occurred during the TLH.
2. Case 30 (year 2) was unable to be ventilated in a sufficiently head down position to allow adequate view of large fibroid uterus.
3. In case 85 (year 4), the uterus was so large that it filled the pelvis completely, leaving limited access to uterine vessels at source and a surgical assistant inexperienced in advanced laparoscopic surgery.

A laparoscopic morcellator was purchased in year 2, and one case required morcellation in year 2, five cases in year 3, eleven cases in year 4 and five in year 5. The median uterine weights in TLH cases increased in consecutive years from 110 g in year1 to 240 g in year 5 (Table 2).

Complications

There was one surgical complication in the TAH group; a patient who was operated on by a specialty doctor sustained

a bladder injury, which was repaired without event. There were no recorded surgical complications in the VH group. In the TLH group, there were 10 surgical complications; four bladder injuries, one bowel injury, two ureteric injuries, two acute haemorrhages and one significant postoperative bleed. Only one complication required immediate conversion to laparotomy as described above (case 13). Two patients were returned to theatre for intra-abdominal bleeding in the immediate postoperative period, one of which was managed by laparotomy by another consultant and the other managed laparoscopically by the author. One complication (ureteric injury) involved return to theatre for reimplantation of ureter and stent insertion. Details of the complications at TLH are shown in Table 3. The overall rate of surgical complication was 0 % for VH, 5.6 % for TAH and 7.2 % for TLH. In the TLH group, there were two complications in the first year (11.8 %), three in the second (13.6 %), one in the third (3.2 %), one in the fourth (2.6 %) and three in the fifth (10.3 %).

Conclusions

This study demonstrates the outcome of offering a TLH to every patient in a general gynaecology clinic that is suitable for an abdominal hysterectomy. It is fundamentally different from many published studies, which examine the outcome of laparoscopic hysterectomy, where the procedure is only performed on selected cases. In this study, the outcomes of all hysterectomy patients are reported so this is a complete data set without selection bias. The study is unique in that the decision to offer all abdominal hysterectomy patients a TLH was made prospectively and then the outcome was studied.

The data show that the success of achieving a TLH increased with time; as cases were unselected, this increase is likely to be due to increase in surgical expertise. Over the whole study, excluding cases where other clinicians chose the surgical route (2 cases), performed the surgery (9 cases) or the patient had a VH (17 cases), 95 % (138/145) of all cases offered a TLH had a TLH. The results show that TLH can justifiably be offered to all patients undergoing non-vaginal hysterectomy as the default procedure providing the surgeon is appropriately experienced in the technique.

Our intraoperative conversion rate to laparotomy was 2.2 %. Both uterine weight and adhesions have been shown as risk factors for conversion of TLH to laparotomy [16]. However, of the three conversions in this study, one was for anaesthetic reasons and one was for surgical assistant shortcomings. The single remaining conversion was for an enlarged uterus fixed in the pelvis and was compounded by an in experienced surgical assistant. It was considered safer to convert than risk a complication. In our current practice, this

Table 2 The range and median uterine weight in grams for vaginal, abdominal and laparoscopic hysterectomy is shown for each year

		VH	TAH	TLH
Year 1	Range	61–85	280–866	58–209
	Median	67.5	561	110
Year 2	Range	42	134–2,793	67–455
	Median	42	1,464	135
Year 3	Range			97–784
	Median			188.8
Year 4	Range			37–1,030
	Median			170
Year 5	Range			70–584
	Median			240

Data obtained from the uterine weight documented at histology

Table 3 Details of complications during total laparoscopic hysterectomy, shown by chronological case number

Patient number	Year	Complication	Result	Conversion	Complicating factors	Uterine dimension (cm^3)	Uterine weight (g)
3	1	Bladder injury	Repaired	No	Endometriosis. 2×LSCS	235	151
13	1	Bowel injury	Repaired	Yes	Severe adhesions	135	Not recorded
31	2	Ureteric injury	Return to theatre. Reimplantation of right ureter and stent insertion	No. Not identified at surgery	Enlarged uterus with adenomyosis	504	Not recorded
32	2	Ureteric injury	Repaired laparoscopically during procedure	No	Endometriosis of both side walls. Dense adhesions (unplanned opening of ureter)	95	128
38	2	Bladder injury	Repaired. Prophylactic right ureteric stent	No	Deep infiltrating endometriosis	189	145
57	3	Bladder injury	Repaired	No	Previous TVT	Not recorded	590
96	4	Bladder injury	Repaired	No	2×LSCS	400	Not recorded
117	5	Bleeding	Return to theatre. Laparotomy. Right uterine artery pedicle. EBL 1000 ml.	No. Not identified at surgery	Multiple adhesions between bowel, ovary and uterus. Previous pelvic sepsis	144	130
124	5	Infection/ Bleeding	Raw area of vault sutured in theatre at 3/52	No	18/40 fibroid uterus. Infection/ bleeding at 3/52 post operation	Morcellated	564
126	5	Bleeding	Return to theatre. Right uterine artery pedicle sutured laparoscopically. EBL 2500 ml	No	16/40 fibroid uterus. 7 cm right broad ligament fibroid adjacent to cervix. Patient on warfarin	Not recorded	375

Uterine dimension was calculated using the height (cm)×width (cm)×depth (cm) documented at histology to produce a modeled uterine volume in cm^3

case would have been offered gonadotrophin releasing hormone agonists preoperatively to reduce the uterine size so that isolation of the uterine arteries could be undertaken as the first surgical step and the appropriate assistance would have been scheduled.

We consider that grossly enlarged uteri or a uterus that is wedged against the pelvic side-wall are likely to be the only remaining surgical reasons for conversion. However, even in these cases, an experienced surgical team with the correct equipment could be expected to achieve TLH in most cases. This is reflected in our data, as only one conversion occurred after the first 50 procedures even though median weight of uteri increased each year.

The primary indication for surgery in all the vaginal hysterectomy cases was uterine prolapse, and the majority of these patients had additional pelvic floor surgery performed. Uterine suspension procedures are now recognised treatment options for women with uterine prolapse [17], and the decline in vaginal hysterectomy with time in this study is explained by the introduction of laparoscopic sacrohysteropexy into the authors practice.

The overall perioperative complication rate for TLH was 7.2 %. Previous studies have shown complication rates of 7.1 % [18] and 5.8 % [19]. Six of the 10 complications occurred in high-risk patients with complicating factors including deep infiltrating endometriosis, previous multiple caesarean section and previous history of pelvic sepsis. This finding demonstrates that if all cases are offered TLH,

including those with surgical comorbidity, the rate of complications is likely to be higher than where the procedure is only offered selectively.

Two complications were cases that were returned to theatre to control postoperative bleeding. In one case, a laparotomy was performed on return to theatre by another consultant where no active bleeding was identified but raw areas in the vault were over-sewn. In this case, it is questionable whether repeat surgery was justified. In the second case, the right uterine artery pedicle was sutured laparoscopically and laparotomy was not required. In the latter case, postoperative bleeding was caused by a uterine artery suture being dislodged when the large, part morcellated, uterus was delivered through the vault. This complication may have been prevented by morcellation to a small residual uterus that could be removed through the vault less traumatically. As surgical experience grows, complications are likely to reduce; however, conversely, it is also likely that more complex cases will be undertaken laparoscopically, which will increase the risk of complication. Thus, predicting how the complication rate should change each consecutive year, when more complex surgery is being undertaken on patients that would have previously been deemed unsuitable for laparoscopic approach is challenging.

Studies have previously shown that even during the learning curve, TLH is safe [20]. With increasing surgical experience, operation length and complication rate are expected to decrease [20]. In a review of 250 laparoscopic hysterectomies, complication rates decreased with time and increasing experience and compared favorably to those expected with open surgery [18]. Identification of procedure numbers needed for complication rates and operating time to plateau in an experienced laparoscopic surgeon have previously been defined as 10 procedures [14]; however, patients were selected for TLH based on a combination of factors including preoperative estimation of uterine size and therefore this is not an assessment of the learning curve in an unselected population.

Similarly, previous studies have described the learning curve with reference to shortening operating time [14]. In this study, where all cases were offered TLH including complex laparoscopic hysterectomy (cases with deep infiltrating endometriosis, adhesions, large uterus or multiple previous operations), comparing the length of operation at the beginning of the study, and in the earlier stage of the learning curve, with the length of the operation at a later stage makes an inaccurate measure, so these data have not been studied.

TLH is associated with shorter length of hospital stay and more rapid recovery [3, 6, 7]. Patient preference and expectation will play an important role in selecting most appropriate route of surgery, and our patients requested the operation that had the shortest recovery time. This is consistent with the evidence that women scheduled for a hysterectomy prefer laparoscopic hysterectomy compared to TAH [21]. We have made no attempt to collect long-term outcome; however, previous authors have reported improved quality of life outcomes at 4 years with laparoscopic hysterectomy compared with abdominal hysterectomy [22]. Women in this study were fully counseled about the risks and benefits of undertaking each route of hysterectomy. All women in this study, who were deemed suitable for TLH, opted for TLH, with the exception of one woman in year 5, who chose a TAH simply to expedite her admission.

A comparison of hospital and indirect costs associated with route of hysterectomy has showed that laparoscopic-assisted vaginal hysterectomy had lower cost to employers on the basis of lost work hours compared with abdominal and vaginal hysterectomy [23]. Further research is needed to establish the true cost of laparoscopic hysterectomy compared to abdominal and vaginal hysterectomy; costs must be compared for the whole patient journey from primary admission until full return to normal activities.

TLH is associated with a low rate of complication and a low conversion rate to laparotomy if performed by an experienced surgeon with the appropriate assistance and equipment. In benign gynaecology, total laparoscopic hysterectomy offers considerable advantages over traditional abdominal hysterectomy and should be offered as the default surgical approach when vaginal hysterectomy is not possible.

Conflict of interest The authors report no conflicts of interest. The authors alone are responsible for the content and writing of the paper.

References

1. Reich H, Decaprio J, McGlynn F (1989) Laparoscopic hysterectomy. J Gynecol Surg 5:213–216
2. Gendy R, Walsh CA, Walsh SR, Karantanis E (2011) Vaginal hysterectomy versus total laparoscopic hysterectomy for benign disease: a meta-analysis of randomized controlled trials. Am J Obstet Gynecol 204(5):388
3. Olsson JH, Ellstrom M, Hahlin M (1996) A randomised prospective trial comparing laparoscopic and abdominal hysterectomy. Br J Obstet Gynaecol 103:345–350
4. National Institute for Health and Clinical Excellence (2010) Laparoscopic hysterectomy (including laparoscopic total hysterectomy and laparoscopically assisted vaginal hysterectomy) for endometrial cancer. IPG356. London: National Institute for Health and Clinical Excellence
5. National Institute for Health and Clinical Excellence (2007) Laparoscopic techniques for hysterectomy. IPG239. London: National Institute for Health and Clinical Excellence
6. Garry R, Fountain J, Mason S, Napp V, Brown J, Hawe J et al (2004) The eVALuate study: two parallel randomised trials, one comparing laparoscopic with abdominal hysterectomy, the other comparing laparoscopic with vaginal hysterectomy. BMJ. doi:10.1136/bmj.37984.623889.F6
7. Jacoby VL, Autry A, Jacobson G, Domush R, Nakagawa S, Jacoby A (2009) Nationwide use of laparoscopic hysterectomy compared with abdominal and vaginal approaches. Obstet Gynecol 114(5):1041–1048
8. Falcone T, Walters MD (2008) Hysterectomy for benign disease. Obstet Gynecol 1(3):753–767
9. Sculpher M, Manca A, Abbott J, Fountain J, Mason S, Garry R (2004) Cost effectiveness analysis of laparoscopic hysterectomy compared with standard hysterectomy: results from a randomised trial. BMJ. doi:10.1136/bmj.37942.601331.EE
10. Bijen CBM, Vermeulen KM, Mourits MJE, de Bock GH (2009) Costs and effects of abdominal versus laparoscopic hysterectomy: systematic review of controlled trials. PLoS One 4(10):e7340. doi:10.1371/journal.pone.0007340
11. Barnett JC, Judd JP, Wu JM, Scales CD, Myers ER, Havrilesky LJ (2010) Cost comparison among robotic, laparoscopic, and open hysterectomy for endometrial cancer. Obstet Gynecol 116(3):685–693
12. Nieboer TE, Spaanderman ME, Bongers MY, Vierhout ME, Kluivers KB (2010) Gynaecologists estimate and experience laparoscopic hysterectomy as more difficult compared with abdominal hysterectomy. Gynecol Surg 7:359–363
13. Ballantyne GH (2002) The pitfalls of laparoscopic surgery: challenges for robotics and telerobotic surgery. Surg Laparosc Endosc Percutan Tech 12(1):1–5
14. Rosen DMB, Cario GM, Carlton MA, Lam AM, Chapman M (1998) An assessment of the learning curve for laparoscopic and total laparoscopic hysterectomy. Gynaecol Endosc 7(6):289–293
15. Perino A, Cucinella G, Venezia R, Castelli A, Cittadini E (1999) Total laparoscopic hysterectomy versus total abdominal hsterectomy: an assessment of the learning curve in a prospective randomized study. Hum Reprod 14(12):2996–2999
16. Park SH, Cho HY, Kim HB (2011) Factors determining conversion to laparotomy in patients undergoing total laparoscopic hysterectomy. Gynecol Obstet Invest 71(3):193–197
17. National Institute for Health and Clinical Excellence (2009) Insertion of mesh uterine suspension sling (including

sacrohysteropexy) for uterine prolapse repair. IPG282. London: National Institute for Health and Clinical Excellence

18. Jones RA (1995) Complications of laparoscopic hysterectomy. Gynaecol Endosc 4(2):95–99

19. Liu CY, Reich H (1994) Complications of total laparoscopic hysterectomy in 518 cases. Gynecol Endosc 3:203–208

20. Vaisbuch E, Goldchmit C, Ofer D, Agmon A, Hagay Z (2006) Laparoscopic hysterectomy versus total abdominal hysterectomy: a comparative study. Eur J Obstet Gynecol Reprod Biol 126 (2):234–238

21. Kluivers KB, Opmeer BC, Geomini PM, Bongers MY, Vierhout ME, Bremer GL et al (2009) Women's preference for laparoscopic or abdominal hysterectomy. Gynecol Surg 6(3):223–228

22. Nieboer TE, Hendriks JC, Bongers MY, Vierhout ME, Kluivers KB (2012) Quality of life after laparoscopic and abdominal hysterectomy: a randomized controlled trial. Obstet Gynecol 119(1):85–91

23. Lenihan JP Jr, Kovanda C, Cammarano C (2004) Comparison of laparoscopic-assisted vaginal hysterectomy with traditional hysterectomy for cost-effectiveness to employers. Am J Obstet Gynecol 190(6):1714

10

Abdominal hysterectomy for benign indications: evidence-based guidance for surgical decisions

Danish S. Siddiqui · Hussain Ali · Kiley A. Bernhard ·
Vincenzo Berghella · Suneet P. Chauhan

Abstract The purpose of this review is to provide evidence-based guidance for surgical decisions during abdominal hysterectomy performed for benign indications. Using combinations of terms "abdominal," "hysterectomy," and "randomized clinical trials (RCT)," we performed Ovid, PubMed, and Cochrane searches for publications between 1988 and 2008. After reviewing over 3,000 abstracts, 19 RCT were identified. There are no grade A recommendations. The only grade B suggestion is use of a bipolar vessel sealing device (LigaSure) for vascular pedicles rather than sutures. Routine closure of peritoneum should be avoided. Evidence behind 71 % (15/21) of surgical steps is insufficient (grade I). Despite its common performance, there are no grade A recommendations that can be made for the technical aspects of abdominal hysterectomy. Since almost 70 % of the surgical steps during abdominal hysterectomy lack randomized clinical trials, adequately designed studies are needed to decrease perioperative morbidity.

Keywords Abdominal hysterectomy · Benign indication · Randomized controlled trials · Evidence-based medicine

D. S. Siddiqui (✉)
Department of Obstetrics and Gynecology, School of Medicine and Public Health, University of Wisconsin,
945 N 12th Street-1K,
Milwaukee, WI 53233, USA
e-mail: danish.siddiqui@aurora.org

H. Ali
St. John's Hospital,
Lebanon, MO, USA

K. A. Bernhard
Aurora Health Care,
Milwaukee, WI, USA

V. Berghella
Jefferson Medical College, Thomas Jefferson University,
Philadelphia, PA, USA

S. P. Chauhan
Eastern Virginia Medical School,
Norfolk, VA, USA

Background

Hysterectomy, or removal of the uterus, is the most common major gynecologic procedure in the USA. Approximately, 600,000 hysterectomies were performed in the USA in the early 2000s [1] and 20 million US women have had their uterus removed [2]. From 1994–1999, the overall hysterectomy rate for US female was 5.5 per 1,000 women who are at least 15 years old [2]. Though the uterus can be removed vaginally, or with laparoscopy, the most common route is with open abdominal hysterectomy (AH). In 2003, there were 538,722 hysterectomies for benign disease, and about two thirds (66 %) of them were performed by abdominal laparotomy [3].

While the mortality with AH for benign indications is 0.25 per 1,000 procedures, morbidity occurs in 3–5 %. The potential complications include infection, blood transfusion, ureteral, bladder or intestinal injury, deep venous thrombosis, and pulmonary embolism [4–6]. One possible way to decrease the surgical complication rate is to ascertain what aspects of the surgery are evidence-based and have been linked with lower morbidity. Additionally, a review of the literature would identify the surgical decisions that are not based on randomized clinical trials (RCT) and potentially encourage properly designed trials.

The purpose of the review article is to provide gynecologists with evidence-based guidance during planned AH regarding operative technique and to identify the steps that need a properly conducted RCT.

Material and methods

Since this is a literature search, an approval from the Institutional Review Board was not obtained. From TeLinde's *Operative Gynecology*, tenth edition [7], a standard textbook for gynecological surgeons, we identified 21 surgical steps for abdominal hysterectomy and sought RCTs for each one. Using combinations of terms "abdominal," "hysterectomy," "randomized clinical trials (RCT)," and each surgical aspect (e.g., minilaparotomy, open vaginal cuff), we performed Ovid, Cochrane, and PubMed searches for articles published between 1988 and 2008. Each publication and Cochrane review was examined, and the pertinent references were obtained. Articles were excluded if they were in foreign language, focused on antibiotics, pain management, cancer, cost-or-decision analysis, laparoscopy, vaginal hysterectomy, or did not discuss technical aspects of abdominal hysterectomy. Additionally, we excluded studies done on cadavers.

All RCTs that focused on a surgical aspect of abdominal hysterectomy were included. If there were no RCTs, non-randomized reports with comparison groups were included in our analysis. Each step of the surgery was reviewed separately, and the evidence levels and recommendations were categorized according to the US Preventive Services Task Force (Tables 1 and 2) [8].

We excluded randomized trials that concurrently compared several steps of surgery because, with such a design, it is not feasible to directly compare the effects of each individual step [9]. We did not specifically review preoperative consideration like prophylactic oophorectomy and perioperative aspects such as prophylactic antibiotics and prevention of venous thromboembolic events for there are ACOG guidelines to inform clinicians [10–12]. Chi-square test for trend was done, and $P<0.05$ was considered significant.

Findings

Our literature search yielded 3,509 abstracts and of these, 3,392 (97 %) were excluded. The two most common reasons for excluding the articles were that the focus of the study was not a surgical aspect of hysterectomy or that it involved patients with cancer. We reviewed 117 articles that met the inclusion criteria (Fig. 1).

Patient position for AH is usually dorsal supine; however, some surgeons prefer lithotomy position so that a second assistant can be placed between the legs [7]. Patient position has not been studied separately in any trial (recommendation I; level of certainty, low).

Skin cleansing is done for the purpose to minimize wound complications and infectious morbidity. This can be performed using a variety of solutions (e.g., povidone-iodine, chlorhexidine gluconate, hexachlorophene). We did not identify any RCT evaluating the efficacy of any of these skin preparations in reducing the infectious wound morbidity (recommendation I; level of certainty, low).

Vaginal preparation involving preoperative cleansing has been advocated to reduce postoperative infectious morbidity. A variety of preparations are available (e.g., povidone-

	Grade	Definition	Suggestions for practice
Table 1 Recommendations according to US Preventive Services Task Force (USPSTF)	A	The USPSTF recommends the service. There is high certainty that the net benefit is substantial.	Offer or provide this service
	B	The USPSTF recommends the service. There is high certainty that the net benefit is moderate or there is moderate certainty that the net benefit is moderate to substantial.	Offer or provide this service
	C	The USPSTF recommends against routine providing of this service. There may be considerations that support providing the service in an individual patient. There is at least moderate certainty that the net benefit is small.	Offer or provide this service only if other considerations support the offering or providing the service in an individual patient.
	D	The USPSTF recommends against the service. There is moderate or high certainty that the service has no net benefit or that the harms outweigh the benefits.	Discourage the use of this service.
	I	The USPSTF concludes that the current evidence is insufficient to assess the balance of benefits and harms of the service. Evidence is lacking, of poor quality, or conflicting, and the balance of benefits and harms cannot be determined.	If the service is offered, patients should understand the uncertainty about the balance of benefits and harms.

Table 2 Level of certainty regarding the net benefit

Level of certainty	Description
High	The available evidence usually includes consistent results from well-designed, well-conducted studies in representative primary care populations. These studies assess the effects on the preventive service on health outcomes. This conclusion is therefore unlikely to be strongly affected by the results of future studies.
Moderate	The available evidence is sufficient to determine the effect of the preventive service on health outcomes, but confidence in the estimate is constrained by such factors as:
	• The number, size or quality of individual studies.
	• Inconsistency of findings across individual studies
	• Limited generalizability of findings to routine primary care practice
	• Lack of coherence in the chain of evidence
	As more information becomes available, the magnitude or direction of the observed effect could change, and this change may be large enough to alter the conclusion
Low	The available evidence is insufficient to assess effect on health outcome. Evidence is insufficient because of:
	• The number or size of studies
	• Important flaws in study design or methods
	• Inconsistency of findings across individual studies
	• Gaps in the chain of evidence
	• Finding not generalizable to routine primary care practice
	• Lack of information on important health outcomes
	More information may allow estimation of effects on health outcomes.

iodine solution or gel, chlorhexidine). Three randomized trials, involving 1,889 patients, studied the preoperative vaginal cleansing using either povidone-iodine solution or gel. While two RCT [13, 14] did not show a decrease in infectious morbidity, Buppasiri et al. [15] noted a significant decrease with febrile morbidity. Specifically, they noted that the relative risk of infectious morbidity was 8 vs. 19 %, with

a risk difference of −10, and 95 % confidence intervals (CI) of −17.8 to −2.2 % (adjusted odds ratio of 0.4; 95 % CI of 0.2–0.9 %). Thus, preoperative vaginal preparation using 1 % povidone-iodine solution may decrease postoperative infectious morbidity. Compliance with the study's protocol (1,000 cc night before and day of surgery) may not be feasible in clinical practice (recommendation C; level of certainty, moderate).

*Skin incision type*s for abdominal hysterectomy have not been studied separately in a trial. The skin incision can be longitudinal or transverse. Many gynecologists choose a Pfannenstiel incision for its cosmetic appeal, which is a low transverse incision (recommendation I; level of certainty, low).

Skin incision length during abdominal hysterectomy can be <6 cm (minilaparotomy) vs. >6 cm (laparotomy). There have been no RCT trials comparing the minilaparotomy vs. laparotomy with transverse or longitudinal skin incision. There is one observational study [32] with 199 patients, comparing the outcome in ≤6 vs >6 cm transverse incision. The investigators conclude that minilaparotomy is an option during AH for benign indications. The study was hampered not only by a nonrandomized design but also by having significantly different uterine sizes in the two groups. Thus, while minilaparotomy may be the clinicians' and patient's preference in certain clinical situations, it cannot be recommended to improve perioperative outcomes (recommendation, I; certainty low)

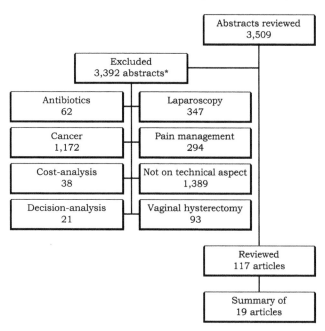

Fig. 1 Results of the literature search

Subcutaneous incision can be made either by a scalpel or electrocautery. One randomized clinical trial [16] with 380 patients was identified which compared electrocautery vs. scalpel in a subcutaneous incision during abdominal hysterectomy. Postoperative wound complications like seroma, hematoma, infection, or dehiscence were not significantly different in the two groups (P=0.4). Thus, the subcutaneous tissue can safely be incised by either electrocautery or scalpel (recommendation, C; certainty, moderate).

Fascial incision has not been studied separately in a trial. In a low transverse Pfannenstiel incision, the fascia is usually incised transversely with the scalpel and then extended with scissors. Some clinicians advocate the use of electrocautery in the cutting mode for the fascial incision [33]. We did not identify any study ascertaining the optimum method to incise the fascia during AH (recommendations, I; certainty, poor).

Rectus fascia dissection of the rectus muscles with transverse fascial incision has not been studied separately during AH (recommendations, I; certainty, poor).

Opening of the peritoneum is achieved with either blunt or sharp dissection. During this surgical step, injury to the underlying organs and bladder inferiorly should be avoided. RCTs have not addressed what is the optimum manner to avoid these potential complications (recommendations, I; certainty, poor).

Retractors are used to improve the exposure during the surgery. The options include self-retaining (Balfour, Kerschner, Bookwalter, Omni-Tract, O'Conner-O'Sullivan, Mobius) or hand-held retractors (Heaney, Deaver, or Richardson). A potential complication with retractor usage is femoral nerve injury [34]. We were unable to identify any study that showed a significant decrease in the rate of this complication. Thus, the selection of the retractor should be based on surgeon's preference (recommendations, I; certainty, poor).

Ureter identification during AH is advocated to avoid injury that tends to occur at the infundibulopelvic ligament where the ovarian vessels are ligated, area of the uterine artery ligation, and the bladder base. The identification may be done by direct visualization of the ureter in the retroperitoneal space on the medial leaf of the broad ligament, palpation, or prophylactic placement of ureteral catheterization. No RCT has addressed the effect and/or optimum method of identification of the ureter to reduce its injury during AH alone (recommendations, I; certainty, low).

Vascular pedicles (involving, uteroovarian/infundibulopelvic ligaments, uterine vessels, and cardinal and uterosacral ligament) can be ligated by suture ligature, staples, or by electrocoagulation. Though an RCT [35] compared staples with suture ligature, we excluded this trial because the investigators did not mention if they used the stapling device for all vascular pedicles, and they used the stapling technique for the closure of vaginal vault. Thus, it is difficult to discern what aspect of surgical technique improved the operative outcome.

We identified two RCTs (n=87) comparing suture ligature vs. bipolar vessel sealing device (LigaSure, Boulder CO) [17, 18]. Compared to suture ligature, use of bipolar vessel sealing device (LigaSure) for vascular pedicles significantly decreased (P<0.01) the postoperative pain during the first three postoperative days [17]. There was no significant reduction in the operating time, blood loss, perioperative complications, and hospital stay [17, 18]. Thus, we recommend use of bipolar vessel sealing device (LigaSure) for vascular pedicles (recommendations, B; certainty, moderate).

Total vs. supracervical hysterectomy involves removal of the uterine body and the cervix in the former, while in the latter, the cervix is kept intact. A Cochrane review [36] summarized three RCT (n=733) (−19, −21) comparing the perioperative outcomes with these two options. The length of surgery (weighted mean difference [WMD] of 11.4 min, 95 % CI 6.6–16.3 min), the estimated blood loss (WMD 85 ml; 95 % CI 27–142 ml), and febrile morbidity (odds ratio [OR] 4.3; 95 % CI 0.25–0.75) were significantly reduced with supracervical hysterectomy. There was, however, no significant difference in the odds of requiring blood transfusion, duration of hospitalization, and return to normal activity. With supracervical hysterectomy, the likelihood of cyclical vaginal bleeding after 1 year was significantly higher when compared to total hysterectomy (11.9 vs. 0.8 %; OR 11.3, 95 % CI 4.1, 31.2). At 2 years, however, there was no significant difference in ongoing bleeding. With 2 years after the surgery, there is no difference in the rate of urinary incontinence, constipation, and measures of sexual function.

One of the RCTs [22] summarized in the Cochrane review published follow-up (mean 9 years, range 7–11 years) of 65 % (181 of 265) of the cohorts that were randomized. There was no long-term difference with total or supracervical hysterectomy with regards to quality of life, mental health, and pelvic organ function. Urinary and bowel function variables did not change significantly.

Thus, for short-term benefit (operative time, blood loss, and febrile morbidity), there is a role for supracervical abdominal hysterectomy in selected women, though there are no long-term advantages (recommendations, C; certainty, high).

Vaginal cuff open vs. closed are the two options once the corpus and the cervix are removed. An open vaginal cuff may provide drainage and potentially prevents infective morbidity. We identified four RCTs (n=612) published between 1992 and1998 [23–26]. Though they differed in how they closed the cuff and the primary outcomes, two of three RCTs noted a significant decrease in the operative time when the cuff was closed, possibly due to the hemostasis at the vaginal cuff obtained during closure with staples or sutures [23, 26]. Using staples to close the cuff [23], there was significant improvement in intraoperative hemostasis and granulation at 6 weeks postoperative. Compared to when the cuff is open, the amount of fluid in the pelvis with a closed cuff is significantly higher on postoperative day 5 [26]. This, however, was not associated with improved febrile morbidity (recommendations, C; certainty, moderate).

Vaginal cuff closure may be achieved with absorbable staples or with sutures. Only one RCT (*n*=60) compared these two options and noted that there was no significant difference in the operative time and febrile morbidity [27]. Thus, there is no clinical advantage of using staples (recommendations, C; certainty, moderate).

Angle stitch consists of reattachment of cardinal and uterosacral ligament to the vaginal cuff with the aim of preventing apical prolapse [37]. Though classical teaching advocates this surgical step, we did not identify either RCT or observational studies (recommendations, I; certainty, low).

Intraabdominal irrigation, done to decrease perioperative morbidity with normal saline before abdominal wall closure, is advised [7]. We did not find any RCTs evaluating irrigation vs. no irrigation (recommendations, I; certainty, low).

Peritoneal closure involves closure of the parietal and visceral peritoneum. We identified three RCTs (*n*=298) comparing closure of the peritoneum with nonclosure in AH. While two trials evaluated either visceral [28] or parietal peritoneal closure [29], one studied the closure of both layers [30]. Nonclosure of the peritoneum, when compared with closure of either single layer or both layers, significantly reduced the operative time in all three trials. The estimated blood loss is also significantly less in the nonclosure group in one trial (45-ml reduction, *P*=0.03). There is no significant difference in the postoperative pain, febrile morbidity, wound infection, and hospital stay between peritoneal closure and nonclosure groups. Thus, routine peritoneal closure is not recommended (recommendations, D; certainty, moderate).

Techniques of fascial closure include use of running or interrupted delayed absorbable sutures. We did not identify any RCT studying facial closure technique in AH for benign pathology (recommendations, I; certainty, low).

Irrigation of the subcutaneous tissue to decrease wound complications in AH has not been evaluated separately by RCT (recommendations, I; certainty, low).

Subcutaneous tissue closure vs. no closure are two options before skin approximation to minimize wound-related morbidity. We identified one RCT (*n*=60) comparing closure with 2-0 polyglycolic acid (Dexon) vs. nonclosure in patients undergoing AH with ≥2.5-cm thickness of the subcutaneous tissue [31]. Mid-line vertical incision was used in 47 %, while the remaining patients had a Pfannenstiel incision. There were fewer seromas, infections, and wound disruptions in the suture group, but statistical significance was not reached. The RCT lacked sample size

calculations and did not perform any statistical analysis (recommendations, C; certainty, low).

Closure of the skin techniques include use of staples, subcuticular suture reinforced with surgical tape (e.g., Steri-Strips), or 2-octyl-cyanoacrylate skin adhesive (Dermabond, distributed by Ethicon, Inc). We did not find any RCTs that address the optimum method of skin closure in AH (recommendations, I; certainty, low).

Comments

In the USA [3], there are 69 hysterectomies performed per hour, and for benign disease, 41 abdominal hysterectomies are done every hour. While the likelihood of postoperative morbidity is about 4 % [4], this rate may decrease further if RCTs with AH demonstrate a clinically significant decline in perioperative complications. A summary of published RCTs would not only allow us to identify the surgical steps that should be performed because of the existing evidence but also encourage investigators to design additional randomized studies.

There are three findings of this review. First, after reviewing over 3,000 abstracts, we identified only 19 RCTs [13–31] that met the inclusion criteria. These trials included 4,129 patients (Table 3). The surgical step with the largest number of cohorts (*n*=1,899) examined the use of vaginal irrigation before AH, and the one with the fewest patients (*n*=60) focused on closing the vaginal cuff with sutures vs. staples [33]. Interestingly, of these 19 studies, only three [16, 20, 27] or 16 % of RCTs were done in the USA. Thus, our evidence-based knowledge of AH is derived from a limited number of studies, with small sample size, done in foreign countries. There is, therefore, an urgent need for additional randomized trials, including in the USA.

The second finding is that 71 % (15/21) of the surgical decisions gynecologists make during AH have insufficient (grade I) evidence. This is understandable considering the limited number of RCTs. About 24 % (5/21) of surgical steps are based on grade C evidence, indicating that these steps should not be done routinely but on an individual basis. We identified only one (5 %) grade D recommendations and that is the peritoneum should not be closed. Using similar analysis, Berghella et al. [9] concluded that with cesarean delivery, neither parietal nor visceral peritoneal layer should be closed (grade D). Though there were no grade A recommendations for AH, there was one grade B suggestion: compared to suture ligature, use of a bipolar vessel sealing device (LigaSure) for vascular pedicles significantly decreases postoperative pain during the first three postoperative days (Table 3). However, this study involved a small sample size of only 57 patients. Thus, if this surgical step is advocated to be done routinely, then an RCT that is compliant with Consolidated Standards of Reporting Trials (CONSORT) guidelines [38] should be conducted.

Table 3 Evidence-based recommendations for abdominal hysterectomy

Technical aspect	RCT	Number	Rec	Certainty	Comment
Patient position	0		I	Low	
Skin cleaning	0		I	Low	
Vaginal preparation	3	1,899	C	Mod	Povidone-iodine vaginal antisepsis may reduce the overall infection morbidity after abdominal hysterectomy. Compliance with protocol (1,000 cc night before and day of surgery) may not be feasible.
Skin incision type			I	Low	
Skin incision length (minilaparotomy)	0		I	Low	
Subcutaneous incision	1	380	C	Mod	Incision of subcutaneous tissue by electrocautery or scalpel does not influence the rate of wound complications.
Fascial incision	0		I	Low	
Rectus fascia dissection	0		I	Low	
Opening peritoneum	0		I	Low	
Retractors	0		I	Low	
Ureter identification	0		I	Low	
Vascular pedicles: suture ligature vs. bipolar vessel sealing device ligature	2	87	B	Mod	Compared to suture ligature, use of bipolar vessel sealing device (LigaSure) for vascular pedicles significantly decreases postoperative pain during first 3 postoperative days.
Total vs. supracervical hysterectomy	4	733	C	High	Compared to total, supracervical hysterectomy is associated with a significant decrease in the duration of surgery, intraoperative blood loss and fever. Postoperative cyclical bleeding up to a year is significantly more common with supracervical than total hysterectomy.
Vaginal cuff open vs. closed (sutures or staples)	4	612	C	Mod	With staples intraoperative time is significantly reduced. Granulation at 6 weeks is significantly less with staples than open.
Vaginal cuff closed suture vs. staples	1	60	C	Mod	No clinical advantage of closing the vaginal cuff with suture or staple.
Angle stitch	0		I	Low	
Intraabdominal Irrigation	0		I	Low	
Peritoneal closure	3	298	D	Mod	Not recommended because peritoneal closure provides no postoperative benefits while unnecessarily increasing surgical time and anesthesia exposure.
Techniques of fascial closure	0		C	Low	
Subcutaneous tissue closure vs. nonclosure	1	60	I	Low	No significant difference in closure vs no closure but the trial design was poor.
Closure of skin with staples vs. subcuticular suture	0		I	Low	
Total	19[a]	4,129			

RCT randomized clinical trial, *Rec* recommendation

[a] The Cochrane review [36] is a summary of three RCTs [19–21]

The third finding of the study focuses on the comparison of evidence for cesarean delivery (CD) vs. AH. The reasons for comparing the two surgeries are that they are the two most common major procedures done by an obstetrician-gynecologist, and it allows us to determine to what extent RCTs have been done to minimize postoperative morbidity. Previously, Berghella et al. [9] reported that, of 44 surgical decisions during CD, 16 % had grade A recommendations compared to none for AH. Overall, the distribution of the recommendations for the two common surgical procedures is significantly different (P=0.029). For CD, 43 % of the recommendations were grade I and for AH, 71 %. Thus, it seems more RCTs have been done for CD than AH. Another difference noted between the different surgical steps of CD and AH is that, in CD, the suture closure and drainage of >2-cm subcutaneous tissue has been recommended as level A [9, 39], whereas in AH, the same recommendation was not observed. This may, again, be due to lack of adequately powered and designed trials.

There are several limitations of this study that should be acknowledged. We used the tenth edition of TeLinde's *Operative Gynecology* to ascertain the technique involved with AH, and there may be surgical steps that were mentioned in earlier editions but are omitted in the latest. Edition 8 [40, 41] for example, described extra- vs. intrafascial AH, and this is not described in the newest version. Though there is an RCT comparing extra- and intrafascial AH [42], we did not include this study in our summary because this step is not mentioned in the tenth edition. We acknowledge that though RCT may show clinical benefit, the recommendation may be difficult to implement in routine practice. Perioperative vaginal irrigation, for example, with 1,000 ml of povidone-iodine vaginal antisepsis on the night before and prior to start of surgery decreased infectious morbidity [15] but seems difficult to implement routinely. While we excluded RCTs that combined AH with other major gynecological surgeries, there may be some useful information from these reports. We excluded manuscripts that focused on other surgeries in conjunction with AH and hysterectomy for cancer because the postoperative outcomes may be different when the surgery is done alone or without underlying cancer. Chou et al. [43] for example, randomized over 3,000 patients to either have or not have bilateral prophylactic ureteral catheter and reported that the likelihood of ureteral injury was similar. This conclusion may be valid with AH but needs confirmation. We did not determine if the RCT trials we included were compliant with the CONSORT statements or not [38]. Compliance with the statements improves the quality of the RCT, and noncompliance with them is associated with an overestimate of the effectiveness of intervention [44].

Conclusion

In summary, though abdominal hysterectomy is the most common major gynecologic surgery, there is a paucity of RCTs that minimize perioperative morbidity. Additionally, evidence with vaginal and laparoscopic hysterectomy needs to be reviewed.

Conflict of interest   The authors report no conflicts of interest. The authors alone are responsible for the content and writing of the paper.

References

1. Whiteman MK, Hillis SD, Jamieson DJ, Morrow B, Podgornik MN, Brett KM et al (2008) Inpatient hysterectomy surveillance in the United States, 2000–2004. Am J Obstet Gynecol 198:34.e1–34.e7

2. Keshavarz H, Hillis SD, Kieke BA, Marchbanks PA (2002) Hysterectomy surveillance—United States, 1994–1999. MMWR 51 (SS05):1–8

3. Wu JM, Wechter ME, Geller EJ, Nguyen TV, Cisco AG (2007) Hysterectomy rates in the United States, 2003. Obstet Gynecol 110:1091–1095

4. McPherson K, Metcalfe MA, Herbert A, Maresh M, Casbard A, Hargreaves J et al (2004) Severe complications of hysterectomy: the VALUE study. BJOG 111:688–694

5. Maresh MJ, Metcalfe MS, McPherson K, Overton C, Hall V, Hargreaves J et al (2002) The VALUE national hysterectomy study: description of the patient and their surgery. BJOG 109:302–312

6. Kafy S, Huang JY, Al-Sunaidi M, Wiener D, Tulandi T (2006) Audit of morbidity and mortality rates of 1792 hysterectomies. J Minim Invasive Gynecol 13:55–59

7. Jones HW. Abdominal Hysterectomy. In Rock AJ, Jones HW (eds) Te Linde's Operative Gynecology, 10th edn. Lippincott Williams & Wilkins, Philadelphia, pp 728–743

8. US Preventive Services Task Force. Agency for health care research and quality. www.ahcpr.gov/clinic/ajpmsuppl/harris3.htm. Last accessed July 12, 2009

9. Berghella V, Baxter JK, Chauhan SP (2005) Evidence-based surgery for cesarean delivery. Am J Obstet Gynecol 193(5):1607–1617

10. American College of Obstetricians and Gynecologists. Elective and risk-reducing salpingo-ophorectomy. ACOG practice bulletin No.89 Jan. 2008

11. American College of Obstetricians and Gynecologists. Antibiotic prophylaxis for gynecologic procedures. ACOG practice bulletin No.104 May 2009

12. American College of Obstetricians and Gynecologists. Prevention of deep venous thrombosis and pulmonary embolism. ACOG practice bulletin No. 84 August 2007

13. Vinkomin V (1995) Vaginal scrub prophylaxis in abdominal hysterectomy. Southeast Asian J Trop Med Pub Health 26:188–192

14. Eason E, Wells G, Garber G, Hemmings R, Luskey G, Gillett P, Martin M (2004) Vaginal Antisepsis For Abdominal Hysterectomy Study Group Antisepsis for abdominal hysterectomy: a randomised controlled trial of povidone-iodine gel. BJOG 111:695–699

15. Buppasiri P, Chongsomchai C, Wongproamas N, Ounchai J, Suwannachat B, Lumbiganon P (2004) Effectiveness of vaginal douching on febrile and infectious morbidities after total abdominal hysterectomy: a multicenter randomized controlled trial. J Med Assoc Thai 87:16–23

16. Hemsell DL, Hemsell PG, Nobles B, Johnson ER, Little BB, Heard M (1993) Abdominal wound problems after hysterectomy with electrocautery vs. scalpel subcutaneous incision. Infect Dis Obstet Gynecol 1:27–31

17. Lakeman M, Kruitwagen RF, Vos MC, Roovers JP (2008) Electrosurgical bipolar vessel sealing versus conventional clamping and suturing for total abdominal hysterectomy: a randomized trial. J Minim Invasive Gynecol 15:547–553

18. Hagen B, Erikson N, Sundset M (2005) Randomized controlled trial of LigaSure versus conventional suture ligature for abdominal hysterectomy. BJOG 112:968–970

19. Gimbel H, Zobbe V, Andersen BM, Filtenborg T, Gluud C (2003) Tabor A randomised controlled trial of total compared with subtotal hysterectomy with one-year follow up results. BJOG 110(12):1088–1098

20. Learman LA, Summitt RL Jr, Varner RE, McNeeley SG, Goodman-Gruen D, Richter HE, Lin F, Showstack J, Ireland CC, Vittinghoff E, Hulley SB, Washington AE (2003) A randomized comparison of total or supracervical hysterectomy: surgical complications and clinical outcomes. Total or Supracervical Hysterectomy (TOSH) Research Group. Obstet Gynecol 102(3):453–462

21. Thakar R, Ayers S, Thakar R, Ayers S, Gerogakapolou, Clarkson P, Stanton S, Manyonda I (2004) Hysterectomy improves quality of life and decreases psychiatric symptoms: a prospective and randomized comparison of total versus subtotal hysterectomy. BJOG 111:1115–1120

22. Thakar R, Ayers S, Srivastava R, Manyonda I (2008) Removing the cervix at hysterectomy: an unnecessary intervention? Obstet Gynecol 112:1262–1269

23. Kalbfleish RE (1992) Prospective randomized study to compare a closed vault technique using absorbable staples at the time of abdominal hysterectomy versus open vault technique. Surg Gynecol Obstet 175:337–340

24. Neuman M, Beller U, Ben Chetrit A, Lavie O, Boldes R, Diamant Y (1993) Prophylactic effect of the open vaginal vault method in reducing febrile morbidity in abdominal hysterectomy. Surg Gynecol Obstet 176:591–593

25. Colombo M, Maggioni A, Zanini A, Rangoni G, Scalambrino S, Mangioni C (1995) A randomized trial of open versus closed vaginal vault in the prevention of postoperative morbidity after abdominal hysterectomy. Am J Obstet Gynecol 173:1807–1811

26. Aharoni A, Kaner E, Levitan Z, Condrea A, Degani S, Ohel G (1998) Prospective randomized comparison between an open and closed vaginal cuff in abdominal hysterectomy. Int J Gynaecol Obstet 63:29–32

27. Stovall TG, Summitt RL Jr, Lipscomb GH, Ling FW (1991) Vaginal cuff closure at abdominal hysterectomy: comparing sutures with absorbable staples. Obstet Gynecol 78:415–418

28. Kucuk M, Okman TK (2001) Non-closure of visceral peritoneum at abdominal hysterectomy. Int J Gynecol Obstet 75:317–319

29. Al-Inany H (2004) Peritoneal closure vs. non-closure: estimation of pelvic fluid by transvaginal ultrasonography after abdominal hysterectomy. Gynecol Obstet Invest 58:183–185

30. Gupta JK, Dinas K, Khan KS (1998) To peritonealize or not to peritonealize? A randomized trial at abdominal hysterectomy. Am J Obstet Gynecol 178:796–800

31. Kore S, Vyavaharkar M, Akolekar R, Toke A, Ambiye VJ (2000) Comparison of closure of subcutaneous tissue versus non-closure in relation to wound disruption after abdominal hysterectomy in obese patients. J Postgrad Med 46:26–28

32. Sharma J, Wadhwa L, Malhotra M, Arora R (2004) Mini laparotomy versus conventional laparotomy for abdominal hysterectomy: a comparative study. Indian J Med Sci 58:196–202

33. Kearns SR, Connolly EM, McNally S, McNamara DA, Deasy J (2001) Randomized clinical trial of diathermy versus scalpel incision in elective laparotomy. Br J Surg 8:41–44

34. Chan JK, Manetta A (2002) Prevention of femoral nerve injuries in gynecologic surgeries. Am J Obstet Gynecol 186:1–7

35. Beresford JM, Moher D (1993) A prospective comparison of abdominal hysterectomy using absorbable staples. Surg Gynecol Obstet 176:555–558

36. Lethaby A, Ivanova V, Johnson NP (2006) Total versus subtotal hysterectomy for benign gynaecological conditions. Cochrane Database Syst Rev 19(2):CD004993

37. Rahn DD, Stone RJ, Vu AK, White AB, Wai CY (2008) Abdominal hysterectomy with or without angle stitch: correlation with subsequent vaginal vault prolapse. Am J Obstet Gynecol 199:669.e1–669.e4

38. Begg CB, Cho M, Eastwood S, Horton R, Moher D, Olkin I et al (1996) Improving the quality of reporting of randomized controlled trials. The CONSORT statement. JAMA 276:637–639

39. Ramsey PS, White AM, Guinn DA, Lu GC, Ramin S, Davies JK et al (2005) Subcutaneous tissue reapproximation, alone or in combination with drain, in obese women undergoing cesarean delivery. Obstet Gynecol 105:967–973

40. Thompson JD, Warshaw, J. Hysterectomy. In Rock AJ, Thompson JD (eds) Te Linde's Operative Gynecology, Eighth edn. Lippincott-Raven, pp 771–85440

41. Kaya H, Sezik M, Ozbasar D, Ozkaya O, Sahiner H (2004) Intrafascial versus extrafascial abdominal hysterectomy: effects on urinary urge incontinence. Int Urogynecol J 15:171–174

42. Kaya H, Sezik M, Ozbasar D, Ozkaya O, Sahiner H (2004) Intrafascial versus extrafascial abdominal hysterectomy: effects on urinary urge incontinence. Int Urogynecol J 15:171–177

43. Chou MT, Wang CJ, Lien RC (2009) Prophylactic ureteral catheterization in gynecologic surgery: a 12-year randomized trial in a community hospital. Int Urogynecol J 20:689–693

44. Moher D, Jones A (2001) Lepage LCONSORT Group. (Consolidated Standards for Reporting of Trials). Use of the CONSORT statement and quality of reports of randomized trials: a comparative before-and-after evaluation. JAMA 285:1992–1995

11

Nociceptive and stress hormonal state during abdominal, laparoscopic, and vaginal hysterectomy as predictors of postoperative pain perception

A. R. H Twijnstra · A. Dahan · M. M. ter Kuile ·
F. W. Jansen

Abstract The primary objective of this study is to compare pain perception during and after surgery between abdominal hysterectomy (AH), laparoscopic hysterectomy (LH), and vaginal hysterectomy (VH). The secondary objective of this study is to investigate whether pain indicators during surgery predict pain perception and demand for analgesics postoperatively. Prospective observational analysis of intraoperative nociceptive state (by means of pulse transit time; PTT), heart rate, and stress hormone levels (adrenalin and noradrenalin) were correlated with postoperative pain scores and stress hormone levels and demand for postoperative analgesics such as morphine. Intraoperative PTT levels and perioperative and postoperative stress hormone levels did not differ significantly between AH, LH, and VH. During the first hours postoperatively, LH patients showed insignificant lower pain scores, compared to AH and VH. One day postoperatively, LH patients reported significantly lower pain scores. High intraoperative stress hormone levels predicted a significant higher demand for morphine postoperatively, accompanied with significant higher pain scores. No differences were found with respect to intraoperative pain indicators well as pain perception during the first hours after surgery between AH, LH, and VH. If VH is not applicable, LH proves to be advantageous over AH with respect to a faster decline in pain scores.

A. R. H. Twijnstra · F. W. Jansen (✉)
Department of Gynecology, Leiden University Medical Center,
PO Box 9600, 2300 RC Leiden, The Netherlands
e-mail: f.w.jansen@lumc.nl

A. Dahan
Department of Anesthesiology, Leiden University Medical Center,
Leiden, The Netherlands

M. M. ter Kuile
Department of Psychosomatic Gynecology and Sexology,
Leiden University Medical Center,
Leiden, The Netherlands

Keywords Hysterectomy · Pain · Pulse transit time · Stress hormones

Background

Almost without exception, surgery is associated with postoperative pain. Also in hysterectomy, women experience postoperative pain to some degree, despite adequate general and or locoregional anesthesia [1].

Among other superior characteristics, vaginal hysterectomy (VH) is particularly known for its short period of postoperative pain and quick recovery, and also therefore considered the *gold standard* in hysterectomy [2]. Over the recent years, some studies stated that laparoscopic hysterectomy (LH) is preferred over VH with respect to lower postoperative pain scores. However, these studies are underpowered [3–5]. When VH is not applicable, LH shows several advantages over abdominal hysterectomy (AH). Firstly, it is generally known that, compared to the abdominal approach, LH is characterized by less intraoperative blood loss, shorter duration of hospital stay, speedier return to normal activities, and fewer wound or abdominal wall infections [2, 6–8]. Secondly, relatively elevated interleukin-6 and C-reactive protein serum levels found in AH suggests that this approach is associated with inclined tissue damage, compared to LH [9–13]. Thirdly, patients claim to prefer LH over AH probably because of the aforementioned findings, combined with esthetical considerations [14]. Lastly, LH patients report to become pain free in a significantly shorter period of time compared to women operated by laparotomy [1, 2, 8, 15].

Surprisingly, a recent study observed that laparoscopic surgery is associated with higher pain scores in the first hours postoperatively [16]. Others described higher nociceptive pain scores during laparoscopic procedures compared to conventional open surgery [17]. These findings are in contrast with the rationale that minimally invasive surgery (MIS), with accompanying less tissue damage, would result in declined perceived pain. Hypothetically, the observed higher pain perception when applying the laparoscopic approach could be the result of peritoneal absorption of insufflated carbon dioxide in laparoscopy, which can cause referred shoulder pain. Another explanation to the reported higher pain scores could be due to a suboptimal analgesic regimen because anesthesiologists assume MIS to be minimally painful as well. Consequently, because of applying thrifty amounts of analgesics, patients could experience more physical stress during and after laparoscopic surgery. However, previous research indicated that MIS is connected with lower intraoperative stress hormone levels [18, 19].

In conclusion, recent research found conventional surgery not superior to MIS with respect to pain perception during surgery and during the first hours postoperatively. These findings cannot be satisfactorily explained yet.

The objective of this study is to compare pain perception during and after surgery between LH, AH, and VH, and whether pain indicators during surgery (nociceptive state, stress hormones) predict pain perception as well as demand for analgesics (e.g., morphine) postoperatively.

Materials and methods

Each consecutive patient scheduled for either AH, LH, or VH at our department was requested to participate in the study. Informed consent was required as several blood samples were to be collected and participation of the patient was needed with respect to completing the questionnaires and assessing pain intensities postoperatively. Exclusion criteria included disturbances of the central nervous system or psychiatric diseases, chemical substance abuse, chronic use of analgesics, chronic pain, cardiovascular, hepatic or renal insufficiency, pregnancy, extended accompanying prolapse or oncologic surgery, and age less than 18 years. In addition, supracervical hysterectomies were excluded from the study as well. The protocol was approved by the local Human Ethics Committee (protocol number P08.100).

After inclusion, plasma catecholamine concentrations (CAMI; norepinephrine and epinephrine levels in nanomoles per liter) were measured at our outpatient department in order to obtain baseline levels. Three more CAMI samples were obtained during surgery (i.e., instantly after intubation, after ligation of the second uterine artery, and after closing the vaginal cuff) and two more samples 4 and 8 h postoperatively, respectively. Each obtained sample consisted of 4 ml venous blood in an EDTA-fuse, instantly stored in a −20 °C environment and analyzed according to protocol within 60 min.

Each patient was asked to assess her pain level using a visual analog scale (VAS) meter (ranging from zero for no pain at all to 10 for intolerable pain) preoperatively (before premedication had been administered) and 4, 8, and 24 h postoperatively, provided she self-rated herself awake (>4 VAS).

In order to correct for catastrophization of pain (exaggerated or extreme negative conception of pain), each patient was provided with a concise validated questionnaire, which was to be filled out on the day prior to surgery [20, 21]. This baseline questionnaire aimed to assess actual pain experience, possible fear of the upcoming surgery, as well as expectations about pain during the first hours after surgery.

A validated mode to assess nociceptive state in patients was by means of measuring the pulse transit time (PTT). Pulse transit time was defined as the interval from the ECG R-wave to the upstroke of the waveform of the pulse oximeter of the same cardiac cycle. Elevation in PTT levels were associated with a low nociceptive stress response, while lowering of PTT indicated elevation in nociceptive stress state.

Pain perception during surgery was measured by continuously assessing nociceptive state as well as by determining stress hormonal levels (i.e., catecholamines, also known as "fight or flight" stress hormones). Perceived pain was assessed during the first 24 h postoperatively.

During surgery, continuous 3-lead ECG and infrared pulse oximeter waveforms were obtained from Cardiocap II and Capnomac Ultima devices (Datex, Helsinki, Finland). These signals were linked to a custom made analog computer (Marc Geerts, Leiden University Medical Center, The Netherlands), which calculated the PTT for each heart beat. The pulse oximeter was attached to the index fingertip of the left arm. PTT and heart rate (HR) values were measured continuously. General anesthesia was induced according to the following guideline: remifentanil at 10 μgkg^{-1}h^{-1}, followed by an induction dose of propofol (2 mg/kg) and atracurium (0.5 mg/kg). The trachea of all patients was subsequently intubated (tube sizes, 8–9) and propofol was continued at an infusion rate of 6–10 μgkg^{-1}h^{-1}. Since this was an observational study, the attending anesthesiologist was allowed to change the drug doses and infusion rates according to his or her own discretion. His or her decisions were based on the routine parameters used to guide anesthesia (heart rate, blood pressure, patient movement, and sudomotor responses).

If patients received general anesthesia combined with epidural anesthesia, epidural anesthesia was continued up to the second day after surgery. Postoperatively, every patient was provided with patient-controlled analgesia (an electronically controlled infusion pump, delivering a prescribed amount of intravenous analgesic when activating the button). The amount of peri- and postoperatively provided analgesics were recorded.

Provided patients undergoing LH experienced more pain during surgery and during the first 8 h postoperatively, compared to AH, we aimed to assess a 30 % mean difference (alpha=0.05) in PTT during surgery, with SD 0.2. Based on results from former research with PTT comparing laparoscopy with laparotomy, 15 patients in each group were needed to achieve a power of 0.90. The VH group primarily acted as a control group as no adequate comparable research on pain perception in vaginal surgery was available.

Data was analyzed using SPSS 17.0 statistical software (Chicago, IL, USA). Variables were tested for normal distribution using the Kolmogorov–Smirnov test. If variables lacked a normal distribution, Spearman's rank correlation coefficients where calculated. Differences between groups were assessed with the chi-square test for proportions and, if normally distributed, Student-independent samples t test for continuous variables. One-way analysis of variance (ANOVA) was used to assess differences between the three groups. 95 % Confidence intervals (95 % CI) and standard deviations were calculated; P values <0.05 were considered statistically significant.

Findings

Patient characteristics were comparable between groups with respect to indication, age, BMI, American Society of Anesthesiologists classification, and preoperative pain perception (Table 1). Perioperative blood loss and amounts of anesthetics administered did not differ between groups, while length of surgery was significantly higher in LH and uterus weight was significantly higher in AH. Patients receiving general anesthesia combined with epidural analgesics were equally distributed in LH and AH. However, VH significantly more often received general anesthesia exclusively.

During the first 90 min of surgery, PTT and HR levels did not differ significantly between AH, LH, and VH (Fig. 1). Perioperative and postoperative stress hormone levels did not differ significantly between groups (Table 2). However, subgroup analysis in patients receiving general anesthesia exclusively showed significant lower noradrenalin levels in LH patients during the first hours after surgery compared to AH.

Analysis of the preoperatively completed questionnaire yielded no differences with respect to actual pain experience, fear of having surgery, and expectations about pain during the first hours after surgery. Preoperative pain scores were comparable between groups (Fig. 2). During the first hours after surgery, LH patients showed insignificant lower pain scores, compared to AH and VH (VAS$_{delta}$ −1.57 (−3.41 to 0.29) and VAS$_{delta}$ −1.66 (−3.54 to 0.23), respectively). About half of the AH and LH patients opted for general anesthesia combined with regional (epidural) anesthesia. In general, patients with postoperative epidural analgesics showed significantly lower pain scores in the first 4 h postoperatively, compared to patients without epidural analgesics (VAS$_{delta}$ −2.17 (−3.32 to −1.02)). However, subgroup analysis of LH patients yielded no difference in pain scores between LH patients with postoperative epidural analgesics compared to LH patients without epidural analgesics (VAS$_{delta}$ −0.40 (−1.66 to 2.44)). One day postoperatively, LH patients reported significantly lower pain scores, compared to AH patients (VAS$_{delta}$ −1.50 (−3.06 to −0.01)). Observed differences in the general anesthesia group mainly contributed to this finding.

High intraoperative CAMI levels predicted a significant higher demand for morphine postoperatively accompanied

Table 1 Study group characteristics

	Total (n=45)	95 % CI	P value	AH (n=15)	LH (n=15)	VH (n=15)
Age (years)	48.2	45.9–50.4	0.129	51.4 (8.5)	46.6 (5.6)	46.7 (7.2)
BMI (kg/m^2)	26.9	25.1–28.7	0.165	28.3 (7.1)	24.5 (4.6)	27.8 (4.7)
Preoperative pain score (VAS)	0.9	0.41–1.35	0.964	0.9 (1.4)	0.9 (1.8)	0.8 (1.5)
ASA I (%)	55.6		0.181	73.3	53.3	40.0
General anesthesia and epidural (%)	40.4		0.027	53.3	53.3	6.7
Length of surgery (min)	107.3	94.7–119.9	0.005	98.7 (37.2)	134.3 (44.7)	89.1 (30.8)
Blood loss (ml)	195.9	131.6–260.2	0.308	230.7 (245.9)	126.0 (150.9)	231.0 (229.9)
Uterus weight (grams)	291.2	202.6–379.7	0.017	446.6 (447.0)	279.6 (135.6)	147.3 (81.9)
BIS (mean values)	39.9	37.3–42.5	0.213	40.1 (4.5)	37.8 (4.9)	43.3 (8.3)
Atracurium dose (mg)	46.8	40.6–53.1	0.084	55.7 (25.6)	42.5 (14.0)	40.5 (8.0)
Remifentanil dose (μm/kg/h)	12.1	9.2–15.1	0.736	5.4 (3.1)	7.4 (4.2)	4.7 (3.9)
Propofol dose (mg/kg/h)	5.9	4.6–7.2	0.187	5.4 (3.1)	7.4 (5.3)	4.7 (4.4)

Values between brackets are standard deviations. Differences between groups were calculated using one-way ANOVA for continuous variables and chi-square for proportions

AH abdominal hysterectomy, *LH* laparoscopic hysterectomy, *VH* vaginal hysterectomy

Fig. 1 Intraoperative PTT and HR levels in total (**a** and **d**), in general anesthesia (**b** and **e**), and general and epidural anesthesia combined (**c** and **f**). *PTT* pulse transit time (microsecond), *HR* heart rate (beats per minute), *AH* abdominal hysterectomy, *LH* laparoscopic hysterectomy, *VH* vaginal hysterectomy. Differences between groups were calculated using one-way ANOVA for continuous variables. *Error bars* represent standard errors of the means

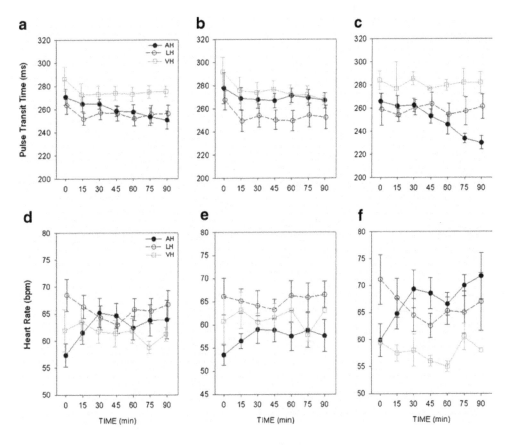

with significant higher pain scores (Table 3). Low mean PTT and high HR levels did not predict a higher demand for postoperative analgesics or pain scores. However, high PTT levels were associated with elevated intraoperative propofol use.

Discussion and conclusions

Pain perception during the first hours after surgery and intra-operative pain indicators are comparable between abdominal, laparoscopic, and vaginal hysterectomy. These outcomes

Table 2 Mean catecholamine (CAMI) levels during and after surgery

		Total (n=45)	95 % CI	P value	AH (n=15)	LH (n=15)	VH (n=15)
Total	Noradrenalin during surgery (nmol/L)	1.66	1.26–2.07	0.658	1.53 (0.88)	1.52 (1.00)	1.92 (1.95)
	Noradrenalin after surgery (nmol/L)	1.05	0.82–1.28	0.517	1.10 (0.75)	0.86 (0.27)	1.17 (0.28)
	Adrenalin during surgery (nmol/L)	0.18	0.09–0.27	0.413	0.12 (0.16)	0.16 (0.30)	0.26 (0.42)
	Adrenalin after surgery (nmol/L)	0.08	0.06–0.09	0.286	0.07 (0.03)	0.07 (0.05)	0.10 (0.09)
					AH (n=6)	LH (n=7)	
No epidural	Noradrenalin during surgery (nmol/L)	1.75	1.16–2.34	0.392	2.01 (1.09)	1.53 (0.87)	
	Noradrenalin after surgery (nmol/L)	1.11	0.67–1.56	0.013	1.62 (0.82)	0.67 (0.20)	
	Adrenalin during surgery (nmol/L)	0.27	0.07–0.46	0.636	0.22 (0.21)	0.31 (0.40)	
	Adrenalin after surgery (nmol/L)	0.09	0.06–0.12	0.355	0.07 (0.03)	0.10 (0.06)	
					AH (n=9)	LH (n=8)	
With epidural	Noradrenalin during surgery (nmol/L)	1.36	0.90–1.82	0.527	1.22 (0.58)	1.51 (1.17)	
	Noradrenalin after surgery (nmol/L)	0.89	0.68–1.10	0.186	0.76 (0.49)	1.03 (0.21)	
	Adrenalin during surgery (nmol/L)	0.04	0.02–0.06	0.355	0.05 (0.04)	0.03 (0.04)	
	Adrenalin after surgery (nmol/L)	0.06	0.04–0.07	0.690	0.06 (0.02)	0.05 (0.04)	

Values between brackets are standard deviations. Differences between groups were calculated using one-way ANOVA for continuous variables; independent samples T tests were applied to calculate differences between two subgroups

AH abdominal hysterectomy, *LH* laparoscopic hysterectomy, *VH* vaginal hysterectomy

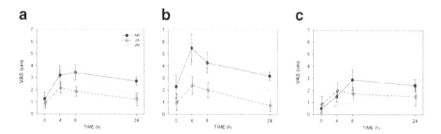

Fig. 2 Baseline and postoperative pain scores in AH, LH, and VH in total (**a**), after general anesthesia (**b**) and general and epidural anesthesia combined (**c**). Preoperative pain scores were comparable between groups. During the first hours after surgery, LH patients showed insignificant lower pain scores, compared to AH and VH (VAS$_{delta}$ −1.57 (−3.41 to 0.29) and VAS$_{delta}$ −1.66 (−3.54 to 0.23), respectively). In general, patients with postoperative epidural analgesics showed significantly lower pain scores in the first 4 h postoperatively, compared to patients without epidural analgesics (VAS$_{delta}$ −2.17 (−3.32 to −1.02)). However,

subgroup analysis of LH patients yielded no difference in pain scores between LH patients with postoperative epidural analgesics compared to LH patients without epidural analgesics (VAS$_{delta}$ −0.40 (−1.66 to 2.44)). One day postoperatively, LH patients reported significantly lower pain scores, compared to AH patients (VAS$_{delta}$ −1.50 (−3.06 to −0.01)). *AH* abdominal hysterectomy, *LH* laparoscopic hysterectomy, *VH* vaginal hysterectomy. Differences between groups were calculated using one-way ANOVA for continuous variables. *$P<0.05$, significant differences. *Error bars* represent standard errors of the means

suggest that an unambiguous anesthetic protocol for both conventional as well as laparoscopic surgery is justified. Minimally invasive surgery is not associated with a minimum of pain perception. This is in contrast with the previously observed minimal tissue damage in MIS. Therefore, MIS patients should be offered a "conventional" anesthetic regime. However, addition of epidural analgesics did not significantly lower postoperative pain scores in MIS patients.

On a patient level, we observed that elevated intraoperative noradrenalin levels predicted elevated postoperative pain scores, accompanied with an increased demand for postoperative rescue analgesia. These findings are solely applicable in a research setting and not clinically relevant, as determination of noradrenalin values is time consuming and rather expensive.

The intraoperative PTT values in our study did not show a significant difference between conventional and MIS procedures,

which was observed in other research [17]. Perhaps, minor heterogeneity in indication for surgery in that former study was causing selection bias. Hypothetically, homogeneity of the patient sample in our study reproduces PTT levels more accurately.

From a scientific perspective, a randomized controlled trial would provide optimal reliable outcomes indicating which approach in hysterectomy is associated with the lowest pain perception. However, from both practical as well as ethical perspective, this design is not feasible anymore, due to two reasons. Firstly, former research provided evidence that VH is superior over AH and LH with respect to many aspects and consequently patients should be offered the best available option [2, 3]. Secondly, with respect to applied amounts of analgesics, no ethical committee would allow a protocol that would not take into account patient specific demand for supplementary analgesics. Therefore, we consider an observational cohort study to be the best available option.

Analysis of intraoperatively administered analgesics yielded no statistically significant differences between groups. Besides, postoperative calls for rescue analgesics were recorded and therefore appropriate for analysis. Furthermore, the observational design of this study facilitates instant applicability in daily practice.

Each previous study on pain perception after hysterectomy mainly focused on the time needed to become pain free [1–3, 8, 22]. One recent study concentrated on pain scores during the first hours after surgery and found higher scores in laparoscopic procedures compared to the conventional approach [16]. However, that study did not take into account the intention-to-treat principle with respect to assessment of pain VAS scores, consequently overrating conscious "laparoscopic" patients while excluding uncooperative, drowsy "abdominal" patients. Also, no correction for amount of administered analgesics was made. In our study, both corrections for consciousness as well as administered analgesics were taken into account.

The few articles, that studied stress hormonal values as an outcome in comparisons between minimally invasive and

Table 3 Correlations between intraoperative and postoperative stress indicators

Principal stress indicators	r_s	P value
PTT and mean postoperative pain VAS	0.04	0.776
PTT and postoperative analgesics use	0.29	0.27
PTT and intraoperative Propofol dose	0.44	0.038
HR and mean postoperative pain VAS	−0.21	0.162
HR and call for postoperative analgesics use	0.13	0.62
Intraoperative NOR and postoperative NOR	0.37	0.005
Intraoperative ADR and postoperative ADR	0.42	0.001
Intraoperative NOR and postoperative pain VAS	0.30	0.046
Intraoperative ADR and postoperative pain VAS	0.37	0.012
Postoperative pain VAS and postoperative analgesics use	0.72	0.029

As parameters lacked a normal distribution, the Spearman's rank correlation coefficient (r_s) was applied to provide a measure of association between principal stress indicators

AH abdominal hysterectomy, *LH* laparoscopic hysterectomy, *VH* vaginal hysterectomy, *PTT* pulse transit time, *VAS* visual analog scale, *HR* heart rate, *NOR* noradrenalin, *ADR* adrenalin

conventional surgery, found lower values in the minimally invasive group [18, 19]. Similar to our study, relatively elevated intraoperative noradrenalin levels were found in the conventional group. The only study researching postoperative hormonal state did determine serum cortisol, a circadian hormone with a long half-life [18]. Our study assessed catecholamines (120 s half-life) at specific time points during and after surgery.

VH and LH, both regarded as true exponents of minimally invasive surgery, are often considered to be minimally painful as well. However, with respect to nociceptive and stress hormonal intraoperative pain indicators, no significant lower values in this study were found, compared to the abdominal approach. These outcomes were confirmed with observed comparable pain scores during the first hours after surgery. As intraoperative and postoperative administered analgesics were corrected, these outcomes are likely to be reliable.

Although not a primary outcome of this study, the added value of epidural analgesics to general anesthesia, with respect to postoperative pain perception in LH patients is questionable. Probably traction on tissue during VH and peritoneal wound healing in AH might explain the differences compared with LH. Also others found lower postoperative pain scores in MIS [3, 4]. This study states that, although LH is preferred over AH with respect to postoperative pain perception, this minimally invasive approach in hysterectomy remains a major surgical procedure. However, perhaps MIS patients are better served in a fast track system without accompanying epidural analgesics, consequently enhancing a quicker recovery [23].

Declaration of interest The authors report no conflicts of interest. The authors alone are responsible for the content and writing of the paper.

References

1. Garry R, Fountain J, Brown J, Manca A, Mason S, Sculpher M et al (2004) EVALUATE hysterectomy trial: a multicentre randomised trial comparing abdominal, vaginal and laparoscopic methods of hysterectomy. Health Technol Assess 8(26):1–154
2. Nieboer TE, Johnson N, Lethaby A, Tavender E, Curr E, Garry R et al. Surgical approach to hysterectomy for benign gynaecological disease. Cochrane Database Syst Rev 2009;(3):CD003677.
3. Ghezzi F, Uccella S, Cromi A, Siesto G, Serati M, Bogani G et al (2010) Postoperative pain after laparoscopic and vaginal hysterectomy for benign gynecologic disease: a randomized trial. Am J Obstet Gynecol 203(2):118
4. Candiani M, Izzo S, Bulfoni A, Riparini J, Ronzoni S, Marconi A (2009) Laparoscopic vs vaginal hysterectomy for benign pathology. Am J Obstet Gynecol 200(4):368–370
5. Gendy R, Walsh CA, Walsh SR, Karantanis E (2011) Vaginal hysterectomy versus total laparoscopic hysterectomy for benign disease: a metaanalysis of randomized controlled trials. Am J Obstet Gynecol 204(5):388
6. Harkki P, Kurki T, Sjoberg J, Tiitinen A (2001) Safety aspects of laparoscopic hysterectomy. Acta Obstet Gynecol Scand 80(5):383–391

7. Makinen J, Johansson J, Tomas C, Tomas E, Heinonen PK, Laatikainen T et al (2001) Morbidity of 10,110 hysterectomies by type of approach. Hum Reprod 16(7):1473–1478
8. Bojahr B, Raatz D, Schonleber G, Abri C, Ohlinger R (2006) Perioperative complication rate in 1,706 patients after a standardized laparoscopic supracervical hysterectomy technique. J Minim Invasive Gynecol 13(3):183–189
9. Malik E, Buchweitz O, Muller-Steinhardt M, Kressin P, Meyhofer-Malik A, Diedrich K (2001) Prospective evaluation of the systemic immune response following abdominal, vaginal, and laparoscopically assisted vaginal hysterectomy. Surg Endosc 15(5):463–466
10. Ellstrom M, Bengtsson A, Tylman M, Haeger M, Olsson JH, Hahlin M (1996) Evaluation of tissue trauma after laparoscopic and abdominal hysterectomy: measurements of neutrophil activation and release of interleukin-6, cortisol, and C-reactive protein. J Am Coll Surg 182(5):423–430
11. Demir A, Bige O, Saatli B, Solak A, Saygili U, Onvural A (2007) Prospective comparison of tissue trauma after laparoscopic hysterectomy types with retroperitoneal lateral transsection of uterine vessels using ligasure and abdominal hysterectomy. Arch Gynecol Obstet 277(4):325–330
12. Ribeiro SC, Ribeiro RM, Santos NC, Pinotti JA (2003) A randomized study of total abdominal, vaginal and laparoscopic hysterectomy. Int J Gynaecol Obstet 83(1):37–43
13. Atabekoglu C, Sonmezer M, Gungor M, Aytac R, Ortac F, Unlu C (2004) Tissue trauma in abdominal and laparoscopic-assisted vaginal hysterectomy. J Am Assoc Gynecol Laparosc 11(4):467–472
14. Kluivers KB, Opmeer BC, Geomini PM, Bongers MY, Vierhout ME, Bremer GL et al (2009) Women's preference for laparoscopic or abdominal hysterectomy. Gynecol Surg 6(3):223–228
15. Perino A, Cucinella G, Venezia R, Castelli A, Cittadini E (1999) Total laparoscopic hysterectomy versus total abdominal hysterectomy: an assessment of the learning curve in a prospective randomized study. Hum Reprod 14(12):2996–2999
16. Ekstein P, Szold A, Sagie B, Werbin N, Klausner JM, Weinbroum AA (2006) Laparoscopic surgery may be associated with severe pain and high analgesia requirements in the immediate postoperative period. Ann Surg 243(1):41–46
17. Sigtermans MJ, Looijestijn J, Olofsen E, Dahan A (2008) Pulse transit time (PTT) measurements during laparoscopic and open abdominal surgery: a pilot study in ASA I–II female patients. Open Anesthesiol J 2:20–25
18. Kataja J, Chrapek W, Kaukinen S, Pimenoff G, Salenius JP (2007) Hormonal stress response and hemodynamic stability in patients undergoing endovascular vs. conventional abdominal aortic aneurysm repair. Scand J Surg 96(3):236–242
19. Thompson JP, Boyle JR, Thompson MM, Strupish J, Bell PR, Smith G (1999) Cardiovascular and catecholamine responses during endovascular and conventional abdominal aortic aneurysm repair. Eur J Vasc Endovasc Surg 17(4):326–333
20. Peters ML, Sommer M, de Rijke JM, Kessels F, Heineman E, Patijn J et al (2007) Somatic and psychologic predictors of long-term unfavorable outcome after surgical intervention. Ann Surg 245(3):487–494
21. Kalkman CJ, Visser K, Moen J, Bonsel GJ, Grobbee DE, Moons KG (2003) Preoperative prediction of severe postoperative pain. Pain 105(3):415–423
22. Lieng M, Lomo AB, Qvigstad E (2010) Long-term outcomes following laparoscopic and abdominal supracervical hysterectomies. Obstet Gynecol Int 2010:989127
23. Lindsetmo RO, Champagne B, Delaney CP (2009) Laparoscopic rectal resections and fast-track surgery: what can be expected? Am J Surg 197(3):408–412

12

A critical review of laparoscopic total hysterectomy versus laparoscopic supracervical hysterectomy

Anwar Moria · Togas Tulandi

Abstract The purpose of our review is to evaluate the perioperative characteristics of laparoscopic total hysterectomy (LTH) and laparoscopic supracervical hysterectomy (LASH) including the hospital stay, hemoglobin concentration, the operative time, postoperative analgesia, intra and postoperative complications. We also examine the quality of life examining general health, sexual satisfaction, dyspareunia and time to first intercourse

Keywords Laparoscopic total hysterectomy · Laparoscopic supracervical hysterectomy

Introduction

Hysterectomy is the most common gynecological procedure. It is estimated that the rate of hysterectomy is 346 per 100,000 women in Canada and 550 per 100,000 women in the United States [1, 2]. These rates are over twofolds of that in Britain, Sweden, the Netherlands and Norway [3]. There are different types of hysterectomy. The most common is abdominal hysterectomy comprising 66% of all hysterectomies followed by the vaginal hysterectomy [4]. Since early nineties, laparoscopic hysterectomy has gained popularity due to its known advantages including short hospital stay, minimal wound related complications and rapid recovery.

Laparoscopic hysterectomy could be divided into laparoscopic assisted vaginal hysterectomy (LAVH), laparoscopic total hysterectomy (LTH) and laparoscopic supracervical hysterectomy (LASH). The proponents of LASH believe that preserving the cervix plays an important role in sexual function, it maintains the pelvic floor support and prevents denervation of bladder and bowel [5–7]. Others feel that there is no strong evidence to support those claims [8–10].

The purpose of our review is to evaluate the perioperative characteristics of LTH and LASH including the hospital stay, hemoglobin concentration, the operative time, postoperative analgesia, intra and postoperative complications. We also examine the quality of life examining general health, sexual satisfaction, dyspareunia and time to first intercourse.

Source of data

We performed a literature search using the keywords "hysterectomy, laparoscopic hysterectomy, total hysterectomy, supracervical hysterectomy and subtotal hysterectomy" and conducted the search in the Medline, OVID, EMBASE and the Cochrane of Database of systematic reviews published between 1990 and 2010. We found two prospective trials, four retrospective analyses, and two quality-of-life analysis (Table 1). The only randomized study was published in Italian language and we could only evaluate its abstract. Table 2 shows the demography of patients who underwent LTH or LASH.

Operating time, hospital stay and blood loss

Table 3 shows the operating time, hospital stay and hemoglobin (Hgb) concentration in women who underwent LASH or LTH.

A. Moria (✉) · T. Tulandi
Department of Obstetrics and Gynecology, McGill University, Montreal, QC, Canada
e-mail: anwar.moria@mail.mcgill.ca

Table 1 Studies comparing laparoscopic total hysterectomy (LTH) and laparoscopic supracervical hysterectomy (LASH)

Authors	Design	Number of patients	Author's conclusion
Morelli et al. 2007 [25]	Randomized trial	71 LASH 70 LTH	No statistically significant difference in surgical complications and clinical outcomes
Harmanli et al. 2009 [11]	Retrospective	566 LASH 450 LTH	Similar overall short-term morbidity Small statistically significant increase risk of urinary tract injury with LTH
Mueller et al. 2009 [12]	Prospective	118 LASH 113 LTH	LTH is comparable to LASH Complication rates might be lower with LASH
Van Evert et al. 2010 [16]	Retrospective	192 LASH 198 LTH	LASH is associated with higher long term complications, while LTH is associated with higher short term complications
Mousa et al. 2009 [13]	Retrospective	122 LASH 105 LTH	LTH is associated with longer operating time, but requires less postoperative analgesia than LASH
Cipullo et al. 2009 [14]	Retrospective	157 LASH 157 LTH	LSH is a valid alternative to LTH Major complications in LASH are significantly less than those in LTH
Kafy et al. 2009 [17]	Retrospective	40 LASH 40 LTH	Both procedures result in similar improvement of general health, body image, sexual function, gastrointestinal and genitourinary functions
Nam et al. 2008 [18]	Prospective	39 LASH 51 LTH	No significant change in quality of sexual life after either procedure

Operating time

Two of the reviewed studies showed no difference in the operating time between LASH and LTH [11, 12]. Perhaps, the time used for suturing of the vaginal opening compensated that for morcellation. However, Mousa et al. [13] and Cipullo et al. found that LTH was longer than LASH (Table 3). The discrepancy between the studies is unclear. In our practice, we often encounter uterus that is too large to be delivered vaginally forcing us to first partially morcellate the uterus. The time spent to morcellate the uterus adds to the operating time of LTH. We also found

Table 2 Demography of patients who underwent laparoscopic total hysterectomy (LTH) or laparoscopic supracervical hysterectomy (LASH)

	Type of procedure	Age (years)	Parity	BMI	Uterine weight (g)
Harmanli et al. 2009 [11]	LASH	43.8±5.9	1.85±1.2	28.5±6.9	190.4±170
	LTH	44.6±7.9	1.92±1.3	27.9±6.6	218.7±196.2
	P value	NS	NS	NS	0.007
Mueller et al. 2009 [12]	LASH	46.7±7.0	NA	25.3±5.1	286.2±209.3
	LTH	46.3±7.5		25.4±4.0	264.8±133.6
	P value	NS		NS	NS
Van Evert et al. 2010 [16]	LASH	44 (28–60)	NA	NA	NA
	LTH	49 (30–81)			
Mousa et al. 2009 [13]	LASH	45.7±0.6	1.6±0.1	26.6±0.4	181±12.0
	LTH	45.9±0.7	1.7±0.1	26.8±1.5	161±11.6
	P value	NA	NA	NA	NS
Cipullo et al. 2009 [14]	LASH	49.5±7.4	NA	27.6±3.5	162.7±112.7
	LTH	50.2±7.8		27.6±4.4	169.7±116.6
	P value	NS		NS	NS
Kafy et al. 2009 [17]	LASH	46.1±7.0	NA	NA	NA
	LTH	46.6±5.3			
	P value	NA			
Nam et al. 2008 [18]	LASH	41.9±4.7	1.8±0.7	22.5±2.4	NA
	LTH	46.3±3.7	1.9±0.7	22.8±3.2	
	P value	NS	NS	NS	

Table 3 Perioperative characteristics of patients who underwent laparoscopic total hysterectomy (LTH) or laparoscopic supracervical hysterectomy (LASH)

	Harmanli et al. 2009 [11]	Mueller et al. 2009 [12]	Mousa et al. 2009 [13]	Cipullo et al. 2009 [14]
Operating time (min)	LTH 168±61	LTH 114±33.8	LTH 136±3.6	LTH 121.7±44.3
	LASH 166±62	LASH 116.5±40	LASH 111±2.9	LASH 111.4±39.1
	NS	NS	$P<0.001$	$P<0.05$
Hospital stay (day)	LTH 1.4±0.7[a]	LTH 5.7±1.1	LTH 1.5±0.7	NA
	LASH 1.2±0.6	LASH 5.3±1.6	LASH 1.8±0.2	
	$P<001$	NS	NS	
Postoperative Hgb difference (g/dl)	LTH 1.9±1.0	LTH 1.6±1.1	LTH 2.1	LTH 2.4±0.9
	LASH 1.9±0.9	LASH 1.5±1.4	LASH 1.9	LASH 2.1±0.9
	NS	NS	NS	$P<0.01$
Postoperative analgesia	NA	*Ibuprofen (g)*	*Morphine (mg)*	NA
		LTH 3.1±0.8	LTH 28±2.9	
		LASH 2.9±0.8	LASH 37.5±3.4	
		NS	$P<0.05$	

NA not available

[a] Recalculated to days

that coagulating and cutting with the same instrument make surgery faster. Clearly, there are many factors that can impact the operating time.

Milad et al. [15] compared the operating time of LASH and LAVH and found that LASH was significantly shorter than LAVH. This could be due to the time used to switch from laparoscopy to the vaginal part of the procedure.

Hospital stay and blood loss

The duration of hospital stay of LASH and LTH is comparable. In one study, the authors found that the hospital stay after LTH was about 5 h longer than LASH [11]. It is statistically different, but clinically does not make much difference.

Estimation of blood loss by laparoscopy is usually difficult and not accurate. Using Hgb level as an index of blood loss, three of four studies showed that there was no difference in the decrease in Hgb level after LASH or after LTH [11–13]. In contrast, Cipullo et al. [14] reported that LTH might be associated more blood loss than LASH. The reason is not clear.

Postoperative pain

Postoperative analgesia requirement after the two types of laparoscopic hysterectomy was evaluated in two studies [12, 13]. Mueller et al. [12] found no difference in ibuprofen requirement after LTH and after LASH. Although the study was prospective, it appears that the length of uterine incisions and the surgical technique of

the surgeons were not standardized. In contrast, Mousa et al. found that the requirement of postoperative analgesia in LTH patients was lower than that in LASH patients [18]. This could be due to a larger incision (≥15 mm) required for the morcellator among women underwent LASH (Table 1).

Postoperative complication

Table 4 shows complications related to hysterectomy including urinary tract injury, cervical stump complication, conversion to laparotomy, reoperation, thromboembolic events, blood transfusion and fever.

Ureter and bladder injury

The incidence of bladder injury was 1.2–2% with TLH and 0–0.2% with LASH [11, 14].This could be related to more extensive separation of the bladder from the cervix in LTH. Yet, in one study the authors found similar incidence of bladder injury with the two hysterectomy techniques [13]. The incidence of ureter injury is comparable between the two techniques.

Cervical Stump complications and reoperation

One of the drawbacks of supracervical hysterectomy is the occurrence of cyclic bleeding from the cervical stump. For example, Van Evert et al. [16] described 6% incidence of vaginal bleeding in the LASH group, and about one-third of

Table 4 Intra- and postoperative characteristics of patients who underwent laparoscopic total hysterectomy (LTH) or laparoscopic supracervical hysterectomy (LASH)

Total	Harmanli et al. 2009 [11]		Mueller et al. 2009 [12]		Van Evert et al. 2010 [16]		Mousa et al. 2009 [13]		Cipullo et al. 2009 [14]	
	LTH 450 n (%) OR (95% CI)[a]	LASH 566 n (%)	LTH 113 n (%)	LASH 118 n (%)	LTH 198 n (%)	LASH 192 n (%)	LTH 105 n (%)	LASH 122 n (%)	LTH 157 n (%)	LASH 157 n (%)
Thromboembolic event	1 (0.2)	0	NA	NA	NA	NA	0	1 (0.8)	0	1 (0.6)
Ureter injury	NA	NA	1 (0.9)	0	0	1 (0.5)	1 (1.0)	0	1 (0.6)	0
Bladder injury	10 (2.2)[b] 4.75 (1.21–18.56)[b]	3 (0.5)[b]	NA	NA	NA	NA	1 (1.0)	2 (1.6)	2 (1.2)	0
Blood transfusion	8 (1.8)	9 (1.6)	NA	NA	NA	NA	1 (1.0)	5 (4.1)	1 (0.6)	0
Reoperation	4 (0.9) NS	1 (0.2)	NA	NA	NA	NA	0	5 (4.1)	2 (1.2)	0
Laparotomy conversion	26 (5.8) 2.25 (1.20–4.22)	23 (4.1)	0	0 NS	3 (1.5)	9 (5)	0	1 (1.0)	NA	NA
Urinary incontinence	NA	NA	NA	NA	2 (1)	2 (1)	0	3 (2.5)	NA	NA
Vaginal bleeding	NA	NA	NA	NA	0	12 (6)	0	1 (0.8)	1 (0.6)	0
Fever	6 (1.3)	5 (0.9)	NA	NA	2 (1)	1 (0.5)	4 (3.8)	2 (1.6)	6 (3.7)	7 (4.4)

NA not available, *NS* not significant

[a] *OR* odds ratio, *CI* confidence interval

[b] Includes both bladder and ureteric injuries

those patients needed subsequent surgical intervention. We previously reported that 4.1% of women after LASH required trachelectomy, mostly due to annoying cyclic vaginal bleeding [13]. This was despite coagulation of the endocervix at the completion of the procedure.

Conversion to laparotomy and other complications

Conversion to laparotomy from LASH or TLH appears to be comparable (Table 3). This is mostly related to technical difficulties, the presence of extensive adhesions and uncontrolled bleeding [11, 16]. The incidence of blood transfusion, thromboembolic events, urinary incontinence and febrile morbidity are also similar.

Quality of life

Table 5 demonstrates the quality of life after LTH and LASH.

General health and dyspareunia

General health or dyspareunia following LTH and LASH are comparable.

Table 5 Quality of Life after laparoscopic total hysterectomy (LTH) or laparoscopic supracervical hysterectomy (LASH)

	Kafy et al. 2009 [17][a]				Nam et al. 2008 [18][b]			
	LTH 40		LASH 40		LTH 51		LASH 39	
	Before	After	Before	After	Before	After	Before	After
General health	2.2±0.4 P<0.001	1.9±0.4 P<0.005	2.3±0.5 NA	2.1±0.6 NA	NA	NA	NA	NA
Self-image	2.2±0.4 P<0.01	2.1±0.4 P<0.006	2.4±0.5 NA	2.1±0.4 NA	NA NA	NA NA	NA	NA
Sexual satisfaction	2.5±0.6 P<0.001	2.2±0.5 P<0.002	2.5±0.7 NS	2.3±0.6 NS	1.98	1.9	2.1	1.95
Dyspareunia	2.4±0.6 P<0.001	1.7±0.5 P<0.002	1.9±0.7 NA	1.6±0.5 NA	2[c]	2	4	1
Time to intercourse	NA NA	NA NA	5.78±1.13 P<0.001	4.92±1.2				

[a] Kafy et al.'s scale: *1* very satisfied, *2* satisfied, *3* somewhat satisfied, *4* unsatisfied, *5* very unsatisfied

[b] Nam et al.'s scale: *1* not satisfied, *2* somewhat, *3* satisfied

[c] Number of patients

Sexual satisfaction and time to first intercourse

Contrary to a previous report of impaired sexual satisfaction after total hysterectomy [7], Kafy et al. could not demonstrate any difference in sexual satisfaction or self image after LTH or LASH [17]. Nam et al. [18] reported earlier resumption of sexual activity in the LASH group compared to LTH group. This might be related to health personnel's advice to avoid sexual contact until 6–8 weeks after surgery. Indeed, early sexual intercourse is one of the predisposing factors for vaginal vault prolapse after total hysterectomy [19].

Conclusions

Besides a slightly increased incidence of bladder injury with LTH and of complications related to cervical retention after LASH, the two laparoscopic techniques appear comparable. Both techniques lead to improvement in dyspareunia. Following the studies demonstrating similar sexual function with and without cervical preservation, we performed mainly LTH. In addition to post-LASH cervical bleeding, retaining the cervix is associated with the concerns of cancer development in the cervical stump. This is especially important in the regions with poor follow-up and lack of annual cervical smears. The risk of developing carcinoma in the cervical stump is less than 0.03% in women who had had previous normal cervical cytology [20].

Other cervical stump complications include obstructive mucocele, infection and sepsis [21, 22]. As there is no risk of vault prolapse, LASH could be followed by early resumption of sexual activity [23, 24]. The issue of retaining or removing the cervix along with the uterine body should be discussed thoroughly with the patient. For those opting for cervical preservation, they should be instructed to have annual cervical smear.

We conclude that LASH is an alternative to total laparoscopic hysterectomy with less incidence of bladder injury and earlier resumption of sexual activity. Cervical preservation carries a small risk of bleeding and malignant transformation that might require further intervention. Total laparoscopic hysterectomy requires less postoperative analgesia, has lower incidence of reoperation and eliminates the complications associated with cervical stump. However, it is associated with increased urinary tract injury and rarely with vault prolapse. The decision to perform either procedure depends on the surgeon's expertise and the preference of both surgeon and the patient.

Conflicts of interest The authors report no conflicts of interest. The authors alone are responsible for the content and writing of the paper.

References

1. The Canadian Institute for Health Information (2006) Health Indicator Reports; Hysterectomy
2. Division of Reproductive Health, National Center for Chronic Disease Prevention and Health Promotion, http://www.cdc.gov/mmwr/preview/mmwrhtml/ss5105a1.htm. Accessed 3 Aug 2010
3. Women's Health Matters (2002) Hysterectomies too Frequent in Canada? http://www.womenshealthmatters.ca/news/news_show.cfm?number=170. Accessed 3 Aug 2010
4. Sokol AI, Green IC (2009) Laparoscopic hysterectomy. Clin Obstet Gynecol 52:304–312
5. Jenkins TR (2004) Laparoscopic supracervical hysterectomy. Am J Obstet Gynecol 191:1875–1884
6. Bojahr B, Raatz D, Schonleber G, Abri C, Ohlinger R (2006) Perioperative complication rate in 1706 patients after a standardized laparoscopic supracervical hysterectomy technique. J Minim Invasive Gynecol 13:183–189
7. Kilkku P, Gronroos M, Hirvonen T, Rauramo L (1983) Supravaginal uterine amputation vs. hysterectomy. Effects on libido and orgasm. Acta Obstet Gynecol Scand 62:147–152
8. Thakar R, Ayers S, Clarkson P, Stanton S, Manyonda I (2002) Outcomes after total versus subtotal abdominal hysterectomy. N Engl J Med 347:1318–1325
9. Gimbela H, Zobbea V, Andersena BM, Filtenborge T, Gluudd C, Taborb A, The Danish Hysterectomy Group (2003) Randomised controlled trial of total compared with subtotal hysterectomy with one-year follow up results. BJOG 110:1088–1098
10. Learman L, Summit R, Varner RE, McNeeley SG, Goodman-Gruen D, Richter HE, Feng L, Showstack J, Ireland C, Vittinghoff E, Helley SB, Washington AE (2003) A randomized comparison of total or supracervical hysterectomy: surgical complications and clinical outcomes. Obstet Gynecol 102:453–462
11. Harmanli OH, Tunitsky E, Esin S, Citil A, Knee A (2009) A comparison of short-term outcomes between laparoscopic supracervical and total hysterectomy. Am J Obstet Gynecol 201(536):e1–e7
12. Mueller A, Renner SP, Haeberle L, Lermann J, Oppelt P, Beckmann MW, Thiel F (2009) Comparison of total laparoscopic hysterectomy (TLH) and laparoscopy-assisted supracervical hysterectomy (LASH) in women with uterine leiomyoma. Eur J Obstet Gynecol Reprod Biol 144:76–79
13. Mousa A, Zarei A, Tulandi T (2009) Changing practice from laparoscopic supracervical hysterectomy to total hysterectomy. J Obstet Gynaecol Can 31:521–525
14. Cipullo L, De Paoli S, Fasolino L, Fasolino A (2009) Laparoscopic supracervical hysterectomy compared. JSLS 13:370–375
15. Milad MP, Morrison K, Sokol A, Miller D, Kirkpatrick L (2001) A comparison of laparoscopic supracervical hysterectomy vs. laparoscopically assisted vaginal hysterectomy. Surg Endosc 15:286–288
16. Van Evert JS, Smeenk JM, Dijkhuizen FP, de Kruif JH, Kluivers KB (2010) Laparoscopic subtotal hysterectomy versus laparoscopic total hysterectomy: a decade of experience. Gynecol Surg 7:9–12
17. Kafy S, Al-Sannan B, Kabli N, Tulandi T (2009) Patient satisfaction after laparoscopic total or supracervical hysterectomy. Gynecol Obstet Invest 67:169–172
18. Nam A, Cho SH, Seo SK, Jeon YE, Kim HY, Choi YS, Lee BS (2008) Laparoscopic total hysterectomy versus laparoscopic supracervical hysterectomy: the effect on female sexuality. Women's Med 1:43–47
19. Agdi M, Al-Ghafri W, Antolin R, Arrington J, O'Kelley K, Thomson AJ, Tulandi T (2009) Vaginal vault dehiscence after hysterectomy. J Minim Invasive Gynecol 16:313–317
20. Storm HH, Clemmensen IH, Manders T, Brinton LA (1992) Supravaginal uterine amputation in Denmark 1978–1988 and risk of cancer. Gynecol Oncol 45:198–201

21. Okaro EO, Jones KD, Sutton C (2001) Long term outcome following, aparoscopic supracervical hysterectomy. BJOG 108:1017–1020
22. Huang JYJ, Ziegler C, Tulandi T (2005) Cervical stump necrosis and septic shock after laparoscopic supracervical hysterectomy. J Min Inv Gynecol 12:162–164
23. Charles JL, Jamse FD (1996) Early outcomes of laparoscopic assisted vaginal hysterectomy versus laparoscopic supra cervical hysterectomy. J Am Assoc Gynecol Laparosc 3:251–256
24. Diaa EM, Wahba MF, Chitranjan LF, Jean MW (2004) Laparoscopic supracervical hysterectomy versus laparoscopic assisted vaginal hysterectomy. J Am Assoc Gynecol Laparosc 11:175–180
25. Morelli M, Noia R, Chiodo D, Mocciaro R, Costantino A, Caruso MT, Cosco C, Lucia E, Curcio B, Gullì G, Amendola G, Zullo F (2007) Laparoscopic supracervical hysterectomy versus laparoscopic total hysterectomy: a prospective randomized study. Minerva Gynecol 59:1–10

13

Laparoscopic hysterectomy in frozen pelvis—an alternative technique of retrograde adhesiolysis

Paul PG · Khan Shabnam · Sheetal Avinash Bhosale ·
Harneet Kaur · Prathap Talwar · Tony Thomas

Abstract Hysterectomy in frozen pelvis is a challenging surgical condition whether done by laparotomy or laparoscopy. We describe an alternative technique of total laparoscopic hysterectomy with retrograde adhesiolysis in patients with frozen pelvis. Total laparoscopic hysterectomy with retrograde adhesiolysis was done in 25 patients with frozen pelvis between October 2003 and May 2012. The mean (standard deviation; 95 % confidence interval) age of patients was 42.6 (6.00; 40.1–45.07). Body mass index was 27.48 (5.06; 25.3–29.57). Twenty (80 %) patients had previous abdominal surgery, and three (15 %) patients had previous failed surgeries for attempted hysterectomy. Twenty-three patients had frozen pelvis due to severe endometriosis, and two patients had severe abdominopelvic adhesions due to multiple previous surgeries. One patient had intraoperative injury to the sigmoid colon and bladder during adhesiolysis, and laparotomy conversion was performed. The median (range) operating time was 210 (120–300) min, and estimated blood loss was 400 (300–600) ml. Length of post-operative stay was 1 (1–6) days, and the post-operative period was uneventful except in two patients who had paralytic ileus. The median (range) follow-up at 1 month and 6 months was 100 and 68 % (17 of 25), respectively. Our technique of laparoscopic hysterectomy with retrograde adhesiolysis and subsequent removal of adnexa is an alternative technique for hysterectomy in frozen pelvis and limits the potential hazards of injury to vital organs; it is associated with fewer complications. We emphasize that adequate surgical experience and expertise still remain the prerequisites for performing hysterectomy in frozen pelvis.

Keywords Retrograde adhesiolysis · Frozen pelvis · Laparoscopic surgery · Severe endometriosis

P. PG (✉) · K. Shabnam · S. A. Bhosale · H. Kaur · P. Talwar
Paul's Hospital, Kochi, Kerala, India
e-mail: drpaulpg@gmail.com

T. Thomas
Walsall Manor Hospital, Walsall, West Midlands, England

Background

Hysterectomy in frozen pelvis is a challenging surgical condition whether done by laparotomy or laparoscopy. Frozen pelvis refers to a surgical condition where reproductive organs and adjacent structures are distorted by extensive adhesive disease and fibrosis, which obscure the normal anatomical landmarks and surgical planes, making dissection extremely difficult and increasing the risk of injury to vital organs [1]. Common causes are infections, endometriosis and multiple previous surgeries, and other causes are ovarian carcinoma and radiotherapy. Surgery in frozen pelvis can result in serious complications like bowel and urinary tract injury. Most of these cases are referred to oncosurgeons who usually perform the surgery by an open retroperitoneal approach [2, 3]. We have been performing a total laparoscopic hysterectomy with retrograde adhesiolysis technique in frozen pelvis for 10 years in selected cases with gross pelvic distortion where the conventional method of laparoscopic hysterectomy is impractical. The concept of hysterectomy in frozen pelvis entails two steps, to perform extensive adhesiolysis first followed by hysterectomy. The highlight of our technique is to perform adhesiolysis sufficient enough to visualize the uterine fundus and cornua and then to proceed with hysterectomy. Difficult posterior bowel adhesions to the uterus and pouch of Douglas are dealt in a retrograde fashion after hysterectomy. Our technique of retrograde adhesiolysis is based on an alternative technique and can be practiced by most gynaecologists.

Material and methods

This is a retrospective case series. We included all patients who had undergone total laparoscopic hysterectomy in frozen pelvis at Paul's Hospital between October 2003 and May 2012. The aim of this study is to find the laparotomy conversion rate, duration of surgery, blood loss, intra- and post-operative complications with this alternate technique. The institutional ethical committee of Paul's Hospital approved the data collection, aggregation, deidentification and analysis for this study. Data regarding patient characteristics like age, body mass index, parity and previous surgeries, and intraoperative details like duration of surgery, complications, estimated blood loss, duration of hospital stay and post-operative events are evaluated. Informed consent is obtained from all patients, and risk of conversion to laparotomy and injury to vital structures is explained. Patients are admitted to hospital on the day of surgery and kept nil per os for 6 h prior to surgery. Bowel preparation is performed using sodium phosphate solution enema. Antibiotic prophylaxis is given at the time of induction of anaesthesia. Procedures are performed under general anaesthesia. Intermittent pneumatic compression device is used for prevention of deep venous thrombosis in all patients. Low molecular weight heparin is administered in high-risk patients.

Patient evaluation

Detailed history is taken regarding severity of abdominal pain, dysmenorrhoea, dyspareunia, dyschezia, haematochezia, diarrhoea, constipation, previous abdominopelvic infections and surgeries. Clinical examination and transvaginal ultrasonography are done by the operating surgeon prior to surgery. MRI is not routinely done.

Surgical technique

Pneumoperitoneum is created using a Veress needle at Palmer's point. Peritoneal entry is done by visual technique using a Ternamian Endotip (Karl Storz, Tuttlingen) at the umbilicus or supraumbilicus in patients with large abdominal masses. Abdominopelvic inspection is done for omental and bowel adhesions and to confirm the preoperative diagnosis (Fig. 1). The three-accessory-port technique is used, two ports in the lower quadrants lateral to the inferior epigastric artery and the third port in the suprapubic area. First, a secondary trocar is inserted under vision in an adhesion-free area, and other ports

are inserted after adhesiolysis. The port position is modified according to the size of the pelvic mass. Omental adhesions on the abdominal wall are released using a monopolar hook, scissors or Harmonic Ace (Ethicon Endosurgery, Cincinnati, OH). Sharp dissection close to the parietal peritoneum is employed to achieve lysis of bowel adherent to the anterior abdominal wall. A Clermont Ferrand uterine manipulator (Karl Storz, Tuttlingen, Germany) with a modified bulger is used. Small-bowel or rectosigmoid adhesions to the uterus and adnexa (Fig. 2) are released by sharp dissection as far as possible. Injection of dilute vasopressin into the myometrium close to bowel adhesions is used to achieve reduction in vascularity. This also facilitates ease of dissection by raising the serosa from the myometrium at the site of adhesion. In dense bowel adhesions, dissection onto the serosa of the uterus is performed. In the majority of cases, complete rectosigmoid adhesiolysis is not possible because of the severity of adhesions and poor accessibility due to the enlarged size of the uterus or adnexa. Enlarged endometriomas, cysts and encysted fluid collections are decompressed for better visibility. Identification of the round ligament and division of the same close to the lateral pelvic wall on both sides are performed. Adnexal adhesions to the uterus are released, and the cornual structures are divided with Enseal or Harmonic Ace. Division of the infundibulopelvic ligament is done at a later stage owing to possible proximity to the ureters. The uterovesical fold is opened and bladder dissection carried out subsequently. The uterine arteries are identified and adhesiolysis done to achieve its safe division. After the uterine arteries were secured, the anterior fornix is opened over the Clermont Ferrand fornix bulger. Once division of the anterior half of the vagina is achieved, the manipulator is removed and the cervix held with a tenaculum and pulled up (Fig. 3). A vaginal blocker is employed to prevent loss of pneumoperitoneum. Circumferential dissection of the vagina is continued to completely separate the cervix from the vagina. Rectal adhesions to the posterior vaginal wall are released by application of traction to the anterior and subsequently posterior lip of the cervix. This helps in safe completion of posterior vaginal wall incision. The posterior lip of the cervix is pulled away from posterior rectal adhesions, and by maintaining traction on the cervix, sharp adhesiolysis is done

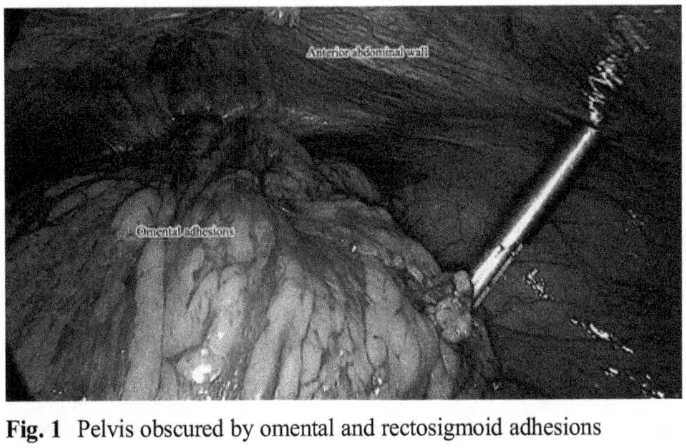

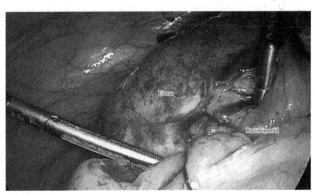

Fig. 1 Pelvis obscured by omental and rectosigmoid adhesions

Fig. 2 Rectosigmoid adhesions to the uterus

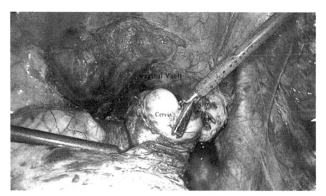

Fig. 3 Pulling up the anterior lip of the cervix to visualize the posterior vaginal wall

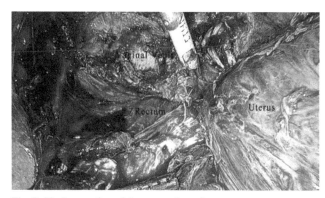

Fig. 5 Final separation of the rectum from the uterus

in retrograde fashion to release the rectum and sigmoid (Figs. 4 and 5). Once the rectum is completely separated from the uterus, retrieval of the specimen is done vaginally with or without morcellation depending on the size of the uterus. A vaginal blocker is used to achieve reinsufflation of the peritoneal cavity. Removal of the uterus creates space to identify the adnexa and helps with their dissection from the lateral pelvic wall. Adnexectomy is done after identifying the ureter, and the specimen is removed vaginally. Endometriotic implants and nodules over the rectal wall are excised. Vault closure is done laparoscopically (Fig. 6). Cystoscopy is done to confirm the integrity of the bladder and urine reflux from both the ureters. The rectum is inflated with air using a no. 16 F disposable suction catheter per anus to check for any inadvertent rectosigmoid injury. A drain is kept in the pelvis through one of the secondary ports and the 10-mm port closed with sutures.

Findings

Total laparoscopic hysterectomy with retrograde adhesiolysis was done in 25 patients with frozen pelvis between October 2003 and May 2012. Patient data are shown in Table 1. The mean (standard deviation (SD); 95 % confidence interval (CI)) age of patients was 42.6 (6.00; 40.1–45.07), and body mass

index was 27.48 (5.06; 25.3–29.57). Twenty (80 %) patients had previous abdominal surgery (laparotomy, laparoscopy), and three (15 %) patients had previous failed surgeries for hysterectomy. Fifteen patients had previous laparotomies, of which eight had one laparotomy, three had two laparotomies, three had three laparotomies and one had five laparotomies. Eleven patients had previous laparoscopic surgeries, of which six had both laparotomy as well as laparoscopy. Fourteen (56 %) patients were nulliparous, and 11 (44 %) were parous, of which five (20 %) had previous caesarean sections. The presenting complaints of patients were dysmenorrhoea in 17 (68 %) and abdominal pain in 8 (32 %). Twenty-three (92 %) patients had frozen pelvis due to severe endometriosis [4]. Out of these 23 patients, seven had fibroid uterus with severe endometriosis, seven had adenomyosis of the uterus with severe endometriosis and nine had severe endometriosis. Two patients had severe abdominopelvic adhesions due to multiple surgeries in the past.

Laparoscopic hysterectomy with retrograde adhesiolysis was successful in 24 (96 %) patients, and one patient had laparotomy conversion. Operative details are mentioned in Table 2. In all the cases, the uterine artery was ligated after complete anterior wall adhesiolysis and before adhesiolysis of the posterior aspect of the uterus. Because of dense adhesions, adnexectomy was done at the end of surgery in all cases. One patient had intraoperative injury to the sigmoid colon and bladder during adhesiolysis, and laparotomy conversion was

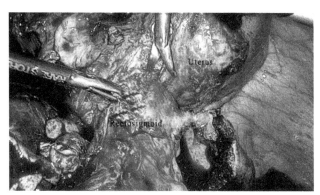

Fig. 4 Retrograde separation of the uterus from the rectosigmoid

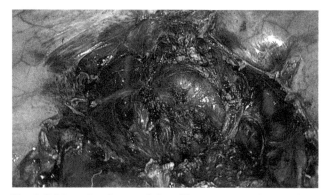

Fig. 6 Pelvic cavity after completion of hysterectomy and adhesiolysis

Table 1 Patient data

Variable	Value[a]
Age	42.6 years
BMI	27.48
Parity median (range)	0 (0–2)
Previous abdominal (laparoscopy + laparotomy) surgery	20 of 25 (80 %)
Previous failed surgeries	3 of 20 (15 %)
Previous laparoscopies only	5 of 20 (30 %)
Previous laparotomy and laparoscopy	6 of 20 (20 %)
Previous laparotomies	15 of 20 (70 %)
Previous 1 laparotomy	8 of 20 (40 %)
Previous 2 laparotomies	2 of 20 (10 %)
Previous 3 laparotomies	3 of 20 (15 %)
Previous 5 laparotomies	1 of 20 (5 %)
Severe endometriosis with fibroid uterus	7 (28 %)
Severe endometriosis with adenomyosis of uterus	7 (28 %)
Severe endometriosis	8 (32 %)
Severe endometriosis with bowel endometriosis	1 (4 %)
Severe abdominopelvic adhesion	2 (8 %)
Follow-up 1 month	25 (100 %)
Follow-up 6 months	17 (68 %)

done with the assistance of a general surgeon; the bladder was repaired in two layers, and since the sigmoid perforation was 2 cm in size with >60 % stricture of a 4-cm segment of the sigmoid colon due to an endometriotic nodule, intestinal

Table 2 Operative data

Variable	Value
TLH BSO	16
TLH USO	4
TLH	3
TLH BSO staging biopsies, omentectomy	1
Laparotomy conversion (TAH BSO with bladder repair and colostomy)	1
Severe endometriosis	22 (88 %)
Severe endometriosis with bowel endometriosis	1 (4 %)
Severe abdominopelvic adhesion	2 (8 %)
Operating time, median (range)	3.5 (2–5) h
Estimated blood loss, median (range)	400 (300–600) ml
Post-op hosp stay, median (range)	1 (1–6) days
Intraoperative complication	1 (4 %)
Post-operative complications	2 (8 %)
Blood transfusion	1 (4 %)

BSO bilateral salpingo-ophorectomy, *USO* unilateral salpingo-ophorectomy, *TLH* total laparoscopic hysterectomy, *TAH* total abdominal hysterectomy

segmental resection and sigmoid colostomy were performed. Two units of blood were transfused. There were no complications related to entry procedures. Post-operative morbidity in the form of paralytic ileus was noted in two (8 %) patients who were managed conservatively. Intraoperative blood transfusion was needed only in one patient. The median (range) operating time was 210 (120–300) min, and estimated blood loss was 400 (300–600) ml. Length of post-operative stay was 1 (1–6) days. The median (range) follow-up visit at 1 month and 6 months was 100 and 68 % (17 of 25), respectively, and was uneventful in all except for one patient who had a localized haemorrhagic collection in the pelvis measuring 4.5× 5 cm; an ultrasonography-guided aspiration was done at 1 month follow-up. A telephonic inquiry at 1 year was done to confirm the well-being of patients and recurrence of symptoms. None of our patients had recurrence of symptoms or occurrence of new symptoms pertaining to endometriosis.

Discussion

Hysterectomy is the commonest major gynaecological procedure [5]. Most hysterectomies can be performed laparoscopically including those with large myomas and severe endometriosis [6–8]. Various techniques have been described previously to tackle difficult hysterectomies, but the level of expertise needed limits the general use of these techniques [9, 10]. Even experienced gynaecologic laparoscopic surgeons find it very difficult to operate in such condition, and the surgery may be abandoned in some cases. In our series, three patients had failed surgeries with attempted hysterectomy and were abandoned due to the operative difficulties. At our centre, total laparoscopic hysterectomy with retrograde adhesiolysis is chosen in all cases of frozen pelvis.

Laparoscopic hysterectomy in frozen pelvis facilitates adnexa removal compared to vaginal hysterectomy as the adnexa may be adherent to surrounding structures that may be extremely difficult to reach transvaginally [9]. The laparotomy conversion rate for laparoscopic hysterectomy in severe endometriosis and large fibroids as described in literature is 4.3 and 7.9 % [8, 11]. In our series, one patient had conversion to laparotomy. This was done to facilitate repair of incidental bladder perforation in a densely adherent bladder and to achieve bowel resection for severe bowel endometriosis with bowel stenosis of greater than 60 % [12]. A study involving 115 patients with severe endometriosis undergoing laparoscopic hysterectomy reported bladder injury in 1 (0.9 %) of 115 cases without any bowel or ureteral injury [8]. In our series, 23 patients had frozen pelvis due to severe endometriosis. Our surgical approach in these patients is focused primarily on symptom-guided approach rather than mandatory oncologic resection [13]. All visible endometriotic lesions were excised and the cul de sac cleared of endometriotic lesions. Considering the rare progressive nature of deep endometriosis, segmental bowel resection was not performed for superficial bowel lesions [14, 15]. We routinely identify the ureter during and after dissection and do cystoscopy at the end of the procedure to confirm the integrity of the bladder and patency of the ureters. Even the most experienced surgeon may encounter bowel injury. The golden rule is early recognition of injury as time of diagnosis is the most important independent factor determining the outcome. A difficult surgical condition can be well anticipated, and the surgeon can arrange for preoperative and, if required, intraoperative surgical or urological assistance. Surgery should be performed in a setting where such facilities are readily available. Paralytic ileus may occur probably due to extensive bowel adhesiolysis and handling; out of 25 patients, two patients developed paralytic ileus in the post-operative period whereas James et al. reported seven cases with paralytic ileus following major gynaecological procedure in 707 patients [16]. The risk of complications depends upon the extent of bowel involvement, adhesions and extent of endometriosis infiltration, surgeon experience and bowel resection [16, 17]. The operating time was 210 min in our study compared to 185±48.7 min mentioned by Chalermchockchareonkit et al., while it was 131 and 147 min in two case reports by Walid et al. [6] in laparoscopic hysterectomy for severe endometriosis [8]. This can be explained by the severity of the disease process and grossly distorted anatomical planes, necessitating meticulous dissection and slow progression. Mean (SD; 95 % CI) weight of the uterus was 390.2 (441.59; 207.91–572.49) g. The mean estimated blood loss in our series was 384 ml whereas Chalermchockchareonkit reported a mean blood loss of 302.6 ml [8], while that reported by Walid et al. was 150 ml in laparoscopic hysterectomy for severe endometriosis [6]. The length of hospital stay was 1.3±1.07 days in our series which is shorter when compared to 3.5±1.1 days reported in the literature [8]. One patient (4 %) required blood transfusion in our series, whereas nine (7.8 %) required blood transfusion out of 115 patients undergoing hysterectomy for severe endometriosis [8].

All procedures have their own limitations, and retrograde adhesiolysis during hysterectomy in frozen pelvis requires adequate surgical experience and expertise to change the course of surgery and manage the complications associated with difficult pelvic surgery. Specialized assistance may be needed to manage the complications. The surgeon should be prepared to modify the surgical technique according to the case. The overall key to success in such cases depends on thorough knowledge of pelvic anatomy and operative experience involving varying degrees of pelvic distortion with or without enlarged uteri. This technique of retrograde adhesiolysis can decrease the complications in difficult hysterectomies with gross pelvic

distortion due to adhesions even in the presence of enlarged uteri. This is a retrospective study, and further evidence is required, preferably by adequately powered well-designed multicentre randomized controlled trials (RCTs) before definitive conclusions can be given.

Conclusion

Even though frozen pelvis is not a common surgical condition, it is not rare to come across such cases in clinical practice. Our technique of initial partial adhesiolysis followed by hysterectomy and retrograde separation of posterior bowel adhesions and subsequent removal of adnexa is an alternative technique. This technique in the hands of a very experienced surgeon might be more appropriate in decreasing the laparotomy conversion rate and the overall complications. This is a retrospective study, and for this rare and difficult situation, it would be impossible and unethical to have a control group; however, adequately powered well-designed multicentre RCTs are required before definitive conclusions can be given.

Conflict of Interest The authors report no conflicts of interest. The authors alone are responsible for the content and writing of the paper.

References

1. Donald PG, Michael JC (2007) Surgical strategies to untangle a frozen pelvis. OBG Management 19(3)
2. Hudson CN (1981) Victor Bonney lecture, 1980. Ovarian cancer—a gynaecological disorder? Ann R Coll Surg Engl 63:118–25
3. Volpi E, Bernardini L, Ferrero AM (2012) The retrograde and retroperitoneal totally laparoscopic hysterectomy for endometrial cancer. Int J Surg Oncol 2012:263850
4. Schenken RS, Guzick DS (1997) Revised ASRM classification for endometriosis: 1996. Fertil Steril 67:820
5. Stovall TG (2007) Hysterectomy. In: Berek JS (ed) Berek & Novak's gynecology, 14th edn. Lippincott Williams & Wilkins, Philadelphia, pp 805–846
6. Walid SM, Heaton RL (2011) Total laparoscopic extirpation of a fixed uterus from benign gynecological disease. Gynecol Surg 8:157–159
7. Sinha R, Sundaram M, Lakhotia S, Mahajan C, Manaktala G, Shah P (2009) Total laparoscopic hysterectomy for large uterus. J Gynecol Endosc Surg 1:34–39
8. Chalermchockchareonkit A, Tekasakul P, Chaisilwattana P, Sirimai K, Wahab N (2012) Laparoscopic hysterectomy versus abdominal hysterectomy for severe pelvic endometriosis. Int J Gynaecol Obstet 116:109–111
9. Pelosi MA III, Pelosi MA (1997) Vaginal hysterectomy for benign uterine disease in the laparoscopically confirmed frozen pelvis. J Laparoendosc Adv Surg Tech 7:345–351
10. Cho FN (2007) A technique to deal with severe adhesions between the uterus and bladder or rectum in laparoscopic-assisted vaginal hysterectomy. J Minim Invasive Gynecol 14:750–751

11. Moon MJ, No JH, Jeon YT, Jee BC, Kim YB (2011) Clinical outcomes of 1,041 total laparoscopic hysterectomies: six years of experience in a single center. Korean J Obstet Gynecol 54:618–622

12. Ferrero S, Camerini G, Maggiore U, Venturini PL, Biscaldi E, Remorgida V (2011) Bowel endometriosis: recent insights and unsolved problems. World J Gastrointest Surg 3:3–38

13. Roman H, Vassilieff M, Gourcerol G, Savoye G, Leroi AM, Marpeau L et al (2011) Surgical management of deep infiltrating endometriosis of the rectum: pleading for a symptom-guided approach. Hum Reprod 26:274–281

14. Koninckx PR, Ussia A, Leila Adamyan L, Arnaud W, Jacques D (2012) Deep endometriosis: definition, diagnosis, and treatment. Fertil Steril 98:564–571

15. Mereu L, Ruffo G, Landi S, Barbieri F, Zaccoletti R, Fiaccavento A et al (2007) Laparoscopic treatment of deep endometriosis with segmental colorectal resection: short-term morbidity. J Minim Invasive Gynecol 14:463–469

16. Donnez J, Squifflet J (2010) Complications, pregnancy and recurrence in a prospective series of 500 patients operated on by the shaving technique for deep rectovaginal endometriotic nodules. Hum Reprod 25:1949–1958

17. Song T, Kim TJ, Kang H, Lee YY, Choi CH, Lee JW, Kim BG, Bae DS (2012) Factors associated with complications and conversion to laparotomy in women undergoing laparoscopically assisted vaginal hysterectomy. Acta Obstet Gynecol Scand 91:620–624

14

Secondary hemorrhage after different modes of hysterectomy

P. G. Paul · Anil Sakhare Panditrao · Shabnam Khan ·
Prathap Talwar · Harneet Kaur · Sheetal Barsagade

Abstract Secondary hemorrhage after hysterectomy is rare but a life-threatening complication. The aim of this study is to estimate the cumulative incidence, patient characteristics, and potential risk factors of secondary hemorrhage after abdominal, vaginal, and laparoscopic hysterectomies. We did a retrospective observational study in which 1,623 cases of total laparoscopic hysterectomy (TLH), 963 cases of total abdominal hysterectomy (TAH), and 1,171 cases of vaginal hysterectomy (VH) were analyzed. Of the total 37 hemorrhages following hysterectomies, 23 were after TLH, 8 following VH, and 6 were after TAH. The cumulative incidence of secondary hemorrhage after any type of total hysterectomies was 0.98 %. TLH was associated with the highest risk of secondary hemorrhage (1.51 %) followed by VH (0.68 %) and TAH group (0.62 %). The relative risk of secondary hemorrhage following TLH compared to TAH and VH were 2.3 and 2.1, respectively. Both were statistically significant. The average size of the uterus in the TLH group was 516.7 g, and in the TAH and VH group, it was 140 and 142.5 g, respectively, which was statistically significant. The median time interval between hysterectomy and secondary hemorrhage was 11 days in TAH and VH group and 13 days in TLH group. Our data suggest that secondary hemorrhage is rare but may occur more often after TLH than after other hysterectomy approaches. Whether it is related to the application of thermal energy to tissues which cause more tissue necrosis and devascularization than sharp colpotomies in the TAH and VH groups is unclear. Large size of uteri, excessive use of energy source for uterine artery, and colpotomy may play a role.

P. G. Paul (✉) · S. Khan · P. Talwar · H. Kaur · S. Barsagade
Paul's Hospital, Kochi, Kerala, India
e-mail: drpaulpg@gmail.com

A. Sakhare Panditrao
Dr.Shankar Rao Chavan, Govt Medical College,
Nanded, Maharashtra, India

Keywords Laparoscopic hysterectomy · Abdominal hysterectomy · Vaginal hysterectomy · Secondary hemorrhage

Background

Secondary hemorrhage after hysterectomy is rare but a life-threatening complication which may require prompt medical and surgical intervention. Although the overall incidence of secondary hemorrhage is low, gynecologists do come across secondary hemorrhage of varying degrees of severity [1]. There are few studies which show the overall incidence of hemorrhage of 0.2–2 % after hysterectomy which includes reactionary and secondary hemorrhage [1–4]. Our centre has been performing laparoscopic hysterectomies since 1994, and we encounter one or two cases of secondary hemorrhage per year in the second or third postoperative week which necessitates hospitalization and active treatment. We believe that this incidence is higher following laparoscopic hysterectomy than the other modes of hysterectomy. The purpose of this study is to estimate the cumulative incidence of secondary hemorrhage resulting from different modes of hysterectomy including abdominal, vaginal, and laparoscopic hysterectomies and to assess whether laparoscopic hysterectomy poses a greater risk.

The second goal of this study is to describe the patient characteristics of those with secondary hemorrhage after hysterectomy and to identify the potential risk factors.

Methods

All women who underwent total laparoscopic hysterectomy (TLH) performed by the first author at Paul's Hospital between January 2004 and April 2012 and all cases of total abdominal hysterectomy (TAH) and vaginal hysterectomy (VH) performed by the second author from February 2010 to May 2012 at various private hospitals in Nanded were included in this study. The medical records of the patients were reviewed to ensure that those patients who had bleeding per vaginum between 24 h to 6 weeks after primary surgery and those requiring some intervention in the form of vaginal packing, vault suturing, laparoscopy, laparotomy, or embolization procedures were included in the analysis.

The institutional review board approved the data collection, aggregation, and analysis for this project. The following data were studied: age, parity, body mass index, indication for hysterectomy, size of uterus, details of surgical procedure, administration of antibiotics, time interval between hysterectomy and secondary hemorrhage, presenting symptoms, hemodynamic status, and type of intervention needed to manage the secondary hemorrhage.

Hysterectomies were categorized as TAH, VH, and TLH. All TLH were type IV E laparoscopic hysterectomies according to the classification system of the American Association of Gynecologic Laparoscopists [5]. TLH procedures were performed by dissecting the entire uterus laparoscopically; uterine arteries were coagulated with bipolar or Enseal (Ethicon Endosurgery, Inc.), and laparoscopic colpotomy was done with monopolar hook at a level above the uterosacral attachment, preserving the uterosacral arch. Vaginal cuff was closed vaginally in a continuous nonlocking fashion with Polysorb, Vicryl, or Dexon 1–0 size. Total abdominal hysterectomies were performed by division and ligation of pedicles with Vicryl 1–0. Uterosacral and cardinal ligament were divided and ligated with the same suture. Vault was sutured transversely with continuous or interrupted sutures while suspending the vault to the uterosacral and cardinal ligament at the angles. Vaginal hysterectomy was performed by clamping, dividing, and ligating the pedicles with Vicryl 1–0; the vault was sutured horizontally with continuous or interrupted sutures while suspending the vault to the uterosacral and cardinal ligament at the angles. All TLH patients received two doses of antibiotics, the first dose intraoperatively and the second dose postoperatively (fluoroquinolones and third generation cephalosporins). They were discharged on postoperative day1. All patients in TAH and VH group received antibiotics preoperatively and continued for 5 days. All TAH patients were discharged on day 7 after hysterectomy, and VH patients were discharged on day 4 which is a hospital protocol. Statistical analyses were performed using chi-square test, Kruskal–Wallis test, and ANOVA. A p value of <0.05 was considered statistically significant.

Findings

A total of 3,757 hysterectomies were performed via all surgical modalities. One thousand six hundred twenty-three had TLH, 1171 had undergone VH, and 963 had TAH. Of the total 37 hemorrhages following hysterectomies, 23 were after TLH, 8 following VH, and 6 were after TAH. The cumulative incidence of secondary hemorrhage due to different modes of hysterectomies were also analyzed (Table 1). The overall cumulative incidence of secondary hemorrhage after any type of total hysterectomies was 0.98 %. TLH was associated with the highest risk of secondary hemorrhage (1.51 %) followed by VH (0.68 %) and TAH group (0.62 %). The relative risk of secondary hemorrhage following TLH compared to TAH and VH were 2.3 and 2.1, respectively. Both were statistically significant with 95 % CI of 0.93 to 5.6 and 0.93 to 4.6. Patient characteristics and clinical presentation were also analyzed (Table 2).

The indications for the hysterectomies are depicted in Table 3 with the main indication being myoma uterus ($n =$ 18). Surgical details of patients are described in Table 4. The average size of the uterus in the TLH group was 516.7 g, and in the TAH and VH group, it was 140 and 142.5 g, respectively, which was statistically significant. In patients with hemorrhage after TLH, bipolar was used in 12 cases, and in the remaining 11 patients, Enseal was used to coagulate the uterine pedicle. The median time interval between hysterectomy and secondary hemorrhage was 11 days in the TAH and VH groups and 13 days in the TLH group.

All patients presented with bleeding per vaginum of varying degrees. Two patients in TAH and VH group had pain abdomen along with bleeding. Three patients in TLH group and three patients in TAH group were in a state of hypovolemic shock at the time of hospitalization. Blood transfusions were needed in five patients in the TLH group and six patients each in the TLH and VH groups (Table 5).

Vaginal packing was sufficient to control bleeding in 14 patients in the TLH group, whereas seven patients required

Table 1 Types of hysterectomy and incidence of secondary hemorrhage

Type of hysterectomy	No. of secondary hemorrhage	Total no. of hysterectomy	Incidence of hemorrhage in % (95 % CI)
TLH*	23	1,623	1.51 (1.01–2.26)
TAH	06	963	0.62(0.25–1.3)
VH	08	1,171	0.68(0.32–1.3)
Total	37	3,757	0.98(0.70–1.34)

*p <0.0001 (TLH vs TAH+VH)

Table 2 Demography of patients with secondary hemorrhage after hysterectomy

Variables	TLH (23)	TAH (06)	VH (08)	Total (37)
Age				
Mean±SD	45.83±4.5	48.83±7.1	48.37±8.5	46.9±5.9
Parity				
Median (range)	2 (1–4)	3.5 (2–4)	4 (3–5)	3.5(3–5)
1	04	0	0	04
≥2	19	06	08	33
Deliveries				
Vaginal	17	05	08	30
Cesarean	06	01	00	07
BMI				
Mean±SD	27.22±3.7	23.1±4.5	26.5±4.8	26.4±4.2

vault suturing. Laparoscopic coagulation of the uterine artery was done in one patient where the source of bleeding could not be identified vaginally. Uterine artery embolization was done twice in one patient to control the bleeding. Three patients each in the VH and TAH group were managed with vaginal packing alone. Four patients in the VH group had vault hematoma which was diagnosed on ultrasound and drained vaginally. In the TAH group, three patients were subjected to laparotomy. Out of the three patients, one had rectus sheath hematoma which had tracked down into the vagina and in the other two patients as the source of bleeding could not be identified; all pedicles were religated. On further evaluation, one of these patients was diagnosed to have chronic idiopathic thrombocytopenic purpura (Table 5).

Resumption of sexual intercourse was not found in any of these patients as all of them presented within 6 weeks after surgery. The period of abstinence advised was 6–8 weeks after TLH and 12 weeks after TAH and VH. Early resumption of regular activities was observed in TLH and VH patients. TAH patients resumed regular activities only after 45 days.

Table 3 Indications for hysterectomy

Indication for hysterectomy	TLH	TAH	VH	Total
Myoma	16	1	1	18
Cervical pathology	0	2	1	3
Myoma with endometriosis	2	0	0	2
Myoma with ovarian pathology	1	0	0	1
Adenomyosis	1	0	1	2
DUB	1	1	1	3
Ovarian pathology	0	1	0	1
Post menopausal bleeding	1	1	0	2
Prolapse uterus	1	0	4	5
Total	23	06	08	37

Discussion

Hemorrhage after hysterectomy is a life-threatening complication [1]. There are few published reports on the incidence of secondary hemorrhage after hysterectomy. In our study of 3,757 hysterectomies, 37 patients (0.98 %) had secondary hemorrhage. TLH had a higher incidence of 1.51 %, whereas VH (0.68 %) and TAH (0.62 %) had a lower incidence.

Donnez et al. in his series of 2,596 laparoscopic hysterectomies including laparoscopic subtotal hysterectomy and TLH had a lower incidence (0.1 %) of hemorrhage [6]. Wattiez et al. in a retrospective comparative study on the effect of learning curve on the outcome of laparoscopic hysterectomy done during 1989–1995 and 1996–1999 on 695 and 952 women, respectively, concluded that there was a substantial decrease in the major complication rates from 5.6 to 1.3 %, excessive hemorrhage from 1.9 to 0.1 % ($p < 0.005$), respectively [7]. Both studies did not specify the type of hemorrhage. Nezhat et al. in his comparative study of laparoscopic-assisted vaginal hysterectomy and abdominal hysterectomy of 20 patients showed that LAVH group had shorter duration of hospitalization (2.4 vs 4.4 days), more rapid recuperation (3 vs 5 weeks) and fewer complications [8]. Canis et al. in a retrospective cohort study on 680 patients found that seven cases (1.03 %) had postoperative hemorrhage following hysterectomy, two cases involved vaginal laceration and five intraperitoneal hemorrhages [9].

Holub et al. reported two cases (0.17 %) of secondary hemorrhage in his series of 1,167 patients with laparoscopic hysterectomy and vaginal hysterectomy [4]. Wilke et al. reported an incidence of 0.23 % of secondary hemorrhage following VH and laparoscopic hysterectomy [1]. In an earlier study by Bhattacharya et al., the incidence of secondary hemorrhage was 0.45 % after vaginal hysterectomies [3]. In our study, the incidence of secondary hemorrhage after TAH and VH is comparable but is higher in the TLH group. Infrequent occurrence of secondary hemorrhage, failure to report to the centre where hysterectomy was performed or nondocumentation of cases may be the possible reasons for lower incidence reported in the literature.

Possible factors which may play a role in secondary hemorrhage are patient characteristics, size of the uterus, surgical techniques, vaginal vault infection, and early resumption of physical activity.

Age and BMI of patients in the three groups were not statistically significant and thus unlikely to contribute to the increased incidence of secondary hemorrhage in the TLH group. In the present study, the size of the uterus was significantly higher among the TLH group. Out of the 18 cases of secondary hemorrhage in the TLH group, 16 had

Table 4 Surgical details

	TLH (23)	TAH (06)	VH (08)	Total (37)
Previous surgeries				
No	13	01	04	18
Yes	10	05	04	19
Total	23	06	08	37
Size of uterus*				
Mean weight±SD	516.7±443.1	140±47.32	142.5±66.9	374.3 ±3 94.2
Energy source of uterine artery				
Bipolar	11	0	0	11
Enseal	12	0	0	12
Suturing	0	06	08	14
Total	23	06	08	37
Energy source for vault				
Monopolar	23	0	0	23
None	00	06	08	14
Total	23	06	08	37
Post-op complications				
Fever	2	0	2	2
Post-op blood transfusions	0	2	3	5
Reactionary hemorrhage	0	0	1	1
Urinary retention	0	0	2	2
Cough/constipation	1	0	1	1
Pain abdomen	0	2	2	4

*p value <0.02

fibroid uterus with mean weight of 516±443. Though TLH is a feasible and safe technique in cases of enlarged uteri, which permits avoidance of laparotomy with evident benefits for the patients [10], high vascularity and large-sized vessels may be responsible for the increased incidence of secondary hemorrhage [11].

Table 5 Clinical presentation and treatment of secondary hemorrhage

	TLH (23)	TAH (6)	VH (8)	Total (37)
Severity of hemorrhage				
Mild ≤200 ml	11	1	3	15
Profuse >200 ml	12	5	5	27
Hemodynamic status				
Stable	20	3	8	34
Hypovolemic shock	3	3	0	3
Treatment				
Blood Transfusion	5	6	6	17
Vaginal packing	14	3	3	20
Vault suturing	7	0	1	7
Laparoscopy	1	0	0	1
Laparotomy	0	3	0	3
Uterine artery embolization	1	0	0	1
Vault hematoma drainage	0	0	4	4

The time interval between hysterectomy and onset of secondary hemorrhage ranged between 3 and 22 days. The median interval for the TLH group was 13 days, and for the TAH and VH groups, it was 11 days. Of the few reported cases in literature, the time interval varied from 3 to 18 days [1, 2, 4].

As the majority of patients could be managed with vaginal packing alone, it implies that the source of bleeding could be from the vaginal cuff. Any obvious vault bleeder can be secured with suture. Laparoscopic surgery in postoperative bleeding after hysterectomy is feasible and may be recommended if the source of bleeding cannot be identified by vaginal examination or if the symptoms indicate that the source of bleeding is intraabdominal [4]. Laparoscopy provides good magnification which allows closer inspection and a more precise use of bipolar coagulation or suturing for management of hemorrhage [1]. In our study, one patient underwent laparoscopic coagulation of uterine artery in the TLH group. Laparotomy may be done where laparoscopic surgical skills are not available [1]. Emergency therapeutic arterial embolization is a safe and effective minimal invasive procedure for patients developing postoperative hemorrhage after gynecological laparoscopic surgery [12]. In our study, one patient with secondary hemorrhage in the TLH group underwent uterine artery embolization twice. Vaginal vault dehiscence is one of the rare complications after hysterectomy [13]. In our study, we did not come across any vaginal vault dehiscence.

The source of bleeding in secondary hemorrhage can be from uterine vessels or descending cervical/vaginal vessels. The source of bleeding was a uterine vessel in two out of 23 cases in the TLH group and two patients in the TAH group. Use of energy source for the uterine vessels is unlikely to increase the incidence of secondary hemorrhage after TLH. Occasionally, uterine artery pseudoaneurysm can cause delayed heavy vaginal bleeding after laparoscopic hysterectomy [14]. Monopolar energy is used for colpotomy in all patients in the TLH group. The use of thermal energy may result in increased tissue damage to the vaginal cuff [2, 15]. Vault bleeding was responsible for secondary hemorrhage in 21 out of 23 cases. Hence, the usage of energy source for the vault may be responsible for higher incidence of secondary hemorrhage after TLH. It may be advisable to minimize the use of thermal energy so that the tissue is not over desiccated [2].

The exact cause for increased incidence of secondary hemorrhage after TLH is unknown. We may hypothesize that the application of thermal energy to tissues may cause more tissue necrosis and devascularization than sharp colpotomies in the TAH and VH groups. Treatment of secondary hemorrhage via vaginal approach in the form of packing, suturing, or drainage of hematoma appears to be feasible as initial intervention to control bleeding. Also, care must be taken while performing TLH in large uteri and limiting the over enthusiastic use of thermal energy. TLH is still recommended over abdominal hysterectomy because of obvious advantages [13, 16, 17].

Limitations of the present study are that it is a retrospective observational study performed in two different places, in two different time periods, and by two different surgeons. Since the incidence of secondary hemorrhage is very low, longer duration was included for the TLH series. So the patient groups were not directly comparable. When the study was started, the first author had 10 years of experience in doing laparoscopic hysterectomy; it is unlikely that the learning curve has affected the outcome. Further prospective randomized control trial studies are needed to validate our results.

Conclusion

Our data suggests that secondary hemorrhage is rare but may occur more often after TLH than after other hysterectomy approaches. Large size of uteri, excessive use of energy source for uterine artery, and colpotomy may play a role. The comparison of different energy sources like ultrasonic (harmonic) or bipolar with scissors for colpotomy in TLH is worth studying. TLH is a feasible and safe technique in cases of enlarged uteri, which permits avoidance of laparotomy with evident benefits for the patients [10].

Conflict of interest On behalf of all the authors, the corresponding author states that there is no conflict of interest. The authors alone are responsible for the content and writing of the paper.

Author's statement of responsibility All the authors of this study were actively involved in the design of the study, data collection and analysis, statistical analysis, and manuscript preparation.

Informed consent Informed consent was obtained from all patients for being included in the study.

References

1. Wilke I, Merker A, Schneider A (2001) Laparoscopic treatment of hemorrhage after vaginal hysterectomy or laparoscopically assisted vaginal hysterectomy (LAVH). Surg Endosc 15:1144–1146
2. Miranda CS, Carvajal AR (2003) Complications of operative gynecological laparoscopy. JSLS 7:53–58
3. Bhattacharya MS, Shinde SD, Narwekar MR (1978) Complications of vaginal hysterectomy (analysis of 1105 cases). J Postgrad Med 24:221–225
4. Holub Z, Jabor A (2004) Laparoscopic management of bleeding after laparoscopic or vaginal hysterectomy. JSLS 8:235–238
5. Olive DL, Parker WH, Cooper JM, Levine RL (2000) The AAGL classification system for laparoscopic hysterectomy. Classification committee of the American association of gynecologic laparoscopists. J Am Assoc Gynecol Laparosc 7:9–15
6. Donnez J, Jadoul P, Donnez O, Squifflet J (2007) What is the preferred route for hysterectomy?—proposition: most uteri can be removed by laparoscopy! In proceedings of the 9th world congress on controversies in obstetrics. Gynecology and Infertility, Barcelona, Spain
7. Wattiez A, Soriano D, Cohen SB, Nervo P, Canis M, Botchorishvilli R et al (2002) The learning curve of total laparoscopic hysterectomy; comparative analysis of 1647 cases. J Am Assoc Gynecol Laparosc 9:339–345
8. Nezhat F, Nezhat C, Gordon S, Wilkins E (1992) Laparoscopic versus abdominal hysterectomy. J Reprod Med 37(3):247–250
9. Canis M, Botchorishvili R, Ang C, Rabischong B, Jardon K, Wattiez A, Mage G (2008) When is laparotomy needed in hysterectomy for benign uterine disease? J Minim Invasive Gynecol 15(1):38–43
10. Fiaccavento A, Landi S, Barbieri F, Zaccoletti R, Tricolore C, Ceccaroni M (2007) Total laparoscopic hysterectomy in cases of large uteri: a retrospective comparative study. J Minim Invasive Gynecol 14:559–563
11. Bonilla DJ, Manis L, Whitaker R, Crawford B, Finan M, Magnus M (2007) Uterine weight as a predictor of morbidity after a benign abdominal and total laparoscopic hysterectomy. J Reprod Med 52(6):490–498
12. Takeda A, Koyama K, Mori M, Sakai K, Mitsui T, Nakamura H (2008) Diagnostic computed tomographic angiography and therapeutic emergency transcatheter arterial embolization for management of postoperative hemorrhage after gynecologic laparoscopic surgery. J Minim Invasive Gynecol 15(3):332–341
13. Hur HC, Guido RS, Mansuria SM, Hacker MR, Sanfilippo JS, Lee TT (2007) Incidence and patient characteristics of vaginal cuff dehiscence after different modes of hysterectomies. J Minim Invasive Gynecol 14:311–317
14. Miligkos DS, Louden K, Page A, Behrens R (2013) Uterine artery pseudoaneurysm following laparoscopic hysterectomy. An

unusual cause of delayed heavy vaginal bleeding. Gynecol Surg. doi:10.1007/s10397-031-0785-5

15. Memon MA (1994) Surgical diathermy. Br J Hos Med 52:403–408

16. Wiser A, Holcroft CA, Tulandi T, Abenhaim HA (2013) Abdominal verses laparoscopic hysterectomies for benign disease: evaluation of morbidity and mortality among 465,798 cases. Gynecol Surg. doi:10.1005/s10397-078-9

17. Karaman YC, Bingol B, Günenç Z (2007) Prevention of complications in laparoscopic hysterectomy: experience with 1120 cases performed by a single surgeon. J Minim Invasive Gynecol 14:78–84

15

Discharge less than 6 hours after robot-assisted total laparoscopic hysterectomy

Jakob Graves Rønk Dinesen · Birgit Hessellund · Lone Kjeld Petersen

Abstract The benefits of fast track regimes, i.e. reduction in hospital stay and minimization of postoperative complications, have led to their widespread use. This study tested the feasibility of a fast track programme based on robot-assisted laparoscopic hysterectomy in which patients were discharged from a day care unit within 6 h after the operation. We enrolled 22 patients. Preoperatively, all patients were carefully informed. All patients except two could be discharged on the same day. Pain during the first 24 h was not a problem. No readmissions occurred within the first 30 days after the surgery. This small series of robot-assisted laparoscopic hysterectomy demonstrates that the postoperative hospital stay could be reduced and that this procedure could be carried out in a day surgery unit. Preparing the patients for surgery in the day unit is an important part of a successful fast track regimen.

Keywords Robot-assisted surgery · Total laparoscopic hysterectomy · Fast track programme

Introduction

The benefits of fast track regimes, i.e. reduction in hospital stay and minimization of postoperative complications, have led to widespread use of the programmes. Many separate factors such as providing the patient with extensive preoperative information, optimal postoperative pain relief, early feeding and mobilization as well as minimal invasive surgical procedures are central features of these programmes.

Hysterectomy is still a very frequently performed gynaecologic procedure. The vaginal approach is considered the most cost effective, [1] but if there is a need for combining the hysterectomy with removal, the fallopian tubes and the ovaries, the vaginal approach may be inappropriate. Consequently, some gynaecologists consider oophorectomy a contraindication to the vaginal hysterectomy [2].

Introducing the laparoscopic hysterectomy solved this problem. Robot-assisted laparoscopic hysterectomy is now widely used even though the operative costs of performing this procedure are significantly higher than those of total laparoscopic hysterectomy [1, 3]. On the other hand, the robotic method seems less traumatic. Postoperative pain is reported the same or reduced in patients, who have undergone a robot-assisted laparoscopic hysterectomy compared to the laparoscopic hysterectomy [4, 5].

The increased costs of the laparoscopic techniques for hysterectomy may be explained by longer operating time and expensive instruments. On the other hand, the benefits of the minimal invasive procedures have reduced the length of hospital stay. Consequently, patients treated by laparoscopic hysterectomy may be discharged within 24 h after the operation [6, 7] and the postoperative setting is redefined to outpatient care.

A day care unit can be defined in different ways, and the working hours differ from day time to 24 h of service. The aim of this study was to test the feasibility of a fast track programme based on robot-assisted laparoscopic hysterectomy in which patients were discharged from a day unit within 6 h after the operation.

J. G. R. Dinesen · B. Hessellund · L. K. Petersen (✉)
Department of Gynecology and Obstetrics,
Aarhus University Hospital, 8200 Aarhus N, Denmark
e-mail: lonpeers@rm.dk

Material and methods

All patients, who were scheduled for a total laparoscopic hysterectomy (TLH) at the department of Gynecology,

University Hospital of Aarhus, were candidates for the robot-assisted total laparoscopic hysterectomy (RTLH) fast track programme. All surgeons are fellowship-trained gynaecologic oncologists. The setup required the use of 5 ports, a 12-mm camera port, three 8-mm ports (robot instruments) and a 12-mm assistant port. Standard robotic monopolar shears and bipolar forceps were used. V-loc suture were used for closing the vaginal cuff. Exclusion criteria were performance status (ASA 3+), age>80. Twenty-two patients were enrolled, and their characteristics are summarized in Table 1. Indications for hysterectomy were persistent dysplasia ($n=5$), prophylactic operation due to genetic predisposition ($n=12$), atypical endometrial hyperplasia ($n=2$), low stage endometrial cancer ($n=2$) and heavy menstrual bleeding ($n=1$).

Preoperatively, all patients were carefully instructed about procedures and the postoperative course. They had metronidazole (1000 mg) for vaginal disinfection the night before the operation and 1000 mg for rectal administration 2 h before the operation.

Patients were walked to the operation room and given general anaesthesia. All were given cefuroxime (1500 mg), dexamethasone (8 mg) and ondansetron (4 mg) intravenously before the operation started and morphine (10 mg) approximately 1 hour before ending the operation. Total intravenous anaesthesia (TIVA), without N2O with propofol/remifentanil, morphine and toradol, was used. A routine RTLH was performed including intraabdominal closure of the vaginal vault. Ropivacaine (50 mg) was injected intraperitoneally before closure of the laparoscopic port incisions, and a total of 20 mg of Ropivacaine were injected in the subcutis and fascia around the ports. Intravenous ketorolac (30 mg) was administrated at the end of the operation. The bladder catheter was removed at the end of the operation

After transmission to the recovery ward, patients rested in bed for 2 h before mobilization was undertaken. Early feeding was encouraged.

Postoperatively, patients were given ibuprofen (400 mg) and paracetamol (1000 mg) four times a day starting 8 h after the operation. All patients had oxycodone hydrochloride (10 mg) and ondansetron (4 mg) as rescue medicine.

All patients were informed about free access to the ward during the week after the operation. They could contact the department by phone at any time, and patients could be readmitted at any time, if necessary. A nurse phoned all patients the day after the operation. Patients were systematically interviewed at this time regarding postoperative nausea and vomiting (PONV), pain and their needs for antiemetics or opoids. At the end of the phone call, they were invited to call the department if any problems should arise within the next week.

Results

The RTLH was combined with bilateral removal of the adnexa in all patients except one.

The operation time is given in Table 1. A body mass index exceeding 40 was associated with markedly longer operation time.

All patients except two could be discharged before the day unit closed. In both patients, the reason for nondischarge was dizziness and a general feeling of anxiety. The patients stayed at the hospital for observation until the next morning without further examinations or treatment.

Pain within the first 24 h was not a problem. All patients completed the recommended pain regime and only three patients needed opoids after discharge. One patient had to continue this treatment for more than 24 h after the operation.

PONV after discharge was reported by 6 patients, but only four patients needed antiemetic medicine during the first 24 h after discharge.

One patient was seen in the out-patient clinic within the first week. An infection over the vaginal vault was diagnosed and treated with antibiotics. When the patients were interviewed by phone on the day after the operation, all felt well, were mobilized and had started eating. All patients were offered second interview within a week after the operation, but no one needed an extra telephone call.

No readmission occurred within the first 30 days after the operation.

Discussion

This small series of robot-assisted total laparoscopic hysterectomy demonstrates that the postoperative hospital stay could be reduced and that this procedure could be carried out in a day surgery unit. Thus, 91 % of the patients could be discharged as planned in less than 6 h after the operation without any readmissions. Although the length of hospital stay has been generally reduced to 1 to 2 days after RTLH [8, 9], this is, to the best of our knowledge, the

Table 1 Patients' characteristics (median (range))

	Median (range)
Age—years	53 (34–73)
Body mass index	25 (19–42)
Operating time "skin-to-skin time" (minutes)	82 (35–170)
Estimated blood loss (mL)	30 (10–100)
Conversion to open surgery	0
Length of hospital stay after the operation (minutes)	225 (150–270)
Readmission	0
Opoid after discharge	3 patients

first report of discharge within a few hours after completion of the operation.

Successful assignment of laparoscopic surgical procedures to day units requires careful selection of patients. One important factor is the risk of conversion to open surgery. Consistent with a meta-analysis demonstrating lower conversion rate in RTLH compared to the TLH [8], conversion was not needed in any patients in our study group. A high body mass index was associated with an increased operating time and a higher conversion rate for open surgery in patients who were treated by radical prostatectomy [10]. Although such factors may normally disqualify a patient from a day surgery unit, obese patients with a high rate of comorbidity may in fact benefit the most from the fast track regimen and the reduced postoperative complication rate.

Whether hysterectomy in day units can be generally undertaken in elderly patients remains to be shown. In our study, the two patients >70 years of age were discharged within the time limits along with younger patients. Similar results have been obtained in general surgery. Thus, there were no significant differences in length of hospital stay or 30-day readmission rate were demonstrated when younger patients were compared to those >70 years [11].

Despite a longer operation time and expensive instruments, the overall hospital costs were significantly lower for robotics compared with hysterectomy performed before the robot era [12]. Thus, the expense of robot-assisted hysterectomies may be balanced by the reduced costs in the postoperative period. The fact that RTLH is associated with a decrease in surgical complications [8] and that fast track regimens are generally associated with a decrease in postoperative complications may positively influence the total expenses.

Preparing the patients for a day surgery unit is an important part of a successful fast track regime. Patients should be informed about normal symptoms in the postoperative period including the high incidence of PONV (80 %) after laparoscopic gynaecologic operations [13]. Apart for the careful information given all patients in our study group, rescue medicine was handed out before discharge—oxycodone hydrochloride and ondasetron for self administration. The low incidence of delayed PONV in this study may at least partly be explained by a low consumption of opoids in the postoperative period combined with an effective antiemetic treatment. Our results were encouraging compared to rates of delayed PONV on 47 % within the period from 2 and 24 h after gynaecologic laparoscopy [14].

The two patients who could not be treated in the day unit were both nervous but without any objective findings. Indeed, no further examinations or treatment was undertaken within the prolonged hospital stay in these two patients.

The low need for readmission or extra visits in the out-patient clinic may indicate well prepared and informed patients. Moreover, the routine nurse phone call on the first postoperative day may prevent readmissions as patients could ask questions and be reassured or guided in case of unexpected symptoms or anxiety. Patients had free access to call the department 24 h a day for 7 days after the operation, but only one patient called once.

In conclusion, discharge within 6 h after robot-assisted total laparoscopic hysterectomy is feasible and does not lead to readmission. Patients must be well informed and prepared carefully in order to secure a successful introduction of this fast track regimen. Follow-up by nurse-led phone calls the day after the operation may add to the patients' feeling of security and prevent readmissions or visits in the out-patient clinic.

Acknowledgments All procedures followed were in accordance with the ethical standards of the responsible committee on human experimentation and with the Helsinki Declaration of 1975, as revised in 2000. Informed consent was obtained from all patients for being included in the study.

Conflict of interest Jakob G.R. Dinesen, Birgit Hessellund and Lone Kjeld Petersen declare that they have no conflict of interest.

References

1. Dayaratna S, Goldberg J, Harrington C, Leiby BE, McNeil JM (2014) Hospital costs of total vaginal hysterectomy compared with other minimally invasive hysterectomy. Am J Obstet Gynecol 210(2):120e1–120e6
2. McCracken G, Lefebvre GG (2007) Vaginal hysterectomy: dispelling the myths. J Obstet Gynecol Can 29:424–428
3. Rosero EB, Kho KA, Joshi GP, Giesecke M, Schaffer JI (2013) Comparison of robotic and laparoscopic hysterectomy for benign gynecologic disease. Obstet Gynecol 122(4):778–786
4. Leitao MM Jr, Malhotra V, Briscoe G, Suidan R, Dholakiya P, Santos K, Jewell EL, Brown CL, Sonoda Y, Abu-Rustum NR, Barakat RR, Gardner GJ (2013) Postoperative pain medication requirements in patients undergoing computer-assisted ("Robotic") and standard laparoscopic procedures for newly diagnosed endometrial cancer. Ann Surg Oncol 20(11):3561–3567
5. El Hachem L et al (2013) Postoperative pain and recovery after conventional laparoscopy compared with robotically assisted laparoscopy. Obstet Gynecol 121(3):547–553
6. Lee SJ, Calderon B, Gardner GJ, Mays A, Nolan S, Sonoda Y, Barakat RR, Leitao MM Jr (2014) The feasibility and safety of same-day discharge after robotic-assisted hysterectomy alone or with other procedures for benign and malignant indications. Gynecol Oncol 133(3):552–555
7. Lassen PD, Moeller-Larsen H, DE Nully P (2012) Same-day discharge after laparoscopic hysterectomy. Acta Obstet Gynecol Scand 91(11):1339–1341
8. Scandola M, Grespan L, Vicentini M, Fiorini P (2011) Robot-assisted laparoscopic hysterectomy vs traditional laparoscopic hysterectomy: five metaanalyses. J Minim Invasive Gynecol 18(6):705–715
9. Orady M, Hrynewych A, Nawfal AK, Wegienka G (2012) Comparison of robotic-assisted hysterectomy to other minimally invasive approaches. JSLS 16(4):542–548
10. Herman MP, Raman JD, Dong S, Samadi D, Scherr DS (2007) Increasing body mass index negatively impacts outcomes following robotic radical prostatectomy. JSLS 11(4):438–442

11. Keller DS, Lawrence JK, Nobel T, Delaney CP (2013) Optimizing cost and short-term outcomes for elderly patients in laparoscopic colonic surgery. Surg Endosc 27(12):4463–4468

12. Lau S, Vaknin Z, Ramana-Kumar AV, Halliday D, Franco EL, Gotlieb WH (2012) Outcomes and cost comparisons after introducing a robotics program for endometrial cancer surgery. Obstet Gynecol 119(4):717–724

13. Eriksson H, Korttila K (1996) Recovery profile after desflurane with or without ondansetron compared with propofol in patients undergoing outpatient gynecological laparoscopy. Anesth Analg 82:533–538

14. Jung WS, Kim YB, Park HY, Choi WJ, Yang HS (2013) Oral administration of aprepitant to prevent postoperative nausea in highly susceptible patients after gynecological laparoscopy. J Anesth 27(3): 396–401

16

Uterovaginal anastomosis for the management of congenital atresia of the uterine cervix

Anish Keepanasseril · S. C. Saha · Rashmi Bagga ·
Sameer Vyas · L. K. Dhaliwal

Abstract Congenital atresia of the cervix is a rare mullerian anomaly. Hysterectomy has been advocated as the management of choice in the early days as the reproductive performance is thought to be low despite successful neo-canal creation. In recent years, conservative surgery is being recommended more frequently in patients with congenital cervical atresia and with total or partial vaginal aplasia and is shown to have a better reproductive performance. The treatment strategy should be tailored to relieve retrograde menstrual symptoms and restore fertility. Here, we report a young girl with congenital cervical atresia with upper vaginal atresia managed with uterovaginal anastomosis and review the management options and reproductive performance in such cases.

Keywords Cervical Atresia · Uterovaginal anastomosis · Mullerian Anomaly

Background

Cervical atresia is an extremely rare and complex mullerian malformation. Unlike most other mullerian anomalies, the initial surgical management of congenital cervical atresia

A. Keepanasseril · S. C. Saha (✉) · R. Bagga · L. K. Dhaliwal
Department of Obstetrics and Gynecology, Postgraduate Institute
of Medical Education and Research (PGIMER),
Sector-12,
Chandigarh, India 160012
e-mail: drscsaha@gmail.com

S. Vyas
Department of Radiodiagnosis, Postgraduate Institute of Medical
Education and Research (PGIMER),
Sector-12,
Chandigarh, India 160012

remains controversial. Total hysterectomy eliminates the symptoms related to hematometra, but loss of reproductive function is irreversible. Hysterectomy should be avoided as first choice and reserved for cases where canalization attempts fail or are impossible. However, canalization procedures, mainly cervical drilling, may be followed by recurrent obstruction of the uterovaginal neo-canal, and persistent infertility. Hence, a majority of clinicians view hysterectomy as the optimal primary surgical management in these patients [1, 2]. Recently, small series have been reported which show an improved reproductive performance after utero-vaginal anastomosis [3, 4]. We report a 16-year-old girl who underwent uterovaginal anastomosis for cervical atresia and review the management options as well as the reproductive performance in such patients.

Method

A 16-year-old girl with primary amenorrhea and cyclic pelvic pain attended our hospital in January 2009. Her clinical examination results showed appropriate general feminization, normal external genitalia; rectal examination results revealed a small uterus with unremarkable adnexa. Trans-abdominal sonography evidenced the presence of uterus ($4.2 \times 2.9 \times 3$ cm) with suspicion of an absent cervix with normal ovaries and kidneys. Magnetic resonance imaging (MRI) revealed that the uterus and endometrial cavity were normal with cervix and the upper end of the vagina suspected to be aplastic (Figs. 1 and 2). The lower vagina was normal and a diagnosis of cervical and upper vaginal atresia was made. Her examination under anesthesia revealed the length of patent lower vagina to be about 6 cm. She underwent uterovaginal anastomosis by an abdomino-perineal approach; adhering to the microsurgical principles.

Fig. 1 Sagittal T2-weighted images (**a, b**) of pelvis showing hypoplasia/atresia of cervix and upper vagina (*black arrow*). Uterine body is normal in contour and shows normal zonal demarcation (*white arrow*)

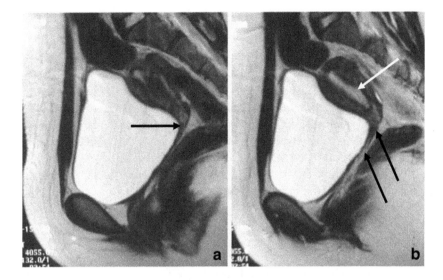

The uterovesical fold of peritomeum was incised and the bladder was reflected down over the atretic cervix (which was about 1.5 cm long) and the upper vagina. A 1-cm transverse incision was made at the uppermost portion of the patent vagina. Next, a 1-cm vertical incision was made in the lower end of the uterine body just above the atretic cervix and the endometrial cavity was opened. A hegar dilator (number 7–8) was introduced into the endometrial cavity through the uterine incision which was extended over the dilator to reach upto the superior limit of the atretic cervix. The dilator was removed and an 18-Fr Foleys catheter was introduced into the vagina from below, made to exit through the vaginal incision and enter into the endometrial cavity through the uterine incision, anterior to and bypassing the atretic cervix. With the Foleys catheter in place, the edges of the uterine incision were sutured to the edges of the vaginal incision. Thus, the lower portion of the uterus was anastomosed to the uppermost part of the patent vagina, bypassing the atretic cervix which was retained as the posterior lip of the neo-cervix, to the neo-uterovaginal canal.

A small endometriotic cyst (2×2 cm) in the left ovary was managed with cystectomy. The post-operative period was normal. Antibiotic treatment was given for 2 weeks in view of the retained Foleys catheter. She was given cyclical low dose contraceptive pills for 6 months. She had normal regular period in the month following surgery. The Foleys catheter was expelled spontaneously after the first menstrual cycle (3 weeks after surgery). Presently, 9 months after surgery, she is having spontaneous and regular menstrual cycles without any dysmenorrhea.

Findings

Atresia or agenesis of the uterine cervix is a rare developmental malformation of the female genital tract. Fujimoto et al. [5] reported 51 cases in the world literature. According to the Buttram and Gibbons [6] classification, cervical agenesis represents a Class I B mullerian anomaly

Fig. 2 Axial T2-weighted images (**a, b**) of pelvis showing uterine body with normal zonal demarcation and endometrial cavity (**a**). Cervix is hypoplastic/atretic (*black arrow*)

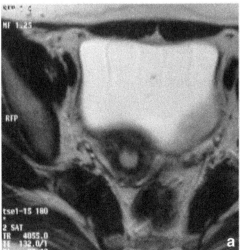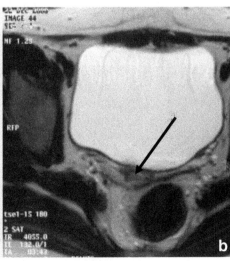

whereas the ASRM classification of 1988 places it in Class II b. In approximately 50% of cases, cervical agenesis is associated with partial or complete vaginal agenesis [5].

Patients usually present with amenorrhea and symptoms of retrograde menstruation plus hematometra. In pubescent girls, pelvic pain in the absence of menstrual bleeding must evoke the suspicion of an obstructive genital syndrome. Clinical examination eliminates vaginal atresia or an imperforate hymen, but it may not always be possible to differentiate cervical atresia from a high vaginal septum. Transabdominal or transperineal sonography may help to identify the level of obstruction but is not so reliable in the diagnosis of cervical atresia [7, 8]. The MRI is a more reliable imaging technique, and may diagnose associated upper genital tract anomalies or problems like hematosalpinx and endometriosis [9, 10]. Laparoscopy allows an exploration of the pelvis with assessment of the internal genital organs. An intravenous pyelography (IVP) can be performed because of the frequency of urinary tract malformations associated with Mullerian ducts anomalies [4]. MRI may be sufficient to obtain a preoperative diagnosis of cervical atresia, as in the present patient. MRI may also diagnose urinary tract malformations; hence an IVP may be omitted.

Unlike most of the other mullerian anomalies, management of congenital cervical atresia is challenging. The earliest reported case of congenital cervical atresia managed by hysterotomy and cervical canalization was described in 1900 [5]. The most successful surgical methods employed involved a transvaginal or transabdominal approach to create a neo-ostium through the dense fibrous cervix and communicate it to the endometrial cavity and vagina. Patency was maintained by application of stents (which were retained postoperatively for varying periods of time), with or without a surrounding full or split-thickness skin graft. However, re-stenosis of fibrous tissue, postoperative severe infection, or septicemia in occasional cases resulted in the recommendation of hysterectomy for this problem [4, 11–13]. However, in recent years, there has been resurgence towards conservative surgery which is now being frequently attempted in congenital cervical atresia associated with total or partial vaginal aplasia, with an aim to preserve the reproductive capability and relieve the menstrual symptoms. A procedure that sustains cyclic menses and does not allow re-stenosis would be optimal. Canalization techniques such drilling are easier to perform, but these are associated with re-stenosis of the cervix and its complications in nearly 40–60%. Hence, the technique of utero-vaginal anastomosis described by Deffarges et al. [4] is now preferred as it has a lower risk of re-stenosis and can be performed even in the presence of associated vaginal aplasia. It reduces the risk of damage to the bladder and rectum and obtains a reliable canalization of uterovaginal canal. They reported only one

patient out of 18 who developed re-stenosis of the uterovaginal canal leading to multiple canalization procedures, and ultimately needed salpingo-oophorectomy for pyosalpinx. Susbequently techniques using laproscopy or with laproscopic assistance have been reported. Novel techniques have been described by El Saman using laproscopic assistance (i.e., endoscopic monitored canaisation under vaginoscopic monitoring and retropubic balloon vagnioplasty). It has the advantages of requiring less laproscopic expertise and with less perineal dissection or extensive [14, 15]. However, the long-term outcome and the reproductive performances after the laparoscopic techniques are yet to be reported.

Due to the risk of retrograde menstruation and subsequent development of endometriosis, creating an outflow tract should be done as early as possible (12–16 years). In cases where hysterectomy needs to be performed for any associated pathology, creation of the neovagina may be delayed up to the age of 18–20 years. In complete aplasia of the vagina, such a two-stage procedure has been carried out successfully [16, 17].

The success of uterovaginal anastomosis depends upon the size of the created ostium, the length of the new endocervical canal, the presence of vaginal mucosa adjacent to the end of the neo-ostium, and the duration of stenting [18]. Laparoscopically assisted utero-vestibular anastomosis is also reported, but data about post procedure reproductive performance is yet not available [19]. The duration of the stenting has been reported to range from 3 weeks to 3 months, but in the series reported by Deffarges et al. [4], it was kept for 2 weeks only, and re-stenosis occurred in only 1/18. In our case, we chose uterovaginal anastomosis, as the long-term outcome and the reproductive performance after this method were reported in the literature. She is currently relieved of her menstrual symptoms. Her stent (Foleys catheter) was expelled spontaneously after 3 weeks, and she is symptom-free 9 months post-procedure.

The likelihood of spontaneous pregnancy occurring as a result of canalization appears to be low. This low fertility rate may be due to the presence of associated endometriosis and pelvis adhesions, plus the lack of normal endocervical canal glandular function. Very few spontaneous pregnancies have been reported after canalization of a completely or partially atretic cervix [4]. Assisted reproductive techniques are usually required to help these patients to achieve a pregnancy. [20, 21]. The need of cervical cerclage is described but is controversial. In series by Deffarges et al. [4], 40% of the women who attempted to conceive had a successful pregnancy, and only one out o ten patients had cerclage. They should be delivered by elective cesarean as the vertical uterine incision may increase the chance of uterine rupture.

Conclusion

In conclusion, a conservative approach may be recommended for women with congenital cervical atresia even in the presence of vaginal agenesis. Uterovaginal anastomosis can be considered as the surgical method of choice in these women. Surgery should be performed as early as possible to avoid complications like endometriosis and its sequelae which may hamper future reproductive performance. In addition, the presence of regular menses has an extremely favorable psychological impact on these young women.

Conflict of interest The authors report no conflicts of interest. The authors alone are responsible for the content and writing of the paper.

References

1. Rock JA, Schlaff WD, Zacur HA, Jones HW Jr (1984) The clinical management of congenital absence of the uterine cervix. Int J Gynaecol Obstet 22:231–235
2. Fliegner JR, Pepperell RJ (1994) Management of vaginal agenesis with a functioning uterus. Is hysterectomy advisable? Aust N Z J Obstet Gynaecol 34:467–470
3. Singh J, Devi YL (1983) Pregnancy following surgical correction of nonfused müllerian bulbs and absent vagina. Obstet Gynecol 61:267–269
4. Deffarges JV, Hadda B, Musset R, Paniel BJ (2001) Utero-vaginal anastomosis in women with uterine cervix atresia: long-term follow-up and reproductive performance. A study of 18 cases. Hum Reprod 16:1722–1725
5. Fujimoto VY, Miller JH, Klein NA, Soules MR (1997) Congenital cervical atresia: report of seven cases and review of the literature. Am J Obstet Gynecol 177:1419–1425
6. Buttram VJ, Gibbons W (1979) Mullerian anomalies: a proposed classification (an analysis of 144 cases). Fertil Steril 32:40–46
7. Graham D, Nelson MW (1986) Combined perineal—abdominal sonography in the evaluation of vaginal atresia. J Clin Ultrasound 14:735–738

8. Meyer WR, McCoy MC, Friz MA (1995) Combined perineal—abdominal sonography in the evaluation of transverse vaginal septum. Obstet Gynecol 85:882–884
9. Reinhold C, Hricak H, Forstner R, Ascher SM, Bret PM, Meyer WR, Semelka RC (1997) Primary amenorrhea: evaluation with MR imaging. Radiology 203:383–390
10. Lang IM, Babyn P, Oliver GD (1999) MR imaging of pediatric uterovaginal anomalies. Pediatr Radiol 29:163–170
11. Olive DL, Henderson DY (1987) Endometriosis and mullerian anomalies. Obstet Gynecol 69:412–415
12. Jacob JH, Griffin WT (1989) Surgical reconstruction of the congenitally atretic cervix: two cases. Obstet Gynecol Surv 44:556–569
13. Hovsepian DM, Auyeung A, Ratts VS (1999) A combined surgical and radiologic technique for creating a functional neo-endocervical canal in a case of partial congenital cervical atresia. Fertil Steril 71:158–162
14. El Saman AM (2009) Combined retropubic balloon vaginoplasty and laparoscopic canalization. Am J Obstet Gynecol 201:333.e1–333.e5
15. El Saman (2010) Endoscopically monitored canalization for treatment ofcongenital cervical atresia: the least invasive approach. Fertil Steril 94:313–316
16. Bugmann P, Amaudruz M, Hanquinet S, La Scala G, Birraux J, Le Coultre C (2002) Uterocervicoplasty with a bladder mucosa layer for the treatment of complete cervical agenesis. Fertil Steril 77:831–835
17. Acién P, Acién MI, Quereda F, Santoyo T (2008) Cervicovaginal agenesis: spontaneous gestation at term after previous reimplantation of the uterine corpus in a neovagina: Case Report. Hum Reprod 23:548–553
18. Gurbuz A, Karateke A, Haliloglu B (2005) Abdominal surgical approach to a case of complete cervical and partial vaginal agenesis. Fertil Steril 84:217
19. Fedele L, Bianchi S, Frontino G, Berlanda N, Montefusco S, Borruto F (2008) Laparoscopically assisted uterovestibular anastomosis in patients with uterine cervix atresia and vaginal aplasia. Fertil Steril 89:212–216
20. Nargund G, Parsons J (1996) A successful in-vitro fertilization and embryo transfer treatment in a woman with previous vaginoplasty for congenital absence of vagina. Hum Reprod 11:1654
21. Anttila L, Penttilä TA, Suikkari AM (1999) Successful pregnancy after in-vitro fertilization and transmyometrial embryo transfer in a patient with congenital atresia of cervix: case report. Hum Reprod 14:1647–1649

17

Robotic surgery in gynecologic oncology

Pierre Lèguevaque · S. Motton · F. Vidal ·
M. Soulé Tholy · J. Hoff · D. Querleu

Abstract The goal of this paper is to review the current data documenting the advantages of robotic surgery over open or laparoscopic surgery. The aim of this study is to compare the complications and perioperative outcome of robotic surgery with open and laparocopic surgery, in gynecologic oncology. The terms radical robotic or robot- assisted hysterectomy in PubMed search lead to 41 references. We excluded one review of literature, ten studies with benign and malignant cases, eight cases reports, one letter to the editor. We kept the prospective studies and comparative studies (total abdominal hysterectomy (TAH) vs. total robotic hysterectomy (TRH), total laparoscopic hysterectomy (TLH) vs. TRH or TAH vs. TRH vs. TLH). The results are separated for endometrial cancers, early cervical cancers, pelvic and paraaortic lymph node dissections, radical parametrectomy and trachelectomy, and pelvic exenteration. The literature on robotic-assisted radical hysterectomy supports its safety and feasibility for the surgical management of early cervical cancer and endometrial cancer. However, the results of a phase III randomized clinical trial testing the equivalence of outcomes after laparoscopic or robotic radical hysterectomy with abdominal radical hysterectomy are expected.

Keywords Robotic · Hysterectomy · Radical · Laparoscopy · Endometrial · Cervical cancer

Background

Total abdominal radical hysterectomy and total abdominal hysterectomy (TAH) has been the standard treatment for early stage cervical and endometrial cancer, respectively, for decades. Advances in laparoscopic instrumentation have made possible to safely perform hysterectomy and radical hysterectomy laparoscopically (total laparoscopic hysterectomy (TLH) and total laparoscopic radical hysterectomy (TLRH)), pelvic and aortic dissection, and even pelvic exenteration [1]

The latest advance in laparoscopic instrumentation has been the development of robotic-assisted surgery. One advantage of the robotic system compared to laparoscopy is the dual lens, 12 mm laparoscope that provides vivid 3-D images. The other advantage is the intra-abdominal articulation of the micro-instruments 2 cm from the tip. These articulations serve the same function of the human wrist and greatly add in the ability to suture and tie knots, and improve tissue dissection. Total robotic hysterectomy (TRH) with lymph node dissection and total robotic radical hysterectomy have been described since 2005 [2–4]. Transperitoneal and extraperitoneal pelvic and aortic lymph node dissection have also been described [5–7].

P. Lèguevaque · S. Motton · F. Vidal · M. S. Tholy · J. Hoff
General and Gynecologic Surgery, CHU Rangueil,
1 Avenue Jean Pouilhès,
31059 Toulouse Cedex 9, France

D. Querleu
Institut Claudius Regaud, Oncological Surgery,
20-24 rue du pont Saint Pierre,
31052 Toulouse Cedex, France

P. Lèguevaque (✉)
Chirurgie Générale et Gynécologique, CHU Rangueil,
1 Avenue Jean Pouilhès,
31059 Toulouse Cedex 9, France
e-mail: leguevaque.p@chu-toulouse.fr

Methods

Objectives

Robotic surgery may overcome many of the difficulties associated with standard laparoscopic surgery of cervical and endometrial cancer. Improved vision, dexterity of instrumentation, and increased control of all instrumentation by the primary surgeon, may provide an advantage during unroofing and dissection of the distal ureter. The robotic-assisted laparoscopic surgery may also be advantageous during lymphadenectomy in some areas, cardinal ligament dissection, and suturing of the vaginal cuff.

However, although the advantages of robotic surgery seem obvious for the surgeon's comfort, the question of patient benefit is still open, considering that the major paradigm shift has been the advent of minimal invasive surgery in the field of oncology. Indeed, two levels of comparison are possible: robotic versus open surgery, robotic versus laparoscopic surgery. The goal of this paper is to review the current data documenting the advantages of robotic surgery over open or laparoscopic surgery.

Data source

A PubMed search has been carried out. The terms radical robotic or robot-assisted hysterectomy lead to 41 references. We excluded one review of literature, ten studies without distinction between benign and malignant cases, eight cases reports, and one letter to the editor. We kept the prospective studies and comparative studies (TAH vs. TRH, TLH vs. TRH or TAH vs. TLH vs. TRH).

Review methods

The evaluation of robotic radical hysterectomy should be complete, with the population characteristics, mean operative time, lymph node count, intra- and postoperative complications, conversion and transfusion rate, estimated blood loss, and length of stay.

Seventeen references were retrieved. Only studies clearly addressing the results by tumor site were included. Ten and seven papers were included for early cervical cancer and endometrial cancer, respectively.

Findings

Radical hysterectomy for early cervix carcinoma

Comparative studies are available (Tables 1 and 2). However, all were historical or open comparisons.

The first robotic hysterectomy was reported in 2005 [2]. Others authors published their early experience [3–8]. Fanning et al. [9] performed robotic radical hysterectomies in 20 consecutive stage IA–IIA cervical cancer patients. Even though the operative time seems to be long compared to other series, Fanning concluded that the improved vision and intra-abdominal articulation of the robot provide an advantage in performing the most difficult steps of radical hysterectomy, such as unroofing and dissection of the distal ureter. A retrospective clinical review of 10 stage Ia2–Ib1 cervical cancer patients who underwent TRH was published by Kim et al. [10] in 2008. The authors concluded that TRH for selected early cervical cancer cases is feasible and associated with low morbidity. Oleszczuk et al. [11] described a technique of vaginal robot-assisted radical hysterectomy in a prospective study in 12 patients. For the authors, the complication rate is lower than in their own TLH series, but the patient number is still relatively small for such conclusions.

Lowe [12] recently published the first multi-institutional study of TRH for early cervical cancer. He summarized the referenced data on TRH as compared to the referenced literature on TLH, and concluded that several surgical outcomes (estimated blood loss, mean operative time, node retrieval, and hospital stay) are equivalent and may be superior in some aspects for patients undergoing a robotic-assisted approach. For the authors, a background in laparoscopy was not a prerequisite to becoming a successful robotic surgeon but may shorten the learning curve in the adoption phase of robotics.

In 2007, a pilot case–control study designed to evaluate the feasibility and efficacy of TRH and bilateral pelvic lymph node dissection for early cervical cancer was reported by Sert et al. [13]. Seven consecutive patients were compared to eight patients treated by conventional TLH. There were no statistically significant differences observed in the two groups in regard of mean operative time, number of lymph nodes, and length of resected parametrial tissues whereas significantly less bleeding and shorter hospital stay were described in the TRH group. However, the small sample size results in a low power of the statistical conclusions in this study. Gradually, the case–control studies showed a larger number of cases [14, 15]. Ko et al. [14] published a TAH/TRH comparison. The mean operative time, estimated blood loss, and length of stay were significantly different with better results in robotic approach. In 2009, Maggioni [15] published a similar comparison with the same results.

Nezhat et al. [16] compared the intra-operative, pathologic, and post-operative outcomes of TRH to TLH in 13 and 21 patients with early stage cervical cancer, respectively. No statistical differences were observed regarding operative time (323 vs. 318 min), estimated blood loss

Table 1 Review of literature: comparative studies of robotic assisted hysterectomy in early cervical cancer: population characteristics, operative time, and lymph nodes count

Authors	Year of publication	Method	Methodology	N	Mean age	Mean BMI	Mean operative time (min)	Lymph nodes
Sert [13]	2007	TLH/TRH	CC	7/8	45/41	22.5/24.6	300/241 (NS)	15/13 (NS)
Ko [14]	2008	TAH/TRH	HC	32/16	41.7/42.3	26.6/27.6	219/290 (S)	17.1/15.6 (NS)
Nezhat [15]	2008	TLH/TRH	PSOC	30/13	46.8/54.8	–	318/323 (NS)	31/25 (NS)
Fanning [16]	2008	TRH	RS	20	44	–	390	18
Kim [17]	2008	TRH	RS	10	49.9	–	207	27.6
Boggess [18]	2008	TAH/TRH	PSOC	49/51	41.9/47.4 (S)	26.1/28.6 (NS)	248/211 (S)	23.3/33.8 (S)
Magrina [19]	2008	TAH/TLH/TRH	CC	35/31/27	50.9/54.9/50	27.3/26.8/27.2	166/220/189 (S)	27.7/25.9/25.9 (NS)
Maggioni [20]	2009	TAH/TRH	CC	40/40	49.8/44.1 (S)	23.6/24.1 (NS)	200/272 (S)	26.2/20.4 (NS)
Oleszczuk [21]	2009	VRARH[a]	PS	12	44	24	356	40
Lowe [12]	2009	MI TRH[b]	PS	42	41	25.1	215	25

TAH Total abdominal radical hysterectomy, *TLH* total laparoscopic radical hysterectomy, *TRH* total robot-assisted radical hysterectomy, *S* significant difference or *NS* no significant difference

[a] Vaginal robot-assisted radical hysterectomy

[b] Multi-institutional total radical robot assisted hysterectomy

(157 vs. 200 ml), and mean pelvic nodes count (25 vs. 31). There were no recurrences in either group with a mean follow-up time of 12 months in the robotic group and 29 months in the laparoscopic group. Their conclusion was that robotic radical hysterectomy appears to be equivalent to TLH with respect to operative time, blood loss, hospital stay, and oncologic outcome.

Boggess et al. [17] published a case–control study of robotic-assisted type III radical hysterectomy with pelvic lymph nodes dissection performed in 51 patients compared with 49 patients who underwent TAH. The results of this study demonstrate that TRH with pelvic lymph node

dissection provides comparables, if not preferable, lymph node dissection over TAH. The robotic approach is associated with lower blood loss and shorter length of stay, in comparison with open approach. Of significant importance is the comparison of the complication rate that was seen in this study of TRH (7.8%) in comparison with the control cohort of TAH (16.3%). The authors give evidence that patients benefits that are associated with TRH and that experience with a laparoscopic approach is not necessary in moving to a robotic approach.

Magrina et al. [14] compared the TAH, TLH, and TRH: the results of this study are consistent with other studies

Table 2 Review of literature: studies of robot assisted hysterectomy in early cervical cancer: complications and outcomes

Authors	Intraoperative complications (%)	Post operative complications (%)	Estimated blood loss (ml)	Transfusion rate (%)	Conversion rate (%)	Length of stay (days)
Sert B [13]	14.3/14.3 (NS)	28.5/14.5 (NS)	160/71 (S)	0/0	0/0	8/4
Ko [14]	3.1/0 (NS)	21.8/18.7	665/82 (S)	31.2/6.3 (NS)	0	4.9/1.7 (S)
Nezhat [15]	6.66/15.4 (NS)	6.6/7.7	200/157 (NS)	–	–	3.8/2.7 (NS)
Fanning J [16]	5	5	300	0	0	1
Kim YT [17]	0	10	355	0	0	7.9
Boggess [18]	7.8%/16.3% (S)	16.3/7.8 (NS)	96.5	0	0	1
Magrina [19]	6/3/0 (NS)	9/6/7 (NS)	208/443/133 (S)	9%/0%/4% (NS)	0/0	2.4/3.6/1.7
Maggioni [20]	12.5/5 (NS)	52.5/30 (NS)	221.8/78 (S)	22.5%/7.5%	0	5/3.7 (S)
Oleszczuk [21]	0	0	123	0	0	4–10
Lowe [12]	4.8	12	50	0	2.4%	1

S significative difference or *NS* no significant difference

demonstrating patients' benefits with the use of laparoscopy as compared to laparotomy for cervical cancer. However, while previous reports demonstrated longer operating times for laparoscopy as compared to laparotomy [18–21], this study showed similar operating times for TRH and TAH, which were significantly shorter as compared to TLH. Two additional differences were noted between TRH and TLH patients: reduced blood loss among patients in the radical subgroup and a shorter hospital stay in the modified radical. Otherwise, laparoscopy and robotic groups compared favorably, and both offered greater patients benefits as compared to laparotomy patients.

Main results

In conclusion, the literature on robotic-assisted radical hysterectomy supports its safety and feasibility for the surgical management of early cervical cancer. Both robotic and laparoscopic radical hysterectomy have been shown to have advantages for patients over the open approach in terms of blood loss, blood transfusions, complications, and length of hospital stay, with the exception of prolonged operation. The available literature suggests that robotic technology may be associated with improved operative outcomes as compared to a traditional laparoscopic approach for radical hysterectomy but no randomized data has been published. Similar recurrence and cure rates have been reported when comparing the results of both techniques. Long-term follow-up data is not available at this time regarding recurrence rates and overall survival. The results of a phase III randomized clinical trial testing the equivalence of outcomes after laparoscopic or robotic radical hysterectomy with abdominal radical hysterectomy in patients with early cervical cancer are expected [22].

Endometrial cancer staging

The first studies were comparative, with historical or open comparison. The open studies presented a low number of patients whereas the case–control studies presented some data with greater statistical power.

Seven publications on TRH and endometrial cancer were selected. The results are presented in Tables 3 and 4.

The first study on endometrial cancer robotic surgery is published by Veljovich et al. [23] in 2008. Analysis of this study suggests that robotic surgery offers the advantages of decreased blood loss and length of stay at the expense of longer operating times. The author anticipates that with more experience with the technology, he will decrease the robotic operative times. The additional 2 h to complete

surgical staging is probably the result of low laparoscopic volume before initiating a robotic program.

Bell et al. [24] published a similar study. Data indicates that robotics or standard laparoscopic staging were about 1 h longer than laparotomy. These data are similar to several other investigators [25, 26] who compared standard TLH to TAH. The perioperative complications are significantly higher for laparotomy procedures than compared to robotic surgery. Furthermore, robotic surgery had resulted in fewer complications than standard laparoscopy [25, 27]. This data demonstrate a significant decrease in hospital stay for both TLH and TRH compared to TAH. The length of stay is directly related to the cost: in this study, both charge data and cost data rank laparotomy as the most expensive modality followed by robotic and laparoscopy.

The study published by Denardis et al. [28] included 56 patients with endometrial cancer who underwent TRH with lymphadenectomy. Robotics data were compared to 106 serially treated patients who were operated by TAH before robotic program. The results are similar to other studies, with a lower rate of perioperative complications, blood loss, transfusion rate, and length of stay. Mean operative time for the TRH cases was more than double that of the open cases, but the TAH mean operative time (79 min) is significantly less than that reported by others authors ranging from 102 to 220 min. Robotic assistance adds a minor amount of time with docking and undocking of the patient-side robotic platform.

Boggess et al. [29] noted a significant reduction in operative time as progress was made through the learning curve, such that the initial robotic surgeries for endometrial cancer required 214 min and the most recent published cases required only 163 min. In a comparative study of three surgical methods for hysterectomy with staging for endometrial cancer (TAH, TLH, and TRH), Boggess concluded that TRH with staging is feasible and preferable over TAH and may be preferable over TLH in endometrial cancer. Further study is necessary to determine long-term oncologic outcomes. Indeed, the TRH and TLH cohorts were comparable with respect to both conversions to TAH and perioperative complications. There were also significantly fewer postoperative complications, when compared with the TAH cohort and a clinically meaningful trend towards fewer post-operative complications, when compared with the TLH cohort. Unlike most studies, Boggess report an increase in the lymph node yield in the robotic cohort compared with both the TAH and TLH cohorts, and a shorter operating time in the robotic cohort, compared with the laparoscopic cohort. For the authors, this in part is due to optimization of port placement that requires a single docking of the robotic instrument and greater ease in overcoming anatomic barriers with robotic assistance, which allows for a more comprehensive lymphadenectomy, such as when

Table 3 Review of literature: studies of robotic assisted hysterectomy in endometrial cancer: population, mean operative time and lymph nodes count

Authors	Year	Methods	Methodology	N	Mean Age (years)	BMI	Mean operative time (min)	Lymph nodes (n)
Veljovich [23]	2008	TAH/TLH/TRH	HC	131/4/25	63/54/59.5	32.2/24.6/27.6	139/255/283	13.1/20.3/17.5 (NS)
Bell [24]	2008	TAH/TLH/TRH	RS	40/30/40	72/68/63	31/31/33	108/171/184 (S and NS)	14.9/17.1/17
Denardis [28]	2008	TAH/TRH	HC	56	63/59	34/29	79/177 (S)	18/19 (NS)
Boggess [29]	2008	TAH/TLH/TRH	PSOC	138/81/103	64/62/61.9	34.7/29/32.9	146/213/191	14.9/23.1/32.9
Hoekstra [30]	2009	TAH/TLH/TRH	HC	26/7/32	56/59/62	37/31/29 (S)	202/270/195 (S)	17/16/17
Lowe P [31]	2009	MI[a] TRH	PS	405	62.2	32.4	170	15.5
Seamon [33]	2009	TLH/TRH	PS and HC	76/105	57/59 (NS)	28.7/34.2 (S)	287/242 (S)	22/21

TAH total abdominal radical abdominal hysterectomy, *TLH* total laparoscopic radical hysterectomy, *TRH* total robot-assisted radical hysterectomy, *S* significative difference or *NS* no significant difference, *CC* case–control study, *HC* historical comparison, *PSOC* prospective study (without randomization) and open comparison, *RS* retrospective study, *PS* prospective study

[a] Multi-institutional total radical robot assisted hysterectomy

obtaining the left periaortic lymph nodes. In the Boggess experience of 103 patients, the surgeons have optimized the port placement to require docking of the robot only once to complete the entire procedure, lymphadenectomy and TRH, thus simplifying the operation, decreasing operative time, and making it more generalizable.

Average estimated blood loss for the TRH group was three times less than that seen in the TAH group and one half that of the TLH group. Patients in the TRH group had a shorter length of stay, when compared with both the TAH and TLH groups. From a clinical standpoint, the estimated blood loss and length of stay results from both the TLH and TRH cohorts were excellent. However, the surgeons in this study had extensive previous laparoscopic experience and still saw significant improvements after the implementation of the robotics program.

In 2009, Hoekstra [30] report the impact of a new robotic surgery program on perioperative outcomes. Median operative time for robotics and laparotomy was significantly less than for laparoscopy. There was no significant difference in lymph nodes yields between the three groups. TRH was associated with significantly less blood loss and lower complication rates compared to the TAH group. Practice management of endometrial cancer transitioned from a predominantly open approach (5.6% TLH, 94.4% TAH) to laparoscopy (11% TLH) and robotics (49% TRH) within 12 months.

The first multi-institutional experience [31] with TRH for endometrial cancer has been recently published by Lowe. The strength of this study is that it allows for analysis and evaluation of data from multiple institutions with surgeons of various levels of experience and expertise

Table 4 Review of literature: studies of robotic assisted hysterectomy in endometrial cancer: complications and outcomes

Authors	Intraoperative complications (%)	Postoperative complications (%)	Estimated blood loss (ml)	Transfusion rate (%)	Conversion rate (%)	Length of stay (days)
Veljovich [23]	–	–	197/75/66[a] (S)(NS)	–	7.4	5.3/1.7
Bell [24]	2.5/3.3/0	25/23/7.5	316/253/166 (S and NS)	15/10/5	–	4/2/2.3[a]
Denardis [28]	20.8/3.6	16.1	241/105 (S)	8.5/0	5.4	3.2/1
Boggess [29]	0.7/3.7/1	28.9/9.9/4.9	266/145/74.5	1.5/2.5/1	−4.9/2.9	4/4/1.2/1[a]
Hoekstra [30]	23/28.5/6.2[a]	46/0/12.5[a]	500/150/50 (S)	–	28.5/3.1	3/1/1[a]
Lowe P [31]	3.5	14.6	87.5	–	6.7	1.8
Seamon [33]	2.6/3.8 (NS)	3.9/1.9 (NS)	88/200 (S)	3/18 (S)	12/26 (S)	1/2

S significant difference or *NS* no significant difference

[a] Significantly different between the open and both robotic and TLH groups, no difference between TLH and TRH groups

with TRH. Each surgeon had performed finally more than 50 robotic surgeries at the time of data analysis. In comparison with the preliminary results of the Lap2 trial of GOG (Walker J), robotic surgery seems at least equivalent if not superior to laparoscopy in several perioperative outcomes. When compared with TAH, a robotic surgical approach has demonstrated an improvement in perioperative outcomes with the exception of operative time in the studies of Boggess, Hoekstra, and Denardis. Although precedent articles primarily represent single institution or single surgeon experiences, the date are very promising and would suggest that a robotic approach is preferable to an open approach and possibly a laparoscopic approach.

The remarkable element of this study [32] is the varying degrees of prior laparoscopic experience among the surgeons before they adopted robotics into their practices. This data suggest that robotic technology may level the playing field between the novice and expert minimally invasive surgeon when applied to complex operations such as endometrial cancer or early cervical cancer staging. Based on these data, the authors feel confident that a strong background in laparoscopy is not a requirement to becoming a successful robotic surgeon.

In that report such as the study of Bell [24], the cost of robotic system was included in the cost analysis for robotic surgery. The total average cost was reported as follows: TAH, $12,943; TLH, $7,569; and TRH, $8,212. There was no statistically significant difference in costs between robotic and laparoscopic approach ($p=0.06$). Both minimally invasive approaches cost significantly less than an open approach ($p=0.001$). However, robotics was associated with less perioperative morbidity and quicker return to normal activity.

Seamon published [33] recently the Ohio State University's experience in TRH for endometrial cancer. The data are similar to precedent studies in term of mean operative time, lymph nodes count, perioperative complications, estimated blood loss, and length of stay. The remarkable element of this study is the report of robotics learning curve. Robotics may offer a shorter learning curve for minimally invasive surgery. When compared with laparoscopy, the robotics platform enables the surgeons to more readily transfer open techniques to a minimal-access setting. For robotic hysterectomy pelvic aortic lymphadenectomy for endometrial cancer, proficiency for Seamon is approximately 20 cases. The most surgeons learning robotic surgery have experience with laparoscopic endometrial cancer staging: unlike the learning curve for laparoscopy [32, 34–36] in which there is a decreased number of lymph nodes as well as an increased estimated blood loss noted during the initial adoption of the procedure, Seamon did not find a statistically significant difference in the robotic

outcomes. The authors noted a significant improvement in times, as experience increased, without compromise in comprehensive staging.

Pelvic and paraaortic lymph node dissection, transperitoneal approach

Laparoscopic pelvic and paraaortic lymph node staging is widely used in patients with advanced cervical cancer prior to initiation of primary chemoradiotherapy [37–40].

An extended pelvic and paraaortic lymphadenectomy can reliably and safely be performed robotically in the management of gynecological malignancies. The robot aids in performing a meticulous dissection and in adhering to sound oncologic principles. For the robotic approach data are available [28, 41, 42] for both pelvic and paraaortic lymphadenectomy performed during staging procedure for endometrial, cervical, or early ovarian cancers. Data are available [37, 43–45] for the laparoscopic approach in terms of safety and feasibility.

The relatively low yield of robotic paraaortic lymphadenectomy with the robot as well as the difficulty of reaching the para-aortic nodes above the inferior mesentery artery must be noticed. No study showed an increased count of lymph nodes in robotic approach in comparison with laparoscopic approach and no randomized data has been published.

Paraaortic lymph node dissection, extraperitoneal approach

Extraperitoneal paraaortic laparoscopic lymphadenectomy is preferable to reduce the risks of adhesions prior to chemoradiotherapy and for obese patients where the transperitoneal approach is sometime impossible. Vergote [46] reported recently on five patients with stage IIb–IIIb cervical carcinoma undergoing robotic retroperitoneal paraaortic lymphadenectomy. For the authors, the procedure was technically easier to perform than with the classical retroperitoneal approach. However, it should be noted that the authors limited the template of dissection to the lower paraaortic area. The number of paraortic lymph nodes removed ranges from 7 to 12, the operating time ranges from 60 to 139 min with one intraoperative complication. In comparison, during a laparoscopic extraperitoneal lymphadenectomy [37], the average duration is 125.9 min and the average number of lymph nodes is 20.7, which is much higher. It must be recalled that the left paraaortic supramesenteric area can be involved alone in cervical and ovarian cancers [47, 48]. Only papers [49] referring to full aortic dissection are potentially relevant.

The main difficulty of robotic approach is the accessibility in one docking to infra- and supra-mesenteric lymph nodes. According to the preliminary experience of Vergote

[46], we believe the da Vinci robot offers advantages due to the steady 3-D visualization, instrumentation with articulating tips that allow for 7° of movement surpassing the human hands mobility, and in addition if needed a downscaling of the surgeons movements without tremor increasing the accuracy and precision.

Narducci et al. [49] published recently their early experience of robotic-assisted laparoscopy for extraperitoneal paraaortic lymphadenectomy up to the left renal vein. Five patients had a left para-aortic lymphadenectomy and one patient had a complete para-aortic lymphadenectomy. The da Vinci surgical system was positioned at the right shoulder of the patient and the assistant stood on the patient's left side. With this position, infrarenal lymph node dissection has been performed by robotic-assisted laparoscopy. The authors concluded that the technique was safe and effective with a short learning period for an experienced oncological team.

Radical parametrectomy

Robotic radical parametrectomy is an option treatment for patients with undiagnosed cervical cancer discovered incidentally on a simple hysterectomy specimen. Traditionally, radical parametrectomy has been performed by laparotomy with few cases described by laparoscopic-assisted vaginal or total laparoscopic approach [50, 51].

Ramirez [52] reported the first five patients treated by robotic radical parametrectomy and pelvic lymphadenectomy. The median operative time was 365 min, estimated blood loss was 100 ml, the median number of pelvic lymph nodes was 14, and there were no conversion to laparotomy. There were two postoperative complications (vesicovaginal fistula and lymphocyst) and one intraoperative complication (cystostomy). The authors concluded this operation is feasible and safe and can be performed with an acceptable complication rate.

Radical trachelectomy

In women with early cervical cancer to preserve fertility, this operation is well established [53–56] and considered to be as safe with laparoscopic pelvic lymphadenectomy. The first report of a robotic radical trachelectomy for fertility sparing in stage Ib1 adenocarcinoma of the cervix was published by Person et al. [57], who reported two cases of robotic radical trachelectomy and pelvic lymphadenectomy performed in two nullipaurous women with early cervical cancer. The duration of the surgeries was 387 and 358 min, respectively. No perioperative complications were observed. The conclusion of Person was that robotic radical

trachelectomy is a safe and feasible alternative to a combined laparoscopic and vaginal approach.

Geisler and Burnett [58, 59] published another case with similar results.

Pelvic exenteration

Minimally invasive surgery may improve the outcome of patients with bulky residual tumors after chemoradiation for locally advanced cervical cancer, and for lateral pelvic wall recurrence. In case of central pelvic recurrence after surgery and adjuvant radiation treatment, pelvic exenteration is the only therapeutic approach with curative goals. The laparoscopy-assisted vaginal pelvic exenteration is feasible [60] with curative intent in selected patients.

Pruthi et al. [61] recently described the technique of robotic-assisted laparoscopic anterior pelvic exenteration performed in 12 women for clinically localized bladder cancer. In all cases, the urinary diversion was performed extracorporeally. Mean operating time was 4.6 h and the mean surgical blood loss was 221 ml. There were two postoperative complications (17%) in two patients.

Conclusions

Potential benefits of robotic technology include 3-D, high-definition optics, instrumentation that allows increased range in motion, precision and scaling, and surgeon autonomy. The mean operating time is longer than laparoscopy but decreases after a short learning curve, even for surgeons with no experience in advanced laparoscopic surgery [12, 31]. One of the favorable effects of the introduction of robotic surgery has been to lead open surgeons to adopt minimal invasive techniques.

However, robotic surgery is basically laparoscopic surgery. Training in standard laparoscopic surgery is definitely required for several reasons: (1) for simple procedures, the cost of robotic surgery is not acceptable; (2) the robot may not be available any time; (3) in case of technical failure, conversion to standard laparoscopic is preferable to conversion to laparotomy; and (4) the assistant must master the spatial orientation characteristic of laparoscopic surgery—that means that the surgeon cannot leave alone this requirement.

The question of the patient benefit and cost-effectiveness of robotic surgery in centers with prior large laparoscopic experience is still open. The results of a prospective randomized trial comparing abdominal, laparoscopic, and open surgery by surgeons equally experienced in all techniques are needed.

Declaration of interest   The authors report no conflicts of interest. The authors alone are responsible for the content and writing of the paper.

References

1. Querleu D, Leblanc E, Ferron G, Narducci F, Rafii A, Martel P (2007) Laparoscopic surgery and gynaecological cancers. Bull Cancer 94(12):1063–1071
2. Beste TM, Nelson KH, Daucher JA (2005) Total laparoscopic hysterectomy utilizing a robotic surgical system. JSLS 9(1):13–15
3. Kho RM, Hilger WS, Hentz JG, Magtibay PM, Magrina JF (2007) Robotic hysterectomy: technique and initial outcomes. Am J Obstet Gynecol 197(1):113–114
4. Advincula AP (2006) Surgical techniques: robot-assisted laparoscopic hysterectomy with the da Vinci surgical system. Int J Med Robot 2(4):305–311
5. Sert BM, Abeler VM (2006) Robotic-assisted laparoscopic radical hysterectomy (Piver type III) with pelvic node dissection—case report. Eur J Gynaecol Oncol 27(5):531–533
6. Reynolds RK, Advincula AP (2006) Robot-assisted laparoscopic hysterectomy: technique and initial experience. Am J Surg 191(4):555–560
7. Fiorentino RP, Zepeda MA, Goldstein BH, John CR, Rettenmaier MA (2006) Pilot study assessing robotic laparoscopic hysterectomy and patient outcomes. J Minim Invasive Gynecol 13(1):60–63
8. Advincula AP, Reynolds RK (2005) The use of robot-assisted laparoscopic hysterectomy in the patient with a scarred or obliterated anterior cul-de-sac. JSLS 9(3):287–291
9. Fanning J, Fenton B, Purohit M (2008) Robotic radical hysterectomy. Am J Obstet Gynecol 198(6):649–4
10. Kim YT, Kim SW, Hyung WJ, Lee SJ, Nam EJ, Lee WJ (2008) Robotic radical hysterectomy with pelvic lymphadenectomy for cervical carcinoma: a pilot study. Gynecol Oncol 108(2):312–316
11. Oleszczuk A, Kohler C, Paulick J, Schneider A, Lanowska M (2009) Vaginal robot-assisted radical hysterectomy (VRARH) after laparoscopic staging: feasibility and operative results. Int J Med Robot 5(1):38–44
12. Lowe MP, Chamberlain DH, Kamelle SA, Johnson PR, Tillmanns TD (2009) A multi-institutional experience with robotic-assisted radical hysterectomy for early stage cervical cancer. Gynecol Oncol 113(2):191–194
13. Sert B, Abeler V (2007) Robotic radical hysterectomy in early-stage cervical carcinoma patients, comparing results with total laparoscopic radical hysterectomy cases. The future is now? Int J Med Robot 3(3):224–228
14. Magrina JF, Kho RM, Weaver AL, Montero RP, Magtibay PM (2008) Robotic radical hysterectomy: comparison with laparoscopy and laparotomy. Gynecol Oncol 109(1):86–91
15. Maggioni A, Minig L, Zanagnolo V et al (2009) Robotic approach for cervical cancer: comparison with laparotomy: a case–control study. Gynecol Oncol 115(1):60–64
16. Nezhat FR, Datta MS, Liu C, Chuang L, Zakashansky K (2008) Robotic radical hysterectomy versus total laparoscopic radical hysterectomy with pelvic lymphadenectomy for treatment of early cervical cancer. JSLS 12(3):227–237
17. Boggess JF, Gehrig PA, Cantrell L et al (2008) A case–control study of robot-assisted type III radical hysterectomy with pelvic lymph node dissection compared with open radical hysterectomy. Am J Obstet Gynecol 199(4):357
18. bu-Rustum NR, Gemignani ML, Moore K et al (2003) Total laparoscopic radical hysterectomy with pelvic lymphadenectomy using the argon-beam coagulator: pilot data and comparison to laparotomy. Gynecol Oncol 91(2):402–409
19. Querleu D (1993) Laparoscopically assisted radical vaginal hysterectomy. Gynecol Oncol 51(2):248–254
20. Frumovitz M, dos Reis R, Sun CC et al (2007) Comparison of total laparoscopic and abdominal radical hysterectomy for patients with early-stage cervical cancer. Obstet Gynecol 110(1):96–102
21. Zakashansky K, Lerner DL (2008) Total laparoscopic radical hysterectomy for the treatment of cervical cancer. J Minim Invasive Gynecol 15(3):387–388
22. Obermair A, Gebski V, Frumovitz M et al (2008) A phase III randomized clinical trial comparing laparoscopic or robotic radical hysterectomy with abdominal radical hysterectomy in patients with early stage cervical cancer. J Minim Invasive Gynecol 15 (5):584–588
23. Veljovich DS, Paley PJ, Drescher CW, Everett EN, Shah C, Peters WA III (2008) Robotic surgery in gynecologic oncology: program initiation and outcomes after the first year with comparison with laparotomy for endometrial cancer staging. Am J Obstet Gynecol 198(6):679
24. Bell MC, Torgerson J, Seshadri-Kreaden U, Suttle AW, Hunt S (2008) Comparison of outcomes and cost for endometrial cancer staging via traditional laparotomy, standard laparoscopy and robotic techniques. Gynecol Oncol 111(3):407–411
25. Frigerio L, Gallo A, Ghezzi F, Trezzi G, Lussana M, Franchi M (2006) Laparoscopic-assisted vaginal hysterectomy versus abdominal hysterectomy in endometrial cancer. Int J Gynaecol Obstet 93(3):209–213
26. Eltabbakh GH, Shamonki MI, Moody JM, Garafano LL (2000) Hysterectomy for obese women with endometrial cancer: laparoscopy or laparotomy? Gynecol Oncol 78(3 Pt 1):329–335
27. Gil-Moreno A, az-Feijoo B, Morchon S, Xercavins J (2006) Analysis of survival after laparoscopic-assisted vaginal hysterectomy compared with the conventional abdominal approach for early-stage endometrial carcinoma: a review of the literature. J Minim Invasive Gynecol 13(1):26–35
28. Denardis SA, Holloway RW, Bigsby GE, Pikaart DP, Ahmad S, Finkler NJ (2008) Robotically assisted laparoscopic hysterectomy versus total abdominal hysterectomy and lymphadenectomy for endometrial cancer. Gynecol Oncol 111(3):412–417
29. Boggess JF, Gehrig PA, Cantrell L et al (2008) A comparative study of 3 surgical methods for hysterectomy with staging for endometrial cancer: robotic assistance, laparoscopy, laparotomy. Am J Obstet Gynecol 199(4):360–369
30. Hoekstra AV, Jairam-Thodla A, Rademaker A et al (2009) The impact of robotics on practice management of endometrial cancer: transitioning from traditional surgery. Int J Med Robot 5(4):392–397
31. Lowe MP, Johnson PR, Kamelle SA, Kumar S, Chamberlain DH, Tillmanns TD (2009) A multiinstitutional experience with robotic-assisted hysterectomy with staging for endometrial cancer. Obstet Gynecol 114(2 Pt 1):236–243
32. Kohler C, Klemm P, Schau A et al (2004) Introduction of transperitoneal lymphadenectomy in a gynecologic oncology center: analysis of 650 laparoscopic pelvic and/or paraaortic transperitoneal lymphadenectomies. Gynecol Oncol 95(1):52–61
33. Seamon LG, Cohn DE, Henretta MS et al (2009) Minimally invasive comprehensive surgical staging for endometrial cancer: robotics or laparoscopy? Gynecol Oncol 113(1):36–41
34. Scribner DR Jr, Walker JL, Johnson GA, McMeekin SD, Gold MA, Mannel RS (2001) Surgical management of early-stage endometrial cancer in the elderly: is laparoscopy feasible? Gynecol Oncol 83(3):563–568
35. Occelli B, Narducci F, Lanvin D, Leblanc E, Querleu D (2000) Learning curves for transperitoneal laparoscopic and extraperitoneal endoscopic paraaortic lymphadenectomy. J Am Assoc Gynecol Laparosc 7(1):51–53

36. Holub Z, Jabor A, Bartos P, Hendl J, Urbanek S (2003) Laparoscopic surgery in women with endometrial cancer: the learning curve. Eur J Obstet Gynecol Reprod Biol 107(2):195–200

37. Querleu D, Dargent D, Ansquer Y, Leblanc E, Narducci F (2000) Extraperitoneal endosurgical aortic and common iliac dissection in the staging of bulky or advanced cervical carcinomas. Cancer 88 (8):1883–1891

38. Kehoe SM, bu-Rustum NR (2006) Transperitoneal laparoscopic pelvic and paraaortic lymphadenectomy in gynecologic cancers. Curr Treat Options Oncol 7(2):93–101

39. Marnitz S, Kohler C, Roth C, Fuller J, Hinkelbein W, Schneider A (2005) Is there a benefit of pretreatment laparoscopic trans-peritoneal surgical staging in patients with advanced cervical cancer? Gynecol Oncol 99(3):536–544

40. Papadia A, Remorgida V, Salom EM, Ragni N (2004) Laparo-scopic pelvic and paraaortic lymphadenectomy in gynecologic oncology. J Am Assoc Gynecol Laparosc 11(3):297–306

41. Magrina JF (2007) Robotic surgery in gynecology. Eur J Gynaecol Oncol 28(2):77–82

42. Holloway RW, Ahmad S, Denardis SA et al (2009) Robotic-assisted laparoscopic hysterectomy and lymphadenectomy for endometrial cancer: analysis of surgical performance. Gynecol Oncol 115(3):447–452

43. Burnett AF, O'Meara AT, Bahador A, Roman LD, Morrow CP (2004) Extraperitoneal laparoscopic lymph node staging: the University of Southern California experience. Gynecol Oncol 95(1):189–192

44. Tillmanns T, Lowe MP (2007) Safety, feasibility, and costs of outpatient laparoscopic extraperitoneal aortic nodal dissection for locally advanced cervical carcinoma. Gynecol Oncol 106(2):370–374

45. Gil-Moreno A, Franco-Camps S, az-Feijoo B et al (2008) Usefulness of extraperitoneal laparoscopic paraaortic lymphade-nectomy for lymph node recurrence in gynecologic malignancy. Acta Obstet Gynecol Scand 87(7):723–730

46. Vergote I, Pouseele B, Van GT et al (2008) Robotic retroperitoneal lower para-aortic lymphadenectomy in cervical carcinoma: first report on the technique used in 5 patients. Acta Obstet Gynecol Scand 87(7):783–787

47. Michel G, Morice P, Castaigne D, Leblanc M, Rey A, Duvillard P (1998) Lymphatic spread in stage Ib and II cervical carcinoma: anatomy and surgical implications. Obstet Gynecol 91(3):360–363

48. edetti-Panici P, Maneschi F, Scambia G, Cutillo G, Greggi S, Mancuso S (1996) The pelvic retroperitoneal approach in the treatment of advanced ovarian carcinoma. Obstet Gynecol 87 (4):532–538

49. Narducci F, Lambaudie E, Houvenaeghel G, Collinet P, Leblanc E (2009) Early experience of robotic-assisted laparoscopy for extraperitoneal para-aortic lymphadenectomy up to the left renal vein. Gynecol Oncol 115(1):172–174

50. Nezhat F, Prasad HM, Peiretti M, Rahaman J (2007) Laparoscopic radical parametrectomy and partial vaginectomy for recurrent endometrial cancer. Gynecol Oncol 104(2):494–496

51. Lee CL, Huang KG (2005) Total laparoscopic radical para-metrectomy. J Minim Invasive Gynecol 12(2):168–170

52. Ramirez PT, Schmeler KM, Wolf JK, Brown J, Soliman PT (2008) Robotic radical parametrectomy and pelvic lymphadenec-tomy in patients with invasive cervical cancer. Gynecol Oncol 111 (1):18–21

53. Shepherd JH, Spencer C, Herod J, Ind TE (2006) Radical vaginal trachelectomy as a fertility-sparing procedure in women with early-stage cervical cancer—cumulative pregnancy rate in a series of 123 women. BJOG 113(6):719–724

54. Diaz JP, Sonoda Y, Leitao MM et al (2008) Oncologic outcome of fertility-sparing radical trachelectomy versus radical hysterectomy for stage IB1 cervical carcinoma. Gynecol Oncol 111(2):255–260

55. Einstein MH, Park KJ, Sonoda Y et al (2009) Radical vaginal versus abdominal trachelectomy for stage IB1 cervical cancer: a comparison of surgical and pathologic outcomes. Gynecol Oncol 112(1):73–77

56. Beiner ME, Hauspy J, Rosen B et al (2008) Radical vaginal trachelectomy vs. radical hysterectomy for small early stage cervical cancer: a matched case–control study. Gynecol Oncol 110(2):168–171

57. Persson J, Kannisto P, Bossmar T (2008) Robot-assisted abdom-inal laparoscopic radical trachelectomy. Gynecol Oncol 111 (3):564–567

58. Burnett AF, Stone PJ, Duckworth LA, Roman JJ (2009) Robotic radical trachelectomy for preservation of fertility in early cervical cancer: case series and description of technique. J Minim Invasive Gynecol 16(5):569–572

59. Geisler JP, Orr CJ, Manahan KJ (2008) Robotically assisted total laparoscopic radical trachelectomy for fertility sparing in stage IB1 adenosarcoma of the cervix. J Laparoendosc Adv Surg Tech A 18(5):727–729

60. Ferron G, Querleu D, Martel P, Letourneur B, Soulie M (2006) Laparoscopy-assisted vaginal pelvic exenteration. Gynecol Oncol 100(3):551–555

61. Pruthi RS, Stefaniak H, Hubbard JS, Wallen EM (2008) Robot-assisted laparoscopic anterior pelvic exenteration for bladder cancer in the female patient. J Endourol 22(10):2397–2402

18

Sun beams on hysterectomies

Liselotte Mettler · Wael Sammur · Thoralf Schollmeyer

Abstract Are hysterectomies still necessary in 2010 and why and how should they be performed? As every now and then a critical evaluation of routine surgical procedure is necessary, there it is: This review follows the "Perspectives on laparoscopic hysterectomy" by Michelle Nisolle (Gynecol Surg 7:105–107, 2010). Hysterectomies performed in the field of obstetrics and gynaecology until the nineteenth century had always a lethal end. In the twentieth century, they were perhaps too frequently performed whereas the twenty-first century has witnessed a steep decline in hysterectomy numbers. It is therefore an opportune time to review the indications for hysterectomies, hysterectomy techniques and the present and future status of this surgical procedure. There is a widespread consensus that hysterectomies are primarily to be performed in cancer cases and obstetrical chaos situations even though minimal invasive surgical technologies have made the procedure more patient-friendly than the classical abdominal opening. Today, minimally invasive hysterectomies are performed as frequently as vaginal hysterectomies, and the vaginal approach is still the first choice if the correct indications are given. It is no longer necessary to open the abdomen; this procedure has been replaced by laparoscopic surgery with multiple and single port entries. Laparoscopic and robotic-assisted laparoscopic surgery can also be indicated for hysterectomies in selected patients with gynaecological cancers. For women of reproductive age, laparoscopic myomectomies and numerous other uterine-preserving techniques are applied in a first treatment step of menometrorrhagia, uterine adenomyosis and submucous myoma. These interventions are only followed by a hysterectomy if the pathology prevails.

Keyword Laparoscopic versus conventional hysterectomies

Background history

In contrast to the twentieth century, hysterectomy is no longer the major gynaecological surgical procedure. How has this change come about? Historical data on the first hysterectomy vary from country to country.

Probably the first documented medical opening of the abdomen took place on December 25, 1809 by Ephraim McDowell (1771–1830). Data relating to the first vaginal hysterectomy go back to the times of Soranus of Ephesus in Greece in the year 120 AD. The first successful abdominal hysterectomies in Europe were performed by Charles Clay on January 3, 1863 and Eugen Köberle on April 3, 1863 in Strasbourg. Both surgeons claimed to have performed the first successful hysterectomy, but this took some time to prove as Clay's first patient in 1843 died soon afterwards. A hysterectomy performed by Conrad Langenbeck on a mentally deficient/retarded patient could not be proved until 26 years later after a postmortem examination.

In the early twentieth century, up until 1945, the subtotal hysterectomy as an abdominal procedure was the universal approach. This type of hysterectomy was associated with less pelvic infections, ureter lesions and other complications in the pre-antibiotic period. After these problems had been

L. Mettler (✉) · T. Schollmeyer
Department of Obstetrics and Gynaecology,
University Hospitals Schleswig-Holstein, Campus Kiel,
Kiel, Germany
e-mail: lmettler@email.uni-kiel.de

W. Sammur
GMC, Dubai Healthcare City,
Dubai, United Arab Emirates

overcome by the development of antibiotics, total hysterectomy was introduced. The main concern was to prevent the occurrence of cervical stump cancer, even though only 0.4% of 6,600 cases were reported in the USA [2] and 0.1% in Finland [3].

Kurt Semm [4] and Tom Lyons [5] published similar data of vaginal cancer following abdominal hysterectomy, yet nobody considered removal of the vagina at hysterectomy as prophylaxis against this.

The Pfannenstiel incision introduced by Johannes Pfannenstiel from Breslau in 1900 proved to be the only real change in the abdominal procedure. This change was from the lower longitudinal abdominal incision to the lower horizontal abdominal incision. The universal acceptance of this incision occurred only after 1970.

Laparoscopic hysterectomies are the achievement of the late twentieth century (see "Laparoscopic hysterectomy" section)

Methods, techniques and findings to resect the uterus in malignant and benign indications

Throughout the world in the US, Germany, Asia, Africa and Australia, gynaecologists have had ample opportunity over the last 40 years to become acquainted with all surgical methods of hysterectomy.

Vaginal hysterectomy

The first hysterectomy performed at the time of Soranus of Ephesus and the newest technique, performed in the twenty-first century under the name of Natural Orifice Surgery, use the vagina as the entrance and exit point. For all gynaecologists and surgeons, there are many ways to perform an operation, but the lex parsimoniae of William Ockham (1235–1350) is always valuable: "If we have different ways to solve a problem, the simplest way is the right one." Surgery is no exception.

When Langenbeck first performed a vaginal hysterectomy in 1813, the discipline of gynaecology was founded. Since then, vaginal access has been the privilege of the gynaecological surgeon.

Austria, with the brilliant schools of Schauta and Wertheim, still has the highest European rate of vaginal surgery. Shiril Sheth 2006 reports on >5,000 vaginal hysterectomies in his Indian experience [6]. Twenty randomized controlled trials (RCTs) comparing total abdominal hysterectomy, vaginal hysterectomy and laparoscopic hysterectomy and 16 RCTs comparing laparoscopic hysterectomies with total abdominal hysterectomies clearly stated that laparoscopic hysterectomy requires greater surgical skill. Vaginal hysterectomy leaves behind no scars

and is the faster operative technique. Vaginal hysterectomy should be performed for the following indications:

1. Uterine prolapse
2. Dysfunctional uterine bleeding
3. Adenomyosis
4. Carcinoma in situ CIN3 of cervix
5. High risk with endometrial cancer
6. Cervical fibroids and uterine polyposis

Operative steps

Vaginal hysterectomy can be performed in six steps according to the situs of the patient [6].

1. Circumcision of the cervix with the scalpel after grasping the cervix with two sutures or cervical clamps. According to Joel-Cohen 1972 [7] and Stark 2006 [8], in patients with uterine prolapse, the incision of the vaginal wall can also start below the orificium urethrae externum. If the cut is deep enough, the vaginal wall can be pushed back with the finger and mobilisation is easy. If necessary, the vaginal wall can be separated from the cervix with scissors.
2. Separation of bladder from uterus and opening of the spatium vesico uterinum or the spatium recto uterinum. If the spatium vesico uterinum cannot be opened easily, it is easier to open the spatium recto uterinum with scissors until the sacrouterine ligaments are visible.
3. Clamping, dissection, suturing or coagulation of the sacrouterine ligaments. The sacrouterine ligaments and paracervical tissue must not bleed. In patients with uterine prolapse, the uterine vessels are directly visible.
4. Identification of the uterine vessels, separation by knife or scissors, suturing or, often today, the use of the biclamp, followed by sharp dissection. If the peritoneum in the area of the vesico-uterine space was not opened, it is now opened by sharp dissection.
5. Extraction of the uterus through the vagina after separation from the round ligaments, the ovarian ligaments or from the infundibulopelvic ligaments. This step is sometimes performed with clamps, dissection and suturing or with the Biclamp® (thermofusion).
6. The peritoneum is left open and only the vagina is closed with individual sutures. If necessary, a reconstruction of the pelvic floor is performed to prevent consecutive vaginal prolapse or formation of a Douglas-cele by placing an extra suture between the two sacrouterine ligaments and the vaginal stump.

According to the data collected by the Center for Disease Control in the USA [9, 10] the mortality rate for a vaginal hysterectomy—excluding cancer patients or obstetrical chaos situations—is 2.7/10,000 compared to 8.6/10,000 for an abdominal hysterectomy.

Abdominal hysterectomy

After the first unintended abdominal supracervical hysterectomies of Charles Clay (1843) and Ellis Burnham (1853), the first deliberate hysterectomy, with the patient surviving, was carried out in 1855 by Kimball. This was an abdominal supracervical hysterectomy. After the introduction of anaesthesia by William Morton on October 16, 1846, there were several reports of abdominal hysterectomy but with a mortality of 25%. Charles Clay performed his first successful hysterectomy with a patient surviving on January 3, 1863 and Eugen Köberle on April 3, 1863. Both of these doctors are considered the fathers of abdominal hysterectomy.

In 1880, T. G. Thomas reported on 365 collected cases of abdominal hysterectomy which revealed a staggering mortality of 70%. In comparison, vaginal hysterectomy had a mortality rate of 15% in 1886. Nevertheless, in 1878, Mikulicz and Wilhelm Alexander Freund [11] provoked progress in abdominal hysterectomy. They placed three ligatures on the broad ligaments, and through the introduction of new techniques for subtotal hysterectomy, the mortality rate went down in the period 1896 until 1906, from 22% to 3.4%.

In the middle of the twentieth century, apart from the change from subtotal which dominated through 1945 with Cutler and Zolenger [2] to total hysterectomy, the only change in the abdominal procedure was the almost universal adoption of the less disfiguring suprasymphysary incision introduced by Johannes Pfannenstiel.

Operative steps

The procedure of abdominal hysterectomy is tailored to the indication. The uterus has to be visualized and freed in the first step. In the second step, the round ligaments are separated from the uterus. In the third step, the adnexa are separated from the uterus or from the pelvic wall. In the fourth step, the parametrium is opened, and the bladder is pushed down in the fifth step. The uterine vessels are clamped, separated and sutured. In the sixth step, the uterus is separated from the vagina trying to preserve the uterine ligament connection. In the seventh step, the vagina is closed and the sacrouterine ligaments are fixed to/through the vagina to prevent Douglas-cele (Moskowitsch technique). In the eighth and last step, after rinsing of the minor pelvis, the visceral peritoneum is left open.

Minilaparotomy hysterectomy

The minilaparotomy procedure may be considered a time-saving technique for total hysterectomy for benign uterine pathology. It offers some of the advantages of a minimally invasive procedure (low morbidity, short hospital stay and good cosmetic results) and the benefits of open access (for example, shorter learning curve than laparoscopy). It is a minimally invasive, feasible option, particularly in countries where laparoscopic hysterectomies are not available. In many reports, minilaparotomy hysterectomy has been compared to laparotomy and laparoscopic-assisted vaginal hysterectomy [12, 13].

Laparoscopic hysterectomy

This technique was developed over the last 25 years. As early as 1984, our teacher, Kurt Semm, was already using laparoscopic assistance in difficult vaginal hysterectomies [14].

He called this technique laparoscopic assistance for vaginal hysterectomies. In fact, many vaginal hysterectomies were performed in Kiel with laparoscopic assistance to dissect the uterus from the round ligaments, the adnexa, the sacrouterine ligaments and the cardinal ligaments. However, worldwide discussion on laparoscopic hysterectomy began after the first published laparoscopic-assisted vaginal hysterectomy by Harry Reich in 1989 [15]. We began to perform supracervical laparoscopic hysterectomy in 1989, but the first publication did not appear until 1991 [4]. Prior to this, a few journals had turned down our submitted papers, referring to the absurdity of such a surgical technique.

Nezhat et al. in the United States described their first radical hysterectomy in 1991, but a publication did not appear until 1992 [16].

Laparoscopic hysterectomies in their different forms have been a provocation for gynaecologists for the last 20 years. Gynaecologists favour the vaginal technique, and today, the only indications remaining for abdominal operations are of a malignant nature. If the operative indication for laparoscopic hysterectomy is given and the surgeon is an experienced laparoscopist, the majority of patients can be spared a laparotomy. Figure 1 gives an overview of the combination possibilities for laparoscopic and vaginal surgery, including parailiacal and paraaortic lymphadenectomies and the subtotal hysterectomies. In comparison to conventional abdominal hysterectomy and vaginal hysterectomy, the following laparoscopic hysterectomy techniques are currently practised [6, 17–19].

1. Laparoscopic-assisted vaginal hysterectomy (LAVH)
2. Total laparoscopic hysterectomy (TLH) or laparoscopic hysterectomy (LH)
3. Intrafascial supracervical hysterectomy (CISH), subtotal or supracervical hysterectomy (LSH)

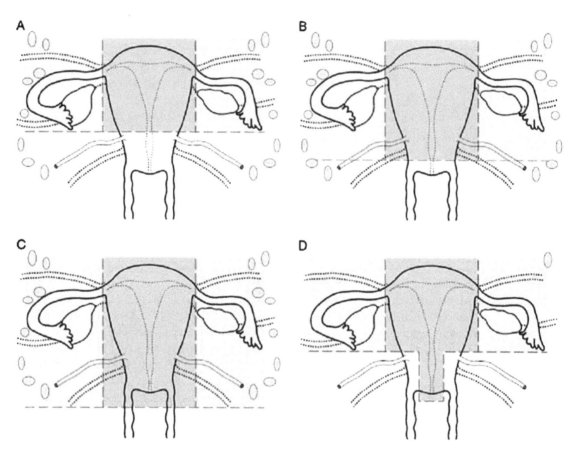

Fig. 1 Variations of laparoscopic hysterectomies (**a**–**d**). In *green* and *blue*, the laparoscopic surgery and in *white*, the vaginal surgery or no further surgery. **a** Laparoscopic resection of the uterus in the region of the round ligament, adnexa and infundibulopelvic ligament from the pelvic side wall above the cardinal ligament with or without lymphadenectomy; the uterus is extracted via the vagina. In case of laparoscopic subtotal hysterectomy (LSH), the uterus is resected above the cervix and the cervical stump remains. Morcellation of the uterus for transabdominal retraction. **b** Laparoscopic resection of the uterus starting from the round ligament up to the infundibulopelvic ligament. Cutting of the uterine vessels and mobilisation of the cervix up to the cervical stump with or without lymph nodes, opening of the paracervical and pararectal spaces and retraction of the uterus through the vagina. **c** Laparoscopic resection of the uterus from the round ligament and infundibulopelvic ligament and uterine artery, visualization of paravesical and pararectal spaces with mobilisation of the uterus, including the upper third of the vagina with or without lymphadenectomy, along with the parametria and retraction of the uterus from the vagina. **d** Classic intrafascial subtotal hysterectomy with coring of the inner cervix and endoscopic resection of the uterus up to above the cardinal ligament. Tying only of ascending branch of the uterine artery without lymphadenectomy (for hysterectomy in benign lesions). Morcellation of the uterus for transabdominal retraction

4. Laparoscopic radical hysterectomy (LRC) according to Wertheim or Schauta, with further specifications according to different schools
5. Robotic assistance in oncologic hysterectomy.

Robotic laparoscopic radical hysterectomy is a variation of LRH. A trachelectomy is performed in lymph node-free cases, whereby the total cervix is dissected and the vagina attached to the uterus.

Laparoscopic-assisted vaginal hysterectomy

In this case, the uterus is mobilised laparoscopically and resected transvaginally. The dissection is carried down to but excluding the uterine vessels which are secured vaginally. Similarly, uterosacral and cardinal ligaments are clamped and transfixed ligated transvaginally. LAVH is performed in four laparoscopic and three vaginal surgical steps [18, 20].

Total laparoscopic hysterectomy or LH

Indications for TLH include benign gynaecological alterations such as fibroids, endometriosis and dysfunctional uterine bleeding in patients for whom vaginal surgery is contraindicated or cannot be performed. TLH may be performed for possible malignant indications such as early endometrial cancer, early localised small cervical cancers (trachelectomy) and also in the early stages of ovarian cancer with lymphadenectomies. The laparoscopic part consists of the preparation of the uterus and the cervix and the complete dissection of the vaginal stump. The individual steps of this procedure are detailed in Fig. 2.

*The intrafascial supracervical hysterectomy
and the laparoscopic subtotal hysterectomy*

In recognition of the CISH technique, performed at the Kiel University Hospital from 1991 to 1995 [21] and still practised with interesting modifications in many countries, we would like to describe the CISH technique and the currently more frequently used LSH technique.

CISH technique Subtotal hysterectomy represents the method of choice in every form of benign uterine disease that affects only the uterus with no cervical abnormality. Annual cervical cytological surveillance is recommended to detect intracervical neoplasia which can occur if the cervix remains intact. Kurt Semm performed subtotal hysterectomy with coring of the inner cervix to totally resect the cylindrical cervical epithelium [4]. The operative steps are detailed in Fig. 3, in a sequence from A till L. The cervix is dissected from the uterine corpus with a LINA loop [6], and the uterus is morcellated transabdominally. It is also now possible to morcellate the

Fig. 2 Total laparoscopic hysterectomy (TLH). **a** Multifibroid uterus, **b** dissection of the left round ligament, **c** preparation of left uterine vessels, **d** presentation of right uterine vessels, **e** ultrasound coagulation and separation of right uterine vessels, **f** ischemic uterus elevated by the uterine manipulator according to Mangeshikar, **g** vaginal delineation line on the ceramic cap of the Mangeshikar manipulator, **h** separation of cervix from vagina using the monopolar hook, **i** the cap becomes visible in the vaginal fornix, **j** continuous dissection of uterus from vagina, **k** extraction of a 210-g uterus from vagina and **l** reinsertion of the manipulator tube with ceramic cap to keep the pneumoperitoneum, closure of vaginal stump with a continuous suture and two corner sutures. To prevent enterocele formation, the sacrouterine ligaments are attached to the vaginal stump

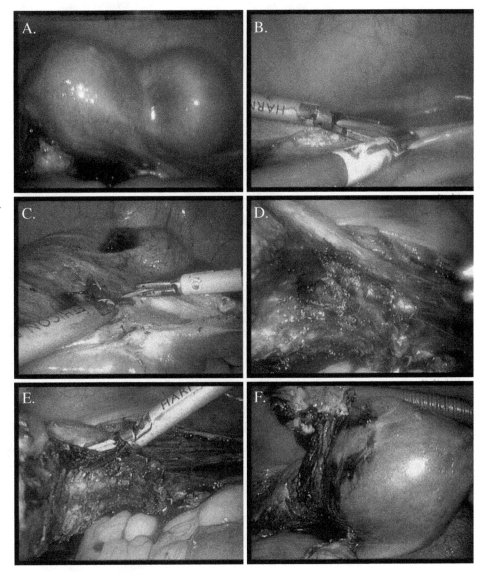

A. Multifibroid uterus
B. Dissection of the left round ligament
C. Preparation of left uterine vessels
D. Presentation of right uterine vessels
E. Ultrasound-coagulation and separation of right uterine vessels
F. Ischemic uterus elevated by the uterine manipulator according to Mangeshikar

Fig. 2 (continued)

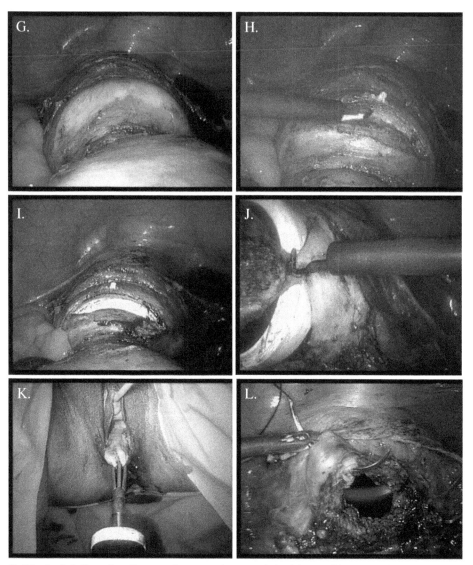

G. Vaginal delineation line on the ceramic cap of the Mangeshikar manipulator
H. Separation of cervix from vagina using the monopolar hook
I. The cap becomes visible in the vaginal fornix
J. Continuous dissection of uterus from vagina
K. Extraction of a 210 g uterus from vagina
L. Reinsertion of the manipulator tube with ceramic cap to keep the pneumoperitoneum,
   closure of vaginal stump with a continuous suture and two corner sutures. To prevent
   enterocele formation, the sacrouterine ligaments are attached to the vaginal stump.

uterus transcervically with the Rotocut (Storz) after coagulation of the ascending branches of the uterine arteries, but without the positioning of Roeder loops.

LSH technique The advantage of the LSH procedure is that it can be performed on nulliparous patients, patients who have not previously had a vaginal delivery and patients who have had previous abdominal surgery. In these cases, the

uterus is morcellated, but no colpotomy is performed. The technique is used mainly for fibroids, therapy-resistant dysfunctional uterine bleeding and adenomyosis. This technique is now practised routinely in Kiel according to the standardised safe minimally invasive technique [22, 23]. In a retrospective study on the clinical significance of adhesions, the effect of SprayShield as an adhesion prophylaxis has been evaluated [24].

Fig. 3 Classic intrafascial subtotal hysterectomy (CISH). **a** Multifibroid uterus, **b** dissection of left adnexa from the uterus with a stapler, **c** opening of the vesico-uterine space, **d** preparation of the bladder, **e** demonstration of the pericervical fascial ring, **f** transcervical and transuterine resection of a 15-mm tissue cylinder including the "transformation zone around an axial guide rod", **g** positioning of a "Roeder loop" as tourniquet to tie the ascending branches of the uterine arteries, **h** sharp dissection of cervix from the uterine corpus with scissors (or a monopolar loop as LINA Loop or Storz cervical loop), **i** further cervical dissection, **j** separation of uterine body from the cervix, **k** morcellation of the uterus and **l** irrigation leaving the visceral peritoneum open

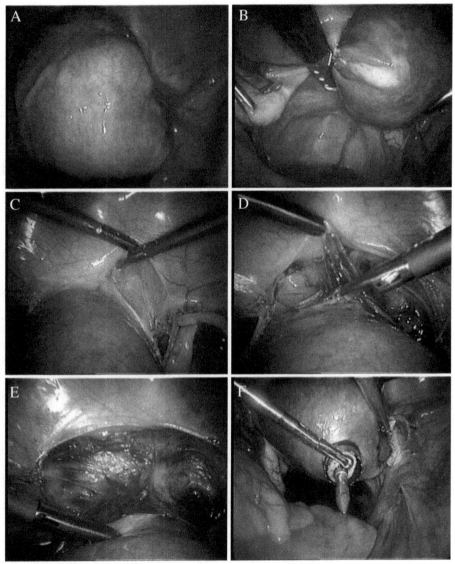

A) Multifibroid uterus
B) Dissection of left adnexa from the uterus with a stapler
C) Opening of the vesico-uterine space
D) Preparation of the bladder
E) Demonstration of the pericervical fascial ring
F) Transcervical and transuterine resection of a 15 mm tissue cylinder including the "transformation zone around an axial guide rod

Laparoscopic radical hysterectomy (Wertheim or Schauta technique)

Following the lead of earlier surgeons, a few skilled European and American gynaecologic surgeons have further refined the technique of radical hysterectomy, partly using robotic assistance. In addition to the Nezhat brothers [16] and Jo Childers [25, 26], who have been propagandists for radical endoscopic surgery worldwide, European colleagues such as

Daniel Dargent [27], Denny Querleu [28], Achim Schneider and Mark Possover [29] have also put intensive work into oncologic endoscopic surgery. However, it is a colleague of the third world, Shailesh Puntambekar, who has successfully brought world attention to the possibility of radical oncological surgery via laparoscopy [30].

In 1986, Dargent already began to perform laparoscopic trachelectomy in cases of small cervical cancers with no iliac lymph node metastases [27].

Fig. 3 (continued)

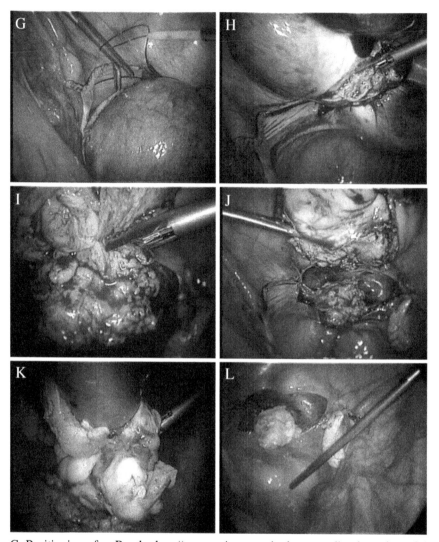

G. Positioning of a „Roeder loop"as tourniquet to tie the ascending branches of the uterine arteries

H. Sharp dissection of cervix from the uterine corpus with scissors (or a monopolar loop as LINA Loop or Storz cervical loop.

I. Further cervical dissection

J. Separation of uterine body from the cervix

K. Morcellation of the uterus

L. Irrigation leaving the visceral peritoneum open

Shailesh Putambekar performs laparoscopic radical hysterectomy not only in endometrial and early cervical cancers, but also for anterior exenteration [31, 32].

A few of us have had the opportunity to work with Shailesh Putambekar in India and in Germany. He performs excellent anterior exenterations endoscopically and proves repeatedly that radical hysterectomies are possible via the endoscopic approach.

The results of radical laparoscopic [33] and radical robotic cancer surgery [34] compare well with the outcome of radical abdominal and vaginal cancer surgery. Radical laparoscopic vaginal hysterectomy according to Schauta is successfully practised in Germany by Schneider et al. and Possover et al.

Endoscopic surgery for malignant alterations has the same chance of success as open surgery, with less surgical trauma. It depends as much on subsequent chemo or radiation therapy as open surgery does. Molecular genetic progress in the therapy of malignant disease will show the real role endoscopic surgery can take.

Robotic assistance in oncologic hysterectomies

The first robotic camera assistant used in endoscopic surgery was the automated endoscopic system for optimal positioning (AESOP; Computer Motion, Goleta, California, USA). This hand, foot or voice-controlled arm allows the surgeon to perform complex laparoscopic surgery faster than with an assistant holding the camera. The next surgical robot was a voice-controlled robot ZEUS (Computer Motion) that consists of AESOP to hold the camera and two additional AESOP-like units, which have been modified to hold the surgical instruments. The modern robot generation named da Vinci surgical system is based on the technologies of Computer Motion and developed by Intuitive Surgical (Mountain View, California, USA). It was approved by the US Food and Drug Administration in May 2005 for clinical use in gynaecology and was first

used in reproductive gynaecology for tubal surgery [35]. There are four main components of the da Vinci surgical system [34].

(1) Surgeon's console: the surgeon sits viewing a magnified three-dimensional image of the surgical field (Fig. 4a–c).
(2) Patient-side cart: this system consists of three instrument arms and one endoscope arm (Fig. 4d).
(3) Detachable instruments (EndoWrist instruments and Intuitive Masters): these detachable instruments allow

Fig. 4 a Da Vinci 2005 steering unit, **b** working position of surgeon, **c** finger movements for robotic action of instruments. Patient-side cart: **d** three-dimensional rapid robotic arms ready to be connected to the three active instruments. Detachable instruments: **e** robotic arm with one working channel. Three-dimensional vision system: **f** abdominal situs at suturing

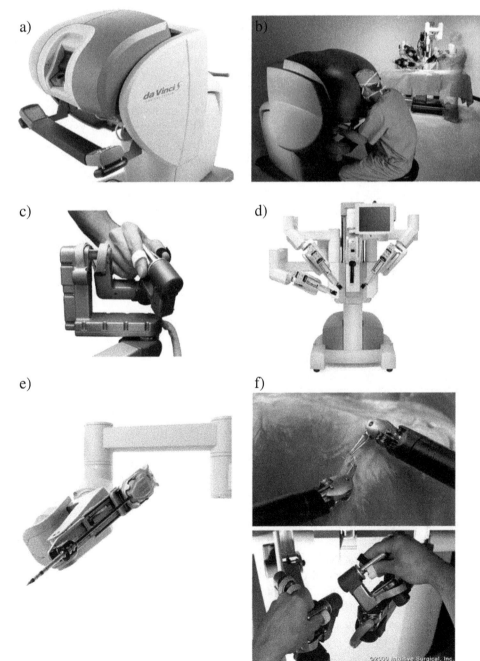

a)

b)

c)

d)

e)

f)

the robotic arms to manoeuvre in ways that simulate fine human movements. There are seven degrees of freedom which offer considerable choice of rotation in full circles. The surgeon is able to control the amount of force applied, which varies from a fraction of a gramme to several kilos. Tremor and scale movements are filtered out. The movements of the surgeon's hand can be translated into smaller ones by the robotic device (Fig. 4e).

(4) Three-dimensional vision system: the camera unit or endoscope arm provides enhanced three-dimensional images with the result that the surgeon knows the exact position of all instruments in relation to the anatomical structures (Fig. 4f).

The patients lie in a horizontal position with both arms tucked alongside their body. Four trocars are placed next to the optic trocar. The surgeon sits at the console and the first surgical assistant is seated in most cases on the patients' left side. This assistant controls the left accessory ports into which the instruments that are used for vessel sealing, retraction, suction, irrigation and suturing are inserted. The middle robotic arm is attached to the optical trocar with two lateral working arms to the right and one to the left. The robotic arms are connected at the beginning of the procedure and disengaged from the trocars at the end of the operation. The incisions are stitched, and the incision lines are reapproximated.

A three-dimensional vision allows the surgeon to perform ultra precise manipulations with intraabdominal-articulated instruments while providing the necessary degrees of freedom [35–42].

Results of robotic-assisted procedures in gynaecological oncology (comparative studies) The team from University of North Carolina reported on 43 robotic-assisted laparoscopic hysterectomies with pelvic and paraaortic lymph node dissection for women with endometrial cancer as a simple case report. There were no conversions to laparotomy in the robotic group compared with 3% in the laparoscopy group. There were significantly more nodes recovered in the robotically staged patients (29.8 versus 23.2). The mean blood loss in the robotic group was 63 ml (25–300), with 45% of patients having no measurable blood loss compared with 142 ml (50–700) in the laparoscopy group. Mean operative time was 163 min compared with 213, and hospital stay was 1.0 compared with 1.2 days, respectively. There were 4.6% major complications in the robotic group compared with 12.8% in the laparoscopy group [43].

The team from Mayo Clinic in Scottsdale compared robotic-assisted surgery, laparoscopic surgery and open laparotomy in patients undergoing radical abdominal hysterectomy with bilateral lymphadenectomy for cervical cancer. They operated on 27 patients robotically with a mean operative time of 189.6 min, 31 patients laparoscopically with a mean operative time of 220.4 min and 34 patients had an open laparotomy, with a mean operative time of 166.8 min; the mean blood loss was 133.1, 208.4 and 443.6 ml, respectively. In this team, robotic lymphadenectomy in 27 patients resulted in a mean of 25.9 excised lymph nodes, and this appeared to be equal to that observed in laparoscopic lymphadenectomy in 31 patients, in which a mean of 25.9 lymph nodes was excised. These results compare well with open abdominal lymphadenectomy, with the mean number of excised lymph nodes being 27.7.

The robotic and laparotomy operating time was significantly shorter as compared with laparoscopy in the subgroup of patients undergoing the modified radical but not the radical technique [44]. In contrast, Boggess and colleagues reported that open abdominal pelvic lymphadenectomy in 48 patients resulted in a mean of 22.3 lymph nodes being excised, which was significantly less than the mean of 38.4 lymph nodes when robotic lymphadenectomy was used in 31 patients. As compared with laparoscopy, patients having robotically assisted surgery experienced reduced blood loss (176 versus 328 ml) and reduced hospitalisation (1.9 versus 2.9 days), though the lymph node count was higher for the laparoscopy group. There were no intraoperative or major postoperative complications in either group [45].

Alternative techniques to hysterectomies

Over the last 10 years, the techniques of uterine artery embolization (UAE) and magnetic resonance imaging (MRI) guidance of focussed ultrasound for uterine leiomyoma treatment have been developed. Descriptions of MRI-guided focussed ultrasound therapy treatment of fibroids indicate that it is an effective treatment for uterine leiomyomata and results in sustained symptomatic relief [46–48].

Uterine artery embolization

Is an alternative to hysterectomy in women seeking treatment for symptomatic uterine myomas [49, 50]. It is associated with a good success rate in properly selected patients, with few major complications [51, 52].

Because of the high risk of infection, women who have had UAE and present with necrotic myoma adjacent to the endometrium should not undergo endometrial biopsy. Routine evaluation of the myoma in relation to the endometrium by means of imaging is recommended.

Endometrium ablation techniques

Endometrium ablation techniques of the first generation= hysteroscopic endometrial resection and coagulation. In long-term studies, a success rate of 80% was achieved in reducing, but not eradicating, dysfunctional bleedings. Hysteroscopic endometrial techniques, such as the YAG laser, the resectoscope and rollerball technique (also a combination of both techniques), cryoablation and microwave techniques are available.

Second-generation methods of endometrial ablation include a number of global ablation techniques. One of the most effective appears to be the NovaSure™ System which was introduced to Germany in 1998 by A. Gallinat [53]. It consists of a bipolar ablation device and a radio-frequency controller that enables endometrial ablation in an average of 90 s.

MRI-guided focussed ultrasound

MRI-guided focussed ultrasound is a non-invasive treatment in which ultrasound energy, focussed on the fibroid in multiple focal spots, raises the temperature of tissue within the focal zone and causes coagulative necrosis. MRI guides and monitors the procedure, thus, providing a closed loop anatomical and thermal feedback. MRI is used to identify tumours or fibroids in the body before they are destroyed by ultrasound. Therapeutic ultrasound is a minimally invasive or non-invasive method to deposit acoustic energy into tissue.

Conclusions and recommendation

Limits for hysterectomies

Are there limits for hysterectomies or for which indications are hysterectomies still recommended? According to present medical standards, malignant disease of the ovaries, tubes and uterus is to be treated by hysterectomy. According to Dargent, trachelectomy can replace hysterectomy in younger women with early cervical cancer (smaller than 2 cm and without lymph node lesions in the cervix).

Contraindications for vaginal hysterectomy are a very large uterus that cannot be vaginally morcellated and non-descent of uterus. In these cases, laparoscopy, in combination with vaginal hysterectomy, can be performed. Abdominal hysterectomy has become less important and is mainly performed for cancer cases. The size of the uterus, multiple adhesions, endometriosis and obstetrical chaos situations can limit the feasibility of laparoscopic hysterectomy. In cases of massive bleeding, abdominal access is still the chosen route. Natural Orifice Surgery, with one instrument panel applied transvaginally, may open new doors for vaginal surgery.

Hysterectomy for benign indications, irrespective of surgical technique, increases the risk for stress urinary incontinence which may occur through damage to nerves, vascular supply or uterine descent [54]. It is also associated with an increased risk for subsequent pelvic organ prolapse leading to enterocele prolapse [55]. LSH or LASH seems to meet best patient satisfaction [56].

Future aspects

Considering how long *Homo sapiens* has inhabited the planet earth, the history of hysterectomy is a short one. This surgical technique began with a high mortality rate and a high morbidity rate, but with technological advances in the twentieth and twenty-first centuries, particularly after antisepsis and antibiotic prophylaxis eradicated infections and safe anaesthesia and infusion therapy decreased the high mortality rates, the procedure has now become very safe, with a mortality rate of approximately 12 per 10,000 [57]. Hysterectomy, with a few exceptions (cancer cases), is increasingly performed to improve quality of life, rather than to save life.

It is difficult to foresee the future, but almost certainly, other alternatives to hysterectomy will continue to evolve. For example, a better understanding of endometriosis has already produced a new therapy basis for this disease. The development of a HPV vaccine, early cervical cancer detection and the effective recognition of endometrium carcinoma also influence therapy. No surgical alternative for ovarian cancer has so far been found, and hysterectomy, in addition to lymphadenectomy and omentum resection, prevails. These techniques, however, can be performed laparoscopically [29, 58].

Summary

In the twenty-first century, abdominal hysterectomy as a surgical intervention for benign indications belongs in the past. With appropriate indications and modern morcellation techniques, even large uteri up to 1 kg and more can be surgically removed with laparoscopic assistance transvaginally or totally laparoscopically. Vaginal hysterectomy is still the favoured route. It should only not be used if symptoms of the patient, the expected morbidity or the inexperience of the surgeon with the vaginal technique demand laparoscopic assistance.

Malignant disease of the vagina, cervix, uterus, tubes or ovaries is the primary indication for abdominal hysterectomy as centres which are able to perform laparoscopic and robotic-assisted laparoscopic techniques for malignant disease are still rare. The further development of laparoscopic vaginal surgery in oncology, as developed by Dargent, remains a challenge for the endoscopic surgeon in the twenty-first century.

Alternative techniques to hysterectomy, such as endometrium ablation, have emerged and should always be considered before a hysterectomy is performed. For benign indications with an intact cervix, no endometriosis and no previous cervical surgery, laparoscopic subtotal hysterectomy leaving the cervix in place (LSH, CISH) provides a minimally invasive alternative to all other methods of total hysterectomy in benign conditions.

However, if the patient cannot have regular controls postoperatively, laparoscopic total hysterectomy is preferable as with subtotal hysterectomy regular pap or thin-prep controls are necessary.

Acknowledgement We highly acknowledge the excellent assistance of our office managers, Dawn Rüther and Nicole Guckelsberger. We thank them for their lasting and continuous support.

Declaration of interest The authors report no conflicts of interest. The authors alone are responsible for the content and writing of the paper.

References

1. Nisolle M (2010) Perspectives on laparoscopic hysterectomy. Gynecol Surg 7:105–107
2. Cutler EC, Zolenger RM (1949) Atlas of surgical operations. McMillan & Co, New York
3. Kilkku P, Gronroos M et al (1985) Supravaginal uterine amputation with peroperative electrocoagulation of endocervical mucosa. Description of the method. Acta Obstet Gynecol Scand 64(2):175–177
4. Semm K (1991) Hysterektomie per laparotomiam oder per pelviscopiam. Geburtshilfe Frauenheilkd 51(12):996–1003
5. Lyons TL (1993) Laparoscopic supracervical hysterectomy. A comparison of morbidity and mortality results with laparoscopically assisted vaginal hysterectomy. J Reprod Med 38(10):763–767
6. Mettler L (ed) (2007) Manual of new hysterectomy techniques. Jaypee Brothers, New Delhi
7. Joel-Cohen SJ (1972) Abdominal and vaginal hysterectomy: new techniques based on time and motion studies. Heinemann, London
8. Stark M, Gerli S et al (2006) The ten-step vaginal hysterectomy. Prog Obstet Gynaecol 17:358–368
9. Sheth SS (2002) Vaginal or abdominal hysterectomy. In: Sheth SS, Studd JW (eds) Vaginal hysterectomy. Martin Dunitz Ltd, London, pp 301–320
10. Sheth SS (2005) Vaginal hysterectomy. Best Pract Res Clin Obstet Gynaecol 19(3):307–332
11. Freund WA (1878) Bemerkungen zu meiner Methode der Uterusextirpation. Zbl Gynäkol 2:497–500
12. Muzii L, Basile S et al (2007) Laparoscopic-assisted vaginal hysterectomy versus minilaparotomy hysterectomy: a prospective, randomized, multicenter study. J Minim Invasive Gynecol 14(5):610–615
13. Royo P, Alcazar JL et al (2009) The value of minilaparotomy for total hysterectomy for benign uterine disease: a comparative study with conventional Pfannenstiel and laparoscopic approaches. Int Arch Arb Med 2(1):11
14. Semm K (1984) Operationslehre für endoskopische abdominalchirurgie. Schattauer, Stuttgart
15. Reich H, DeCaprio J et al (1989) Laparoscopic hysterectomy. J Gynecol Surg 5:213–216
16. Nezhat CR, Burrell MO et al (1992) Laparoscopic radical hysterectomy with paraaortic and pelvic node dissection. Am J Obstet Gynecol 166(3):864–865
17. Mettler L, Semm K (1994) Pelviscopy and its secrets to detect and treat genital endometriosis. In: Coutinho E, Spinola P, Hanson de Moura L (eds) Progress in the management of endometriosis. Parthenon, New York, pp 327–333
18. Mettler L, Ahmed-Ebbiary N et al (2005) Laparoscopic hysterectomy: challenges and limitations. Minim Invasive Ther Allied Technol 14(3):145–159
19. Mettler L (ed) (2006) Manual for laparoscopic and hysteroscopic gynecological surgery. Jaypee Brothers, New Delhi
20. Mettler L (ed) (2002) Endoskopische Abdominalchirurgie in der Gynäkologie. Schattauer, Stuttgart
21. Semm K (1993) Hysterectomy by pelviscopy; an alternative approach without colpotomy (CASH). In: Garry R, Reich H (eds) Laparoscopic hysterectomy. Blackwell Scientific Publications, Oxford, pp 118–132
22. Salfelder A, Lueken RP et al (2005) A prospective multicenter study by the VAAO. Geburtshilfe Frauenheilkd 65:396–403
23. Bojahr B, Raatz D et al (2007) Laparoscopic supracervical hysterectomy: a standardised safe minimal invasive technique. In: Mettler L (ed) Manual of new hysterectomy techniques. Jaypee Brothers, New Delhi
24. Mettler L, Alhujeily M (2007) Role of laparoscopy in identifying the clinical significance and cause of adhesions and chronic pelvic pain: a retrospective review at the Kiel School of Gynecological Endoscopy. JSLS 11(3):303–308
25. Childers JM, Surwit EA (1992) Combined laparoscopic and vaginal surgery for the management of two cases of stage I endometrial cancer. Gynecol Oncol 45(1):46–51
26. Childers JM, Brzechffa PR et al (1993) Laparoscopically assisted surgical staging (LASS) of endometrial cancer. Gynecol Oncol 51(1):33–38
27. Dargent D (1987) A new future for Schauta's operation through pre-surgical retroperitoneal pelviscopy. Eur J Gynaecol Oncol 8:292–296
28. Querleu D (1989) Transvaginal hysterectomy. Sub-serous technic. J Gynecol Obstet Biol Reprod 18(4):515–518
29. Kamprath S, Possover M et al (2000) Laparoscopic sentinel lymph node detection in patients with cervical cancer. Am J Obstet Gynecol 182(6):1648
30. Puntambekar SP (2007) Atlas of laparoscopic surgery in gynecologic oncology. Jaypee Brothers, New Delhi
31. Puntambekar SP, Kudchadkar RJ et al (2002) Role of pelvic exenteration in advanced and recurrent pelvic tumours. J Pelvic Surg 8(5):241–245
32. Puntambekar SP, Kudchadkar RJ (2006) Laparoscopic pelvic exenteration for advanced pelvic cancers: a review of 16 cases. Gynecol Oncol 102(3):513–516
33. Querleu D (1993) Laparoscopically assisted radical vaginal hysterectomy. Gynecol Oncol 51(2):248–254
34. Mettler L, Schollmeyer T et al (2008) Robotic assistance in gynecological oncology. Curr Opin Oncol 20(5):581–589
35. Degueldre M, Vandromme J et al (2000) Robotically assisted laparoscopic microsurgical tubal reanastomosis: a feasibility study. Fertil Steril 74(5):1020–1023

36. Sung GT, Gill IS (2001) Robotic laparoscopic surgery: a comparison of the Da Vinci and Zeus systems. Urology 58(6):893–898

37. Reynolds RK, Burke WM et al (2005) Preliminary experience with robot-assisted laparoscopic staging of gynecologic malignancies. JSLS 9(2):149–158

38. Advincula AP (2006) Surgical techniques: robot-assisted laparoscopic hysterectomy with the da Vinci surgical system. Int J Med Robot 2(4):305–311

39. Reynolds RK, Advincula AP (2006) Robot-assisted laparoscopic hysterectomy: technique and initial experience. Am J Surg 191(4):555–560

40. Nezhat C, Saberi NS et al (2006) Robotic-assisted laparoscopy in gynecological surgery. JSLS 10(3):317–320

41. Advincula AP, Song A (2007) The role of robotic surgery in gynecology. Curr Opin Obstet Gynecol 19(4):331–336

42. Kho RM, Hilger WS et al (2007) Robotic hysterectomy: technique and initial outcomes. Am J Obstet Gynecol 197(1):113, e1–4

43. Boggess JF, Fowler WC Jr et al (2007) Robotic assistance improves minimally invasive surgery for endometrial cancer. 38th Annual Meeting of the Society of Gynecologic Oncologists, San Diego, 3–7 Mar 2007 (Abstract no. 265)

44. Magrina JF, Kho RM et al (2008) Robotic radical hysterectomy: comparison with laparoscopy and laparotomy. Gynecol Oncol 109(1):86–91

45. Schafer A, Boggess JF et al (2006) Type III radical hysterectomy for obese women with cervical carcinoma: robotic versus open. 37th Annual Meeting of the Society of Gynecologic Oncologists, Palm Springs, 22–26 Mar 2006 (Abstract no. 49)

46. Stewart EA, Gedroyc WM et al (2003) Focused ultrasound treatment of uterine fibroid tumors: safety and feasibility of a noninvasive thermoablative technique. Am J Obstet Gynecol 189(1):48–54

47. Stewart EA, Rabinovici J et al (2006) Clinical outcomes of focused ultrasound surgery for the treatment of uterine fibroids. Fertil Steril 85(1):22–29

48. Stewart EA, Gostout B et al (2007) Sustained relief of leiomyoma symptoms by using focused ultrasound surgery. Obstet Gynecol 110(2 Pt 1):279–287

49. Ravina JH, Herbreteau D et al (1995) Arterial embolisation to treat uterine myomata. Lancet 346(8976):671–672

50. Ravina JH, Aymard A et al (2003) Uterine fibroids embolization: results about 454 cases. Gynécol Obstét Fertil 31(7–8):597–605

51. Spies JB, Spector A et al (2002) Complications after uterine artery embolization for leiomyomas. Obstet Gynecol 100(5 Pt 1):873–880

52. Mehta H, Sandhu C et al (2002) Review of readmissions due to complications from uterine fibroid embolization. Clin Radiol 57(12):1122–1124

53. Gallinat A (2007) Endometrial ablation contra hysterectomy: who takes the decision? In: Mettler L (ed) Manual of new hysterectomy techniques. Jaypee Brothers, New Delhi, pp 1116–1120

54. Altman D, Granath F et al (2007) Hysterectomy and risk of stress-urinary-incontinence surgery: nationwide cohort study. Lancet 370(9597):1494–1499

55. Altman D, Falconer C et al (2008) Pelvic organ prolapse surgery following hysterectomy on benign indications. Am J Obstet Gynecol 198(5):572, e1–6

56. Kafy S, Al-Sannan B, Kabli N, Tulandi T (2009) Patient satisfaction after laparoscopic total or supracervical hysterectomy. Gynecol Obstet Investig 67:169–172

57. Bachmann GA (1990) Hysterectomy. A critical review. J Reprod Med 35(9):839–862

58. Querleu D, Ferron G et al (2008) Pelvic lymph node dissection via a lateral extraperitoneal approach: description of a technique. Gynecol Oncol 109(1):81–85

19

Abdominal versus laparoscopic hysterectomies for benign diseases: evaluation of morbidity and mortality among 465,798 cases

Amir Wiser · Christina A. Holcroft · Togas Tulandi · Haim A. Abenhaim

Abstract Hysterectomy is the most common major gynecological surgery performed in women. The aim of this study was to compare major morbidity and mortality between abdominal hysterectomy (AH) and laparoscopic hysterectomy (LH) for benign diseases. We performed a retrospective cohort study using the data from Health Cost and Utilization Project Nationwide Inpatient Sample. Women were admitted for hysterectomy for benign diseases between the years 2002 and 2008. In-hospital morbidities and mortalities were identified using the diagnostic and procedural codes classified according to the *International Classification of Disease, Ninth Revision, and Clinical Modification*. Logistic regression analysis was used to estimate the relationship between the type of hysterectomy and the development of major morbidity and mortality. Of a total 465,798 cases, 389,189 women (83.6 %) underwent AH and the remainders underwent LH (76,609, 16.4 %). The LH group was younger and more likely to be Caucasian than those who underwent AH. Although major morbidities and mortalities were rare, women who underwent LH were less likely to develop thromboembolic events (0.68 % vs. 0.84 %, odds ratio (OR) 0.85 (0.77–0.93)), require blood transfusions (2.4 % vs. 4.7 %, OR 0.58 (0.55–0.61)), and sustain bowel perforation (0.07 % vs. 0.13 %, OR 0.56 (0.42–0.74)). The mortality rate was also lower in the LH group (0.01 %) compared with the AH group (0.03 %, OR 0.48 (0.24–0.95)). Our conclusion was that for benign diseases, laparoscopic hysterectomy is associated with a lower complication rate than abdominal hysterectomy. When possible, hysterectomy performed for benign diseases should be performed with minimally invasive technique.

Keywords Laparoscopic hysterectomy · Abdominal hysterectomy · Morbidity · Mortality

Background

Hysterectomy is the most common major gynecological surgery performed in women [1]. The majority of patients undergo hysterectomy for benign conditions including uterine leiomyoma, pelvic organ prolapse, or menorrhagia [2]. The surgical indication for hysterectomy has remained unchanged over time; however, the medical and surgical options for treatment of benign gynecological diseases have evolved considerably. The traditional approaches for hysterectomy were by laparotomy (abdominal hysterectomy (AH)) or vaginally [1].

Reich et al. reported the first case of total laparoscopic hysterectomy (LH) in 1989 [3]. This approach is associated with shorter hospitalization, faster recovery, and fewer postoperative infections compared to abdominal hysterectomy [4]. It appears that laparoscopic hysterectomy is preferable than abdominal hysterectomy [5, 6]. The benefits of LH versus AH include early return to daily activities, less intraoperative blood loss, and fewer wound or abdominal wall infections [6]. The single complication that was found to be increased after laparoscopic surgery was urinary tract injury [5, 6]. However, despite substantial evidence regarding the advantages of LH, most hysterectomies are still performed via laparotomy [2]. The purpose of our study was to compare the morbidity and mortality between abdominal and laparoscopic hysterectomies for benign diseases.

A. Wiser · C. A. Holcroft · T. Tulandi (✉) · H. A. Abenhaim
Department of Obstetrics and Gynecology, McGill University, 687 Pine Avenue West,
Montreal, Quebec H3A 1A1, Canada
e-mail: togas.tulandi@mcgill.ca

T. Tulandi
Centre for Clinical Epidemiology and Community Studies, Jewish General Hospital, Montreal, Quebec, Canada

Abdominal versus laparoscopic hysterectomies for benign diseases: evaluation of morbidity...

123

Materials and methods

We performed a retrospective cohort study using the data from the Healthcare Cost and Utilization Project Nationwide Inpatient Sample (HCUP-NIS) from 2002 to 2008. Each annual data set contains approximately 7 million records of hospitalized patients including demographic data, discharge diagnosis, procedure codes, and vital status at discharge for each respective admission. Records included in the data sets are representative samples of approximately 20 % of admissions to the US hospitals. Diagnostic and procedural codes are classified according to the *International Classification of Diseases, Ninth Revision, Clinical Modification* (ICD-9).

We defined our cohort as records indicating both benign diseases and hysterectomy procedures from 2002 to 2008. Benign disease was defined as ICD-9 codes 626.2, 626.6, 626.8, and 627.0 (menorrhagia) and 218x and 219x (leiomyomas) in any of the 15 diagnostic variables associated with hysterectomy. All of the 15 procedure codes were examined for ICD-9 codes to define hysterectomy. Any hysterectomy was identified by codes 68.3 (subtotal abdominal hysterectomy) and 68.4 (total abdominal hysterectomy). Within the hysterectomies, the subgroup of laparoscopy procedures was defined as code 68.51 or any other laparoscopy procedure (54.21, 65.01, 65.31, 65.41, 65.53, 65.63, or 65.64). The remaining hysterectomies were defined as abdominal hysterectomy.

Patient characteristics that were included in the analysis included age, race, income group (combined variables for median household income categories and median household income quartiles for patient's zip code which were defined in different years), insurance type (Medicare, Medicaid, private, or others), hospital type (rural, urban non-teaching, and urban teaching), and elective vs. non-elective admission (combining a *type* and *elective* variables defined in different years). Comorbidities have been incorporated in the HCUP-NIS database since 2002 and are calculated with the Agency for Healthcare Research and Quality software (www.ahrq.gov/data/hcup). We included congestive heart failure, chronic pulmonary disease, diabetes (complicated or uncomplicated), hypertension (complicated or uncomplicated), lymphoma, and peripheral vascular disorders.

We identified several hospital outcomes as potentially associated with the type of hysterectomy. Death and length of stay were available in the NIS database. The 15 diagnostic code variables were checked for any code indicating deep vein thrombosis (453.4 or V12.51), pulmonary embolism (415.1 or V12.51), acute myocardial infarction (410), bowel perforation (569.8, other specified disorders of intestine), and bladder injury (665.5, other injury to pelvic organs). Transfusion of blood and blood components was defined as any procedure code 99.0.

Descriptive statistics were used to analyze baseline characteristics among women undergoing a hysterectomy by abdominal approach and by laparoscopic approach. Logistic regression analysis was used to examine the association between hysterectomy type and each clinical outcome using odds ratios with adjustment for age, race, median household income, insurance type, hospital type, procedural elective status, and comorbidities. Analyses were conducted using SAS statistical software (SAS Enterprise, Cary, NC, USA). Ethical approval for the use of the data set was obtained from the Director of Professional Services of Jewish General Hospital in keeping with the provincial requirements for the use of hospital databases.

Findings

A total of 465,798 women in the HCUP-NIS database underwent hysterectomy for benign diseases between 2002 and 2008. This includes 389,189 (83.6 %) women who underwent AH and 76,609 (16.4 %) who underwent LH.

Figure 1 shows a linear reduction in the total number of hysterectomies performed from 2002 to 2008. In 2002, almost 80,000 hysterectomies were included in the database compared to less than 60,000 in 2008, a decrease of more than 30 %. The decrease was noted in the rate of AH only; although the rate of LH vs. AH increased, the total number of LH procedures remains almost constant.

The baseline characteristics of the women are summarized in Table 1. The proportion of younger women (<35 years of age) in the LH group was higher compared to the AH group (11 % vs. 8 %, respectively). The proportion of Caucasian women was also higher among the LH group, while women identified as African-American were more likely to have an AH procedure.

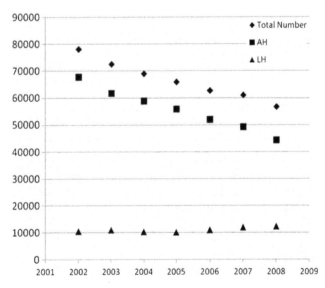

Fig. 1 Number of inpatient abdominal and laparoscopic hysterectomies between the years 2002 and 2008 in the USA

Table 1 Baseline characteristics of 465,798 patients who underwent laparoscopic vs. abdominal hysterectomies for benign disease

Baseline characteristic	Abdominal hysterectomy ($n=389,189$)	Laparoscopic hysterectomy ($n=76,609$)
Age (year)		
<35	29,792 (8 %)	8,107 (11 %)
35–39	56,658 (15 %)	12,295 (16 %)
40–44	106,817 (27 %)	19,256 (25 %)
45–49	110,282 (28 %)	20,301 (27 %)
≥50	85,399 (22 %)	16,606 (22 %)
Race		
Caucasian	170,001 (44 %)	43,174 (56 %)
African-American	62,291 (16 %)	5,963 (8 %)
Hispanic	31,295 (8 %)	4,569 (6 %)
Others	17,100 (4 %)	2,627 (3 %)
Unknown	108,492 (28 %)	20,276 (26 %)
Median income (US$)		
<35,000	95,202 (24 %)	15,921 (21 %)
35,000–44,999	97,967 (25 %)	19,278 (25 %)
≥45,000	187,998 (48 %)	39,707 (52 %)
Insurance type		
Medicare	21,399 (6 %)	3,668 (5 %)
Medicaid	34,267 (9 %)	5,207 (7 %)
Private	304,072 (78 %)	63,140 (82 %)
Others	28,726 (7 %)	4,456 (6 %)
Hospital type		
Rural	50,239 (13 %)	10,455 (14 %)
Urban, non-teaching	177,299 (46 %)	36,546 (48 %)
Urban, teaching	161,324 (41 %)	29,570 (39 %)
Admission		
Elective	338,668 (87 %)	48,453 (12 %)
Non-elective	68,361 (89 %)	7,898 (10 %)
Comorbidities[a]		
Congestive heart failure	1,539 (0.4 %)	125 (0.2 %)
Chronic pulmonary disease	26,585 (7 %)	5,100 (7 %)
Diabetes	21,998 (6 %)	3,159 (4 %)
Hypertension	79,065 (20 %)	12,028 (16 %)
Lymphoma	265 (0.07 %)	40 (0.05 %)
Peripheral vascular disorder	499 (0.1 %)	68 (0.09 %)

[a]Missing comorbidity data in 5,324 records

The mode of hysterectomy and the risks of major mortality and morbidity rates are listed in Table 2. Overall, the rates of complications were very low. Even so, the patients who underwent LH had lower morbidity (deep vein thrombosis, pulmonary embolism, requirement for blood transfusion, and acute myocardial infarction) as well as less mortality compared to women in the AH group.

Discussion

The most common approach for hysterectomy is the open abdominal hysterectomy [1]. Compared to AH, our study shows lower morbidity and mortality after minimally invasive approach with LH even after adjusting for age, race, median household income, insurance type, hospital type, procedural elective status, and comorbidities.

Figure 1 shows a decrease in the number of hysterectomies for benign diseases of more than 30 % from 2002 to 2008. This has been described in other studies [4, 7]. The decline is probably in part due to an increase in alternative medical treatments such as the levonogestrel IUD [4, 8] and minimally invasive procedures such as endometrial ablation [4]. More recent procedures include magnetic resonance-guided focused ultrasound and uterine artery embolization. These procedures are performed as outpatient interventional radiologic treatment

Table 2 Effect of hysterectomy approach on the risk of major morbidities and mortality

Outcome	Abdominal hysterectomy	Laparoscopic hysterectomy	OR (95 % CI)	P value
DVT	2,879 (0.74 %)	502 (0.66 %)	0.88 (0.80–0.96)	0.04
PE	3,099 (0.8 %)	522 (0.68 %)	0.85 (0.77–0.93)	0.006
DVT or PE	3,281 (0.84 %)	529 (0.69 %)	0.48 (0.24–0.95)	0.0004
Blood transfusion	18,124 (4.7 %)	1,805 (2.4 %)	0.56 (0.42–0.74)	0.0001
Bowel perforation	490 (0.13 %)	52 (0.07)	N/A	0.0001
Bladder injury	17 (<0.01 %)	0 (0 %)	0.29 (0.27–0.31)	N/A
Acute MI	133 (0.03 %)	13 (0.02 %)	0.58 (0.55–0.61)	0.2
Length of stay >6 days	15,917 (4.1 %)	804 (1.1 %)	0.29 (0.27–0.31)	0.0001
Death	123 (0.03 %)	9 (0.01 %)	0.69 (0.39–1.2)	0.036

DVT deep vein thrombosis, *PE* pulmonary embolism, *MI* myocardial infarction, *N/A* not available

of uterine leiomyomas, which can replace the traditional hysterectomy for the management of fibroid-related symptoms. These non-invasive alternatives are especially beneficial for women who prefer to avoid hysterectomy, as well as for those with high surgical risks [9]. All these non-surgical options offer alternatives to women with benign diseases.

One of the most important elements of our study was to define the study population as patients who underwent hysterectomy specifically for benign diseases. We chose to exclude patients who underwent hysterectomy for malignant disease since those patients are at higher risk of adverse outcome. They undergo more complicated hysterectomy due to the lymph node sampling and higher risk for DVT [10]. To ensure that only patients with benign disease would be included, we chose the diagnosis codes of leiomyomas and menorrhagias since these are the most common benign indications for hysterectomy. This method of selection of patients with benign disease has preliminarily been described [11]. These inclusion criteria ensured a specific patient population that would allow us to analyze the operative complications without the potential bias of hysterectomies performed for malignancy.

We found that the patients in the LH group had fewer complications (Table 2). These findings of decreased complication rates after LH concur with all major recent meta-analyses [1, 5, 6, 12, 13]. The only significant complication that was described in some studies as more prominent in LH patients compared to AH was urinary tract injuries. The last Cochrane database [6] reviewed 34 randomized trials and found a higher rate of urinary tract injuries after LH. In contrast Brummer et al. [12] described a lower rate of urinary tract injuries in LH patients compared to AH patients. Our large study confirmed the findings of Brummer et al. and also showed that the rate of bladder injury as well as bowel injury was lower among the LH group.

Other major complications, deep vein thrombosis, and pulmonary embolism (PE) were also lower in patients who

underwent LH. Immobility is a known risk factor for DVT and PE [14], and short hospitalization was described as beneficial in preventing PE [15]. The LH group had a significantly shorter length of stay in the hospital (Table 2) which may explain the lower rate of DVT and PE. However, this shorter length of stay in the hospital could be a bias. The "postoperative" period for DVT and PE is not well defined, neither for diagnosis of these complication nor for prophylaxis [10]. It ranges in different studies, for prophylaxis from 24 h up to 5 days or until discharge, and for diagnosis from 30 until 42 days postoperation [10]. It is possible that women in the LH groups had a DVT or PE after discharge and were diagnosed as outpatients; in such cases, these patients would not be included as a complication of the LH procedure. Since the LH group had shorter length of stay, it could be that more patients were diagnosed as outpatient cases and decrease the real number of PE and DVT cases.

Our study has several limitations. First, our data does not contain information about the extent of pathology which can affect the type of the surgery and the possible complications. A very large myoma, for example, could be a technical limitation of laparoscopic intervention or be associated with a higher rate of complications during the procedure. Therefore, it could be argued that the patients who underwent LH are "easier" cases compared to the AH patients. In a large registry of 3,139 patients undergoing uterine artery embolization, the investigators noted that the presence of five or more myomas was more commonly observed among African-American women as compared to Caucasians (37 % vs. 28 %) [16]. Abenhaim et al. [11] showed that African-Americans were less likely to undergo LH as compared with Caucasians, based on the same database from the years 1998 to 2002. Our study shows a similar trend in the years 2002–2008; the rate of African-Americans who underwent AH was double the rate of patients who underwent LH (16 % vs. 8 %, respectively). It is possible that the higher rate of African-American women in the AH group of our study reflects more difficult cases with larger leiomyomas and could in part explain the higher complication rate among the AH group.

An additional limitation is the procedural coding, which does not enable us to identify women who started initially with laparoscopic approach and were converted to laparotomy. Although this would probably be more likely in difficult cases, we hypothesize that this has a minor confounding effect only, since the overall conversion rate has been estimated at approximately 8 % [17]. While this rate of conversion was published in 2005, we believe that at this time, given advanced proficiency after the period of learning curve, it is likely to be even lower. Another potential limitation is the lack of information on important potential confounding variables such as obesity. Obesity has been shown to be associated with both socioeconomic class and surgery performed [18]. We do not have the data regarding patients' BMI, and it is possible that the AH group had more obese patients and as a result higher complication rate. It is also possible, however, that this confounder would shift the effect towards more laparascopic cases as it is believed by many that in obese women, a laparoscopic approach is easier.

In our study, we did not have the data about vaginal hysterectomy (VH) to compare between all three options of hysterectomy for benign disease. Brummer et al. [12] reported that VH was the most common hysterectomy performed, at 44 % of patients with benign disease in Finland. LH and VH comprised 76 % of the national operations. No significant differences in major complications were found between these two approaches. A major complication will occur in 3–4 % of patients, and VH is also considered as a safe option for hysterectomy.

However, our study has a number of strengths. First, it is a population-based sample of all US admissions. This important aspect of our study population allows appropriate generalizations to balance any confounder that could be encountered such as economic, racial, and ethnic differences. Data analyzed in this study is less than 10 years old (2002–2008) and thus reflects the current standard of care. This study is the largest study that can reflect the era following the learning curve associated with laparoscopic hysterectomy [8]. Finally, the data sample is extremely large allowing us to identify important associations in rare outcomes such as death and acute myocardial infarction that would perhaps not be able to be detected in a smaller, single-center experience study.

Conclusion

In conclusion, AH and LH performed for benign diseases are procedures with low complication rates. LH appears to be associated with a lower complication rate than AH as well as a lower overall mortality. Our findings suggest that, when possible, surgeons should be encouraged to consider LH over AH for benign diseases.

Conflict of interest The authors report no conflict of interest. The authors alone are responsible for the content and writing of the paper.

References

1. Warren L, Ladapo JA, Borah BJ, Gunnarsson CL (2000) Open abdominal versus laparoscopic and vaginal hysterectomy: analysis of a large United States payer measuring quality and cost of care. J Minim Invasive Gynecol 16:581–588
2. Wu JM, Wechter ME, Geller EJ, Nguyen TV, Visco AG (2007) Hysterectomy rates in the United States, 2003. Obstet Gynecol 110:1091–1095
3. Reich H (1992) Laparoscopic hysterectomy. Surg Laparosc Endosc 2:85–88
4. Candiani M, Izzo S (2010) Laparoscopic versus vaginal hysterectomy for benign pathology. Curr Opin Obstet Gynecol 22:304–308
5. Johnson N, Barlow D, Lethaby A, Tavender E, Curr L, Garry R (2005) Methods of hysterectomy: systematic review and meta-analysis of randomised controlled trials. BMJ 330:1478
6. Nieboer TE, Johnson N, Lethaby A, Tavender E, Curr E, Garry R et al (2009) Surgical approach to hysterectomy for benign gynaecological disease. Cochrane Database Syst Rev 3:CD003677
7. Brummer TH, Jalkanen J, Fraser J, Heikkinen AM, Kauko M, Makinen J et al (2009) FINHYST 2006—national prospective 1-year survey of 5,279 hysterectomies. Hum Reprod 24:2515–2522
8. Vilos GA, Marks J, Tureanu V, Abu-Rafea B, Vilos AG (2011) The levonorgestrel intrauterine system is an effective treatment in selected obese women with abnormal uterine bleeding. J Minim Invasive Gynecol 18:75–80
9. Sasa H, Kaji T, Furuya K (2012) Indications and outcomes of uterine artery embolization in patients with uterine leiomyomas. Obstet Gynecol Int 2012:920831
10. Einstein MH, Pritts EA, Hartenbach EM (2007) Venous thromboembolism prevention in gynecologic cancer surgery: a systematic review. Gynecol Oncol 105:813–819
11. Abenhaim HA, Azziz R, Hu J, Bartolucci A, Tulandi T (2008) Socioeconomic and racial predictors of undergoing laparoscopic hysterectomy for selected benign diseases: analysis of 341487 hysterectomies. J Minim Invasive Gynecol 15:11–15
12. Brummer TH, Jalkanen J, Fraser J, Heikkinen AM, Kauko M, Makinen J et al (2011) FINHYST, a prospective study of 5279 hysterectomies: complications and their risk factors. Hum Reprod 26:1741–1751
13. Kluivers KB, Ten Cate FA, Bongers MY, Brölmann HA, Hendriks JC (2011) Total laparoscopic hysterectomy versus total abdominal hysterectomy with bilateral salpingo-oophorectomy for endometrial carcinoma: a randomised controlled trial with 5-year follow-up. Gynecol Surg 8:427–434

14. Brasileiro AL, Miranda F Jr, Ettinger JE, Castro AA, Pitta GB, de Moura LK et al (2008) Incidence of lower limbs deep vein thrombosis after open and laparoscopic gastric bypass: a prospective study. Obes Surg 18:52–57

15. Cotter SA, Cantrell W, Fisher B, Shopnick R (2005) Efficacy of venous thromboembolism prophylaxis in morbidly obese patients undergoing gastric bypass surgery. Obes Surg 15:1316–1320

16. Myers ER, Goodwin S, Landow W, Mauro M, Peterson E, Pron G et al (2005) Prospective data collection of a new procedure by a specialty society: the FIBROID registry. Obstet Gynecol 106:44–51

17. Leonard F, Chopin N, Borghese B, Fotso A, Foulot H, Coste J et al (2005) Total laparoscopic hysterectomy: preoperative risk factors for conversion to laparotomy. J Minim Invasive Gynecol 12:312–317

18. Hakim RB, Benedict MB, Merrick NJ (2004) Quality of care for women undergoing a hysterectomy: effects of insurance and race/ethnicity. Am J Public Health 94:1399–1405

20

Primary intent vaginal hysterectomy: outcomes for common contraindications to vaginal approach hysterectomy

Malcolm W. Mackenzie · Jeffrey D. Johnson

Abstract The objective of this study is, within a broadly inclusive selection strategy for benign vaginal hysterectomy, to determine whether the most commonly invoked "contraindications" to vaginal hysterectomy—fibroid enlargement >14 weeks, prior cesarean, need for oophorectomy—result in increased risk of complications. This study is of retrospective design within a rural community hospital. All vaginal hysterectomies performed by a single practitioner over an 11-year-period (1998–2009) were used as samples in this study. With few exclusions, all candidates for benign hysterectomy underwent vaginal hysterectomy. Comparison was made between vaginal cases without enlargement >14 weeks, prior cesarean, or need for oopherectomy defined as "Standard" and those with contraindications defined as "Non-standard." Intraoperative complications and morbidity, including conversion to abdominal route, and postoperative morbidity, including return to the OR, transfusions, and length of hospital stay, were the main outcome measures. Of 325 hysterectomies attempted vaginally during the study period, 165 were classified as "Standard" and 160 classified as "Non-standard." Hysterectomy was completed vaginally in 311 (95.7%) patients, while 14 (4.3%) required abdominal conversion; more common for the non-standard group (8.1% vs. 0.6%, $p<0.05$). Complications not requiring conversion were not different. Only operative time, EBL, and uterine weight were increased for the non-standard group ($p<0.05$). No differences were seen in length of stay, early, or late postoperative complications. Uterine enlargement >14 weeks, prior cesarean, or oophorectomy conventionally contraindicates vaginal hysterectomy; a primary intent vaginal hysterectomy strategy using broad inclusion criteria results in a high vaginal hysterectomy rate, and low complication rates no greater for vaginal hysterectomies performed with contraindications than for those performed without such contraindications.

Keywords Vaginal hysterectomy · Contraindications · Fibroid · Cesarean · Oophorectomy

M. W. Mackenzie (✉) · J. D. Johnson
Department of Obstetrics and Gynecology,
Cheshire Medical Center/Dartmouth Hitchcock,
Keene, NH, USA
e-mail: mmacken1@mah.harvard.edu

M. W. Mackenzie · J. D. Johnson
Department of Obstetrics and Gynecology,
Mount Auburn Hospital,
330 Mount Auburn St,
Cambridge, MA, USA

Present Address:
M. W. Mackenzie
836 Nelson Rd,
Nelson, NH 03457, USA

Introduction

In the USA, over 600,000 hysterectomies are performed annually, making it second only to cesarean delivery among surgeries performed on women [1]. The abdominal approach, the most commonly performed [2], carries the highest complication rate [3] and imposes the greatest recovery burden and highest cost [4]. Laparoscopic hysterectomy, potentially a less invasive alternative to abdominal hysterectomy, has suffered from slow skill development [5] and higher complication rates [6] and cost as compared to the vaginal approach [7]. Vaginal hysterectomy, with its lowest rate of complications, recovery burden, and costs [8, 9], might be considered the optimal approach. Mindful, the American College of Obstetricians and Gynecologists, in its November 2009 Committee Opinion #444 regarding hysterectomy route for benign indications states, "evidence demonstrates that, in general, vaginal hysterectomy is associated with better outcomes and fewer complications than laparoscopic or abdominal hysterectomy" concluding "vaginal hysterectomy is the approach of choice whenever feasible, based on its well-documented advantages and lower complication rates" [10].

Many are the claimed "contraindications" to a vaginal approach hysterectomy; any complexity beyond the normal sized, unscarred, descended uterus, without indication for oophorectomy dissuades many practitioners from attempting vaginal hysterectomy. The clinical reality is that conditions which constitute for many surgeons "contraindications" to vaginal hysterectomy—fibroid enlargement, prior cesarean delivery or pelvic surgery, and need for oophorectomy—are commonly present in the hysterectomy candidate. In consequence, rates of vaginal hysterectomy, despite being an optimal approach by all criteria, are low— no greater than 20–25%—a fact bemoaned by those promoting a best practice standard of 75–80% vaginal hysterectomy rate [11, 12].

We report the outcomes of a hysterectomy strategy that preferentially and primarily pursues a vaginal approach where neither fibroid enlargement to 18-week size, prior history of cesarean delivery, or need for oophorectomy (much less prior pelvic surgery, known adhesions, endometriosis, nulliparity, obesity, or absence of uterine descent) are considered dissuasive from initiating vaginal hysterectomy and to determine whether any greater risk of complications accrues to vaginal hysterectomies challenged by such "contraindications" than to vaginal hysterectomies not so challenged.

Methods

Following approval from Dartmouth Hitchcock Medical Center's Committee for Protection of Human Subjects, all hysterectomies performed by one gynecologic surgeon at The Cheshire Medical Center/Dartmouth Hitchcock-Keene were identified for the dates February 1, 1998 to February 28, 2009.

Patients undergoing abdominal approach hysterectomies (open and laparoscopic) were identified and their charts reviewed to determine the indication for the abdominal approach. For the remaining necessarily vaginal hysterectomies—performed, following standard bowel prep and protocol-driven antibiotic prophylaxis, with standard technique notable for intrafascial dissection and delayed peritoneal entry—inpatient and outpatient records were reviewed. All measures bearing on the feasibility of and those bearing on the morbidity potentially consequent upon a vaginal approach were extracted: preoperative data including patient age, body mass index (BMI), gravida, para, number of vaginal deliveries, number of cesarean deliveries, preoperatively estimated uterine size (in weeks), hemoglobin and hematocrit, presence and degree of uterine descent (traditional grading system grade 0–4), presence and degree of coincidental pelvic floor abnormalities (cystocele/rectocele), prior pelvic surgeries with or without known intrapelvic adhesive disease, and preoperatively identified indication(s) for hysterectomy: fibroid-related symptoms (bleeding, mass effect, pain), non-fibroid bleeding, non-fibroid pain, non-fibroid dysmenorrhea, known endometriosis, known adenomyosis, and pelvic floor dysfunction/prolapse. Intraoperative events were recorded: estimated blood loss (EBL), total operative time (OR) from first cut to finish of surgery, concomitant procedures (oophorectomy, pelvic floor repairs including anterior and posterior repairs and sacrospinous ligament suspension), method of anesthesia, intraoperative complications, need for conversion to abdominal route, and uterine weight. Postoperative events were identified: immediate (during hospitalization), early (discharge to 3 months postoperative) and late (3 to 12 months postoperative) complications including returns to the OR, transfusions, ICU admissions, and hospital readmissions. Also recorded were length of hospital stay (LOS), years of follow-up, and the occurrence/recurrence of symptomatic prolapse.

Averages with standard deviations were calculated for continuous variable data while rates and percentages were calculated for categorical or binary data.

Based upon preoperative criteria, and focusing on commonly invoked contraindications to vaginal route hysterectomy, patients were then divided into two groups:

Standard: vaginal hysterectomies without "contraindication" (size less than 15 weeks, no history of cesarean, no oophorectomy)

Non-standard: vaginal hysterectomies performed despite "contraindications" (size 15 weeks or greater, and/or prior cesarean, and/or oophorectomy)

Utilizing Excel (Microsoft Corp, USA), comparison between these "Standard" and "Non-standard" hysterectomy groups was conducted in terms of preoperative, intraoperative, and postoperative criteria. Comparative rates with significance for non-continuous data were calculated using Yates' chi-squared analysis. Significance testing utilizing two-tailed Student's t test was applied to the comparison of continuous data.

An additional analysis, intended to identify the morbidity consequent upon intraoperative conversion to abdominal route, compares "Non-standard" hysterectomies that resulted in a conversion to abdominal route against the group of "Non-standard" hysterectomies that were completed vaginally.

Results

There were 405 hysterectomies performed during the study period. For 80 hysterectomies, no vaginal approach was attempted: 17 for known or suspected malignancy, 13 for uterine size ≥19 weeks, seven for uterine size <19 weeks but with fibroid distortion of the ureter/uterine artery nexus, nine for laparoscopic supracervical hysterectomy (no total laparoscopic hysterectomies nor laparoscopically assisted vaginal hysterectomies were performed), 18 where planned urogynecologic procedure directed an abdominal approach, and three for history of severe sexual abuse out of concern for consequent posttraumatic stress. Amongst general surgical indications, abdominal hernia repair, small bowel obstruction, and pelvic abscess directed an abdominal approach in 13 other cases.

For 325 patients, primary intent vaginal approach hysterectomy was attempted. Demographic and outcome data for this primary intent vaginal hysterectomy group is seen in Table 1.

Preoperative data

Of these 325 primary intent vaginal hysterectomies, 80 (24.6%) had a history of C/S (27 (8.3%) with one cesarean delivery, 37 (11.4%) with two cesareans, 11 (3.4%)with three, and five (1.5%) with four). Eighty-nine (27.4%) patients registered body mass indices in the range of 30–39.9 kg/m [2] (obesity) and 37 (11.4%) patients evidenced a BMI in excess of 40 kg/m [2] (morbid obesity). Twenty-five (7.7%) patients were nulligravid. One hundred (30.1%) patients had preoperatively identified uterine enlargement: 60 (18.5%) had enlargement that was assessed as 8–12 weeks and 40 (12.3%) assessed at a 13–18-week size, of which 17 (5.2%) were 15 weeks or greater. One hundred fifty-seven (48.3%) patients had a prior history of some type of pelvic surgery of which 48 (14.8%) were major surgeries. Pelvic adhesions were known to be present in 33 (10.1%) patients. Amongst the standard indications for hysterectomy, the most common was non-fibroid bleeding (29.8%).

Intraoperative data

There were 14 (4.3%) conversions to abdominal approach—utilizing laparoscopy (2) or laparotomy (12)—for reasons including intraoperative discovery of occult malignancy (2), bleeding from adnexa (2), technical inability to complete hysterectomy(5), technical inability to complete adnexectomy (4), and cystotomy (1) unable to be repaired vaginally. During the period of study, one additional cystotomy and no ureteral injuries occurred for a total urologic injury rate of 0.6%. Average blood loss for the total group of patients was 140 cm³. Average operating time was 105 min (range 39–332 min); this included in all patients hysterectomy, cul-de-

sac obliteration, McCall, and round ligament resuspension, in addition to concomitant adnexectomy and pelvic reconstructive procedures. Ninety (27.7%) hysterectomies also involved some manner of unilateral or bilateral oophorectomy. Obviating the performance of McCall culdoplasty, sacrospinous ligament suspension was performed in 21 (6.5%) cases. Spinal anesthesia was utilized in 53 (16.3%) patients with conversion to general anesthesia necessary in ten (3.1%) patients.

Postoperative data

Immediate postoperative complications involved two (0.6%) patients returning to the OR for laparoscopy, both for infundibulopelvic bleeding. The only transfusions were for these same two patients. No ICU admissions were necessary in any of the 325 patients. Median length of hospital stay for all patients was 1 day, range 0–7 days. The total post-discharge (early and late) complication rate was 2.5% involving eight patients. Early postoperative complications included one readmission for pyelonephritis on day 5 post-operative, one readmit at 2 weeks postoperative for vaginal apex bleeding requiring oversewing of the cuff. One patient required readmission for pain control 3 days following surgery and this same patient was readmitted on day 10 for *Clostridium difficile* colitis. *C. difficile* colitis necessitated admission for one other patient at day 10 postoperative. Pelvic abscess requiring laparotomy and drainage was seen in one patient 2 weeks postoperative. Late postoperative complications included one fatal myocardial infarction in a 72-year-old 10 months postoperative and one death from non-gynecologic carcinoma. One patient with ovarian remnant required laparoscopic excision at 8 months following hysterectomy. Mean uterine weight for all patients was 157 g (range 23–913 g). An average of 4.3 years of follow-up was achieved in 304 patients with 15 (5.0%) patients evidencing symptomatic recurrent or new prolapse.

"Standard" vs. "Non-standard"

From this group of 325 vaginal hysterectomy patients, 160 were designated as non-standard cases—based upon the presence of at least one of the contraindications of prior cesarean, uterine enlargement greater than 14 weeks, and planned adnexectomy—with the remaining 165 patients without such contraindication designated standard. Comparison between these groups and statistical analysis is presented in Table 2.

In terms of preoperative criteria, significant differences in patient age, uterine descent or other pelvic floor defects, pelvic adhesions, fibroid uterus, and endometriosis were evident. Endometriosis was a very common indication for hysterectomy (necessarily with BSO), significantly more

Table 1 All vaginal hysterectomies (*n*=325)

	Avg.	SD	Present	%
Preoperative:				
Age (years)	44.9	11.9		
BMI (kg/m^2)	29.6	7.9		
Gravida #	2.5	1.4		
Para. #	2.2	1.2		
Vag delivery: # of pts. with any Vag. Del.			239	73.5
Cesarean delivery: # of pts. with any C/S			80	24.6
Hgb (mg/dl)	13.2	1.4		
Hct (%)	40	21.1		
Any uterine descent			131	40.3
Other pelvic floor defects			44	13.5
Prior major pelvic surgeries			48	14.8
Prior minor pelvic surgeries (1)			109	33.5
Pelvic adhesions known present			33	10.1
Pelvic adhesions known absent (2)			23	7.1
Fibroids			79	24.3
Non-fibroid bleeding			97	29.8
Non-fibroid pain			20	6.2
Non-fibroid dysmenorrhea			49	15.1
Endometriosis			47	14.5
Adenomyosis			50	15.4
Prolapse			67	20.6
Other			24	7.4
Intraoperative:				
Conversion to abdominal route #			14	4.3
EBL (cm^3)	140	152		
Complications w/out conversion			1	0.3
OR time (min)	105	45		
LSO or RSO			30	9.2
BSO			60	18.5
Anterior repair			1	0.3
Posterior repair			23	7.1
Anterior and posterior repair			9	2.8
Sacrospinous ligament suspension			21	6.5
Any pelvic floor repair			37	11.4
Anesthesia:				
GET			230	70.8
GLMA			52	16
Spinal			53	16.3
Uterine weight (g)	157	140		
Postoperative:				
Return to OR			2	0.6
Transfusion			2	0.6
ICU admit			0	0
Hospital LOS (days)	1.5	0.7		
Early and late postoperative complications			8	2.5
Follow-up: >1 year (3)			258	79.4
Length of long-term follow-up (years)	4.3	2.6		
Apical descent in pts. with any follow-up			15	4.9

Table 1 (continued)

	Avg.	SD	Present	%
(1) No prior surgeries: 168 (51.7%)				
(2) Adhesions unknown: 269 (82.8%)				
(3) Follow-up: <1 year=46 (14.2%); None=21 (6.5%)				

common (26.9%) in the non-standard group than in the standard group (2.4%).

The rate of conversion to abdominal route was higher, operative time longer—though with comparable ranges of 47–331 min vs. 39–332min—and average uterine weight greater in the non-standard as compared to the standard group. The use of spinal anesthesia and pelvic reconstructive procedures were more common in the standard group. Excluding intraoperatively discovered occult malignancy as the indication for conversion (n=2), the rate of conversion for the non-standard group recalculates to a rate of 6.7% still significantly (p<0.05) higher than in the standard group. Aside from conversion to abdominal route, no intraoperative complications were encountered in the standard group while a cystotomy repaired vaginally occurred in the non-standard group; the total intraoperative complication rate—both those necessitating conversion and those not—were significantly lower in the standard group (0.6%) than in the non-standard group (8.7%). Though both urologic injuries occurred in the non-standard group, the calculated rates of urologic injury were not significantly different (p=0.47). There were significant differences between the two groups in terms of average operative time: for the standard and for the non-standard vaginal hysterectomies, 96 and 114 min, respectively. Significantly more pelvic reconstructive procedures were performed in the standard group (19.4%) than the non-standard group (3.1%).

The 1.5-day average length of hospital stay was identical between groups. An equal number and rate (0.6%) of immediate postoperative complications (requiring transfusion and return to the OR) occurred in each group. Neither was there significant difference in the combined (immediate, early, and late) postoperative complication rate between the standard (1.2%) and non-standard (5%) groups. The single early complication in the standard group involved bleeding from the vaginal apex (requiring oversewing of the cuff) encountered 2 weeks postoperative. All remaining and previously identified complications occurred in the non-standard group. Long-term follow-up beyond 1 year was known for 153 (92.7%) of the standard group and 105 (66%) of the non-standard group (p<0.05) with the average interval to follow-up similar. For those with known follow-up beyond 1 year, recurrent or new symptomatic vault descent

occurred significantly more often (compare 8.5% to 1.9%) in the standard than in the non-standard group.

Finally, to determine whether certain risk factors for conversion to abdominal route can be identified from preoperative conditions and whether there are significant differences in postoperative outcomes, non-standard hysterectomies were separated according to whether conversion to abdominal route was necessary or not; this data appears in Table 3. As indications for hysterectomy, non-fibroid pelvic pain and an absence of uterine descent and were significantly more common in the group for whom conversion was necessary. Intraoperative complications (bleeding or bladder injury) were significantly more common in the conversion group (23.1%) as compared to the non-conversion group (0.6%). Not surprisingly, OR time, EBL, and LOS were all significantly greater for cases involving conversion than for cases successfully completed vaginally.

Discussion

This study reports the outcomes of one practitioner's strategy of preferentially pursuing vaginal approach for benign hysterectomy; a selection strategy driven by inclusive primary intent rather than exclusionary contraindications. By attempting a vaginal approach to hysterectomy despite commonly invoked contraindications—uterine enlargement >14 weeks, concomitant oophorectomy, or prior cesarean delivery—one of the highest published vaginal hysterectomy rates was achieved. We demonstrate that vaginal hysterectomy cases challenged by contraindications evidence slightly higher rates of conversion to abdominal approach than those cases not so challenged; we also identify no other significant differences in morbidity of clinical import. In conclusion, the three most commonly invoked contraindications to vaginal approach hysterectomy need not be dissuasive to primarily attempting a vaginal approach.

Many authors identify that, utilizing certain techniques, completion of vaginal hysterectomy is possible even for fibroid enlarged uteri over a range of sizes, with cutoffs set at 12 [11], 14 [13], 16 [12], or even 20 [14]-week size. Some authors also attest to the ease of transvaginal

Table 2 Vaginal hysterectomies: "Non-Standard" vs. "Standard"

	p	Non-standard (n=160)				Standard (n=165)			
		Avg	SD	Present	%	Avg	SD	Present	%
Preoperative:									
Age (years)	<0.01	42.8	11			46.9	12.4		
BMI (kg/m^2)	NS	30.4	7.9			28.8	7.8		
Gravida #	NS	2.5	1.3			2.6	1.5		
Para #	NS	2.2	1.1			2.3	1.2		
Hgb (mg/dl)	NS	13.1	1.4			13.3	1.4		
Hct (%)	NS	38.8	3.6			41.3	29.4		
Any uterine descent	<0.001			43	26.9			88	53.3
Other pelvic floor defects	<0.001			6	3.8			38	23
Prior pelvic surgeries: major	NS			23	14.4			25	15.2
Prior pelvic surgeries: minor	NS			52	32.5			57	34.5
Intrapelvic adhesions known present	<0.05			24	15			9	5.4
Intrapelvic adhesions known absent				12	7.5			11	6.7
Fibroids	<0.05			48	30			31	18.8
Non-fibroid bleeding	NS			45	28.1			52	31.5
Non-fibroid pain	NS			13	8.1			7	4.2
Non-fibroid dysmenorrhea	NS			26	16.2			23	13.9
Endometriosis	<0.001			43	26.9			4	2.4
Adenomyosis	NS			26	16.3			24	14.5
Pelvic floor dysfunction or prolapse	<0.001			11	6.9			56	33.9
Other	NS			9	5.6			15	9.1
Intraoperative:									
Conversion to abdominal route	<0.05			13	8.1			1	0.6
EBL (cm^3)	<0.05	166	172			115	125		
Complications w/out conversion	NS			1	0.6			0	0
OR time (min)	<0.001	114	47			96	42		
Any pelvic floor repair	<0.001			5	3.1			32	19.4
Uterine weight (g)	<0.001	185	167			130	101		
Postoperative:									
Transfusion	NS			1	0.6			1	0.6
Hospital LOS (days)	NS	1.5	0.7			1.5	0.8		
Return to OR	NS			1	0.6			1	0.6
Early and late postoperative complications	NS			7	4.4			1	0.6
Length of long-term follow-up (years)	NS	4.3	2.6			4.3	2.6		
Descent in pts. with >1 year follow-up	<0.05			2	1.9			13	8.5

oopherectomy [15, 16] and some identify a history of cesarean delivery and the consequent scarring of cystouterine dissection planes as being of no impediment to vaginal hysterectomy [17]. They argue that singly each of these contraindications should not dissuade otherwise skilled surgeons from vaginal approach. The clinical reality however is that multiple contraindications are often present in candidates for hysterectomy. The data presented here argues for a selection strategy for vaginal approach most broadly applicable even when overlapping contraindications apply.

This study extends the work of previous authors who also challenge commonly invoked contraindications to vaginal approach: enlarged uteri >180 g, functional or actual nulliparity, and previous cesarean or pelvic laparotomy [18]. In our study, however, we chose the most commonly invoked contraindications to vaginal route—oopherectomy, prior cesarean delivery, and uterine enlargement >14 weeks. We did not address less commonly invoked contraindications to vaginal hysterectomy—nulliparity, obesity, absence of uterine descent or vaginal access, history of

Table 3 Nonstandard hysterectomies: no abdominal conversion vs. conversion

	p	No conversion (n=146)				Conversion (n=14)			
		Avg	SD	Present	%	Avg	SD	Present	%
Preoperative:									
Age (years)	NS	42.4	10.7			47.2	13.1		
BMI (kg/m²)	NS	30.2	7.9			32.8	8.4		
Grav. #	NS	2.5	1.3			2.5	1.3		
Para. #	NS	2.2	1.1			2.2	1		
Vag delivery # per	NS	1.2	1.3			1.3	1.3		
Cesarean delivery # per	NS	1	1.1			0.8	1.3		
History of any cesarean	NS			75	46.4			5	38.4
Hgb (mg/dl)	NS	13.1	1.4			13.5	1.2		
Hct (%)	NS	38.6	3.7			40.3	2.9		
Any uterine descent	<0.001			39	26.5			4	30.8
Other pelvic floor defects	NS			5	3.4			1	7.7
Prior pelvic surgeries: major	NS			23	15.6			0	0
Prior pelvic surgeries:minor	NS			50	32.7			4	30.8
Intrapelvic adhesions known present	NS			22	15			2	15.3
Intrapelvic adhesions known absent	NS			10	6.8			2	15.4
Fibroids	NS			42	28.6			6	46.2
Non-fibroid bleeding	NS			42	28.6			3	23.1
Non-fibroid pain	<0.01			9	6.1			4	30.8
Non-fibroid dysmenorrhea	NS			26	17.7			0	0
Endometriosis	NS			40	27.2			3	23.1
Adenomyosis	NS			25	17			1	7.7
Pelvic floor dysfunction or prolapse	NS			11	7.5			0	0
Other	NS			8	5.4			1	7.7
Intraoperative:									
EBL (mg/dl)	<0.01	141	119			448	357		
Complications w/out conversion	<0.05			1	0.6			3	23.1
OR time (min)	<0.001	107	40.4			191	47		
Any adnexectomy	NS			79	53.7			11	84.6
Any pelvic floor repair	NS			4	2.7			1	7.7
Uterine weight (gms)	NS	177	155			278	254		
# pts. with uterine weight >200 g	NS			113	76.9			8	62
Postoperative:									
Transfusion	NS			1	0.6			0	0
ICU admit				0	0			0	0
Hospital LOS (days)	<0.05	1.41	0.62			2.2	0.9		
Return to OR	NS			1	0.6			0	0
Late postoperative complications	NS			5	3.4			2	15.4

prior major pelvic surgery, and known or unknown adhesive disease. Though such lesser contraindications were not differentially represented between the two comparative groups, neither were they dissuasive against a primary intent vaginal approach.

A uterine size cutoff of greater than 18 weeks was chosen as the limit of this practitioner's intent to perform hysterec-tomy vaginally. The 18-week cutoff however extends most previously published cutoffs as proof of the validity of more liberal criteria for inclusion vs. exclusion from vaginal approach.

Suggested here, the broadest applicability of a vaginal approach to hysterectomy challenges practitioners to exam-ine what skills are required for a primary intent vaginal approach to hysterectomy. This has been answered by recent authors who point out that "attitude" [12] or "physician-level factors" [19] have perhaps greater influence on the choice of hysterectomy route than does actual "aptitude"; gynecologic surgeons have the requisite skill set and can, with a change of "attitude" or focus on evidence-based approaches [20, 21], increase substantially their vaginal hysterectomy rate. Additionally, by this study we extend the challenge to include an even larger group of patients for whom vaginal hysterectomy is entirely appropriate. That this group of patients with all ranges of uterine size, need for oophorectomy, and history of cesarean delivery—not to mention conditions of nulliparity, obesity, absence of descent, history of prior major pelvic surgery with known or unknown adhesive disease, etc. that we did not focus on at all—was treated successfully with vaginal hysterectomy implies then the concept of a "trial of vaginal hysterectomy" rate as a measure of quality different than the rate of "vaginal hysterectomy": for this study the former "trial" rate is calculated to be 80.2% and the latter rate of "completion" is calculated as a "vaginal hysterectomy" rate of 95.7%.

This study evaluated the broadest range of relevant outcomes to hysterectomy including rarely identified longer-term outcomes such as later pelvic floor dysfunction or prolapse. We did not however include sexual function, quality of life outcomes, or time to return to full function/work.

We recognize that despite this study being one of the largest single practitioner studies comparing vaginal hysterectomy outcomes, unlike multi-practitioner studies, our comparison of morbidity between subgroups demonstrates a rarity of complications making it difficult to identify true differences that this study, less powered, might otherwise have clarified. Nevertheless, this study, representing a single practitioner, community-based data set, appropriately represents the conditions, circumstances, and potential outcomes for many gynecologic surgeons facing the challenge of increasing their vaginal hysterectomy rate.

We do not address the potentially doubly confounding influence on outcomes represented by either the presence of prolapse or the corrective procedures often performed for it in addition to hysterectomy. Cases where prolapse is the indication for hysterectomy may benefit in terms of outcome due to the associated technical ease of access to the uterus and cervix. More common in the standard group, prolapse could also result however in higher morbidity where adjunct resuspension procedures are necessarily performed

In our analysis, comparing non-standard hysterectomy cases requiring conversion to those without conversion, neither fibroid enlargement, oopherectomy or prior cesare-an were clearly predictive of conversion, nor did conversion to abdominal route of itself result in significant morbid sequelae; for the 13 Non-standard cases which necessitated conversion to abdominal route, prolonged OR time, an increased EBL without transfusion and a slightly prolonged LOS were the only significant differences. Indeed in the properly counseled patient, conversion need not represent a regrettable outcome. Going forward, we can also see the increased role of laparoscopy in those rare situations in which conversion might become necessary—a "laparoscopic assist" only, as some authors suggest, when necessary and not as precondition for a vaginal approach [22]. We do understand that statistical analysis within the subset of cases converted to abdominal route lacks the power to make particularly strong conclusions.

This study is not of prospective design. Arguably, the retrospective comparison between groups is simply one of convenience and of no import. Not formally prospective, this study nevertheless represents a retrospective analysis of a prospective intent to perform with few exceptions all cases vaginally and thus approaches the rigor of a truly prospective study. Our comparison therefore is not one of convenience but one that, as credible as a prospective analysis might be, indicates that performing vaginal hysterectomy in patients with one or more of prior cesarean, enlarged uteri >14 weeks, or need for oophorectomy while possibly fraught with increased difficulty is nevertheless not fraught with more complications or greater real morbidity.

Conclusion

This study identifies the relative safety and acceptability of an inclusive strategy for selection of vaginal route hysterectomy and challenges the three most common contraindications to vaginal hysterectomy. By such a strategy, we have achieved a rate of vaginal hysterectomy beyond 95% with the only clinically significant complications being a very low rate of conversion to abdominal route that, without greater morbid sequelae, is preferable to primarily choosing an abdominal or laparoscopic route for all.

Acknowledgments This work was done under the auspices of Dartmouth Hitchcock/Cheshire Medical Center, Keene, NH, USA.

Disclosure of interests No conflict of interest.

Contribution to authorship Substantial writing, editing, literature review, and data analysis were contributed by Dr. Johnson. Study concept, clinical work, data extraction, data entry, statistical analysis, and majority writing and editing were contributed by Dr. Mackenzie.

Funding   There was no funding.

Declaration of interest   The authors report no conflicts of interest. The authors alone are responsible for the content and writing of the paper.

References

1. Wu JM, Wechter ME, Geller EJ, Nguyen TV, Visco AG (2007) Hysterectomy rates in the United States, 2003. Obstet Gynecol 110:1091–1095

2. Whiteman MK, Hillis SD, Jamieson DJ, Morrow B, Podgornik MN, Brett KM et al (2008) Inpatient hysterectomy surveillance in the United States, 2000–2004. Am J Obstet Gynecol 198:34.3e1–34e7

3. Garry R, Fountain J, Mason S, Hawe J, Napp V, Abbott J et al (2004) The eVALuate study: two parallel randomized trials, on comparing laparoscopic with abdominal hysterectomy, the other comparing laparoscopic with vaginal hysterectomy. BMJ 328:129–138

4. Lumsden MA, Twaddle S, Hawthorn R, Traynor I, Gilmore D, Davis J et al (2000) A randomised comparison and economic evaluation of laparoscopic-assisted hysterectomy and abdominal hysterectomy. BJOG 53:214–219

5. Reich H, Roberts L (2003) Laparoscopic hysterectomy in current gynaecological practice. Rev Gynaecol Pract 3:32–40

6. Altgassen C, Michels W, Schneider A (2004) Learning laparoscopic assisted hysterectomy. Obstet Gynecol 104:308–313

7. Kovac SR (2000) Hysterectomy outcomes in patients with similar indications. Obstet Gynecol 95:787–793

8. Van Den Eeden SK, Glasser M, Mathias SD, Colwell HH, Pasta DJ, Kunz K (1998) Quality of life, health care utilization, and costs among women undergoing hysterectomy in a managed-care setting. Am J Obstet Gynecol 178:91–100

9. Mulholland C, Harding N, Bradley S, Stevenson M (1996) Regional variations in the utilization rate of vaginal and abdominal hysterectomies in the United Kingdom. J Public Health Med 18:400–405

10. Choosing the route of hysterectomy for benign disease (2009) ACOG Committee Opinion No. 444. Obstet Gynecol 114 (5):1156–1158

11. Kovac SR (1995) Guidelines to determine the route of hysterectomy. Obstet Gynecol 85:18–23

12. Varma R, Tahseen S, Lokugamage AU, Kunde D (2001) Vaginal route as the norm when planning hysterectomy for benign conditions: change in practice. Obstet Gynecol 97:613–616

13. Davies A, Vizza E, Bournas N, O'Connor H, Magos A (1998) How to increase the proportion of hysterectomies performed vaginally. Am J Obstet Gynecol 179:1008–1012

14. Magos A, Bournas N, Sinha R, Richardson RE, O'Connor H (1996) Vaginal hysterectomy for the large uterus. British J Obstet Gynecol 103:246–251

15. Hoffman MS (1991) Transvaginal removal of ovaries with endoloop sutures at the time of transvaginal hysterectomy. Am J Obstet Gynecol 165:407–408

16. Kovak SR, Cruikshank SH (1996) Guidelines to determine the route of oopherectomy with hysterectomy. Am J Obstet Gynecol 175:1483–1488

17. Hoffman MS, Jaeger M (1990) A new method for gaining entry into the scarred anterior cul-de-sac during transvaginal surgery. Am J Obset Gynecol 162:1269–1270

18. Doucette RC, Sharp HT, Alder SC (2001) Challenging generally accepted contraindications to vaginal hysterectomy. Am J Obstet Gynecol 184:1386–1391

19. Tu FF, Beaumont JL, Senapati S, Gordon TEJ (2009) Route of hysterectomy influence and teaching hospital status. Obstet Gynecol 114:73–78

20. Dunn TS, Weaver A, Wolf D, Goodard W (2006) Vaginal hysterectomies performed in a residency program: can we increase the number? J Reprod Med 51:83–86

21. Kovac SR (1999) Determining the route and method of hysterectomy. Key Clinical Decision Series—Ethicon Endo-Surgery ISBN 0-9673302-0-3

22. Richardson RE, Bournas N, Magos AL (1995) Is laparoscopic hysterectomy a waste of time? Lancet 345:36–41

21

Two-port method for laparoscopically assisted vaginal hysterectomy: approach and outcomes

Jong Woon Bae · Un Suk Jung · Joong Sub Choi ·
Jung Hun Lee · Chang Eop Son · Seung Wook Jeon ·
Jin Hwa Hong

Abstract The aim of our study was to assess the feasibility and efficacy of laparoscopically assisted vaginal hysterectomy (LAVH) with the two-port method. One hundred seventy-six women with uterine diseases underwent LAVH using the two-port method. We reviewed the medical records of the patients' age, parity, body mass index, history of previous abdominal surgery, operative indications, histopathological diagnosis, operating time, weight of the removed uterus, change in the hemoglobin levels, hospital stay, and occurrence of any complications. The median age of the patients was 46 years (range, 33–60 years), the median parity was 2 (range, 0–5), and the median body mass index was 23.4 kg/m² (range, 17.6–29.6 kg/m²). Forty-two patients (23.9%) had previous abdominal operative history. The most common operative indication was menorrhagia, and the most common histopathological diagnosis was leiomyoma. The median operating time was 58 min (range, 30–150 min), and the median weight of the removed uterus was 230 g (range, 60–660 g). The median change in the hemoglobin level was 1.7 g/dL (range, 0.1–3.8 g/dL). The median hospital stay was 3 days (range, 2–7 days). An ileus occurred postoperatively in one patient, which was managed conservatively. No additional port was required in any of the cases. No operation was converted to an abdominal hysterectomy. LAVH using the two-port technique with the aid of a 5-mm telescope and an endoscopic stapler is both feasible and efficient.

Keywords Hysterectomy · Laparoscopy · Surgical stapler · Port

Jong Woon Bae and Un Suk Jung contributed equally to this work.

U. S. Jung
Department of Obstetrics and Gynecology, Konyang University Hospital, Konyang University College of Medicine, Daejeon, Republic of Korea

J. W. Bae · J. S. Choi (✉) · J. H. Lee · C. E. Son · S. W. Jeon · J. H. Hong
Division of Gynecologic Oncology and Gynecologic Minimally Invasive Surgery, Department of Obstetrics and Gynecology, Kangbuk Samsung Hospital,
Sungkyunkwan University School of Medicine,
108, Pyung-dong, Jongno-gu,
Seoul 110-746, Republic of Korea
e-mail: yjjy.choi@samsung.com

Background

Laparoscopically assisted vaginal hysterectomy (LAVH) is one of the most frequently performed gynecologic operations, and numerous authors have demonstrated the safety and feasibility of LAVH [1]. Researchers have performed LAVH on variously sized uteri with broad indications and have successfully introduced methods that reduce morbidity [2–4]. The three- or four-port method with various port-placement systems is used in most laparoscopic hysterectomies. The aim of our study was to evaluate the feasibility and efficacy of LAVH with the two-port method using a 5-mm telescope and endoscopic staplers.

Materials and methods

Eight hundred seventy-nine women with various uterine diseases underwent LAVH at Kangbuk Samsung Hospital from December 2005 to June 2009. Among those, 176 women (19.2%) underwent LAVH utilizing the two-port method. For the rest, including 18 single-port method, either the three-port method or the four-port method was used [2]. All patients underwent preoperative assessments that included a detailed medical history, pelvic examination, pelvic ultrasonogram, and Pap smear. When indicated, a colposcopically directed cervical biopsy, conization of the uterine cervix, or endometrial biopsy was performed preoperatively. Information such as age, parity, body mass index, the number of previous abdominal surgery, operative indications, histopathological results, weight of the extracted uterus, operating time, hemoglobin level, and operative complications were collected by investigating surgical and anesthetic records. Operating time was defined as the time from the first umbilical incision to the skin closure. Informed consents were obtained in all the cases.

Patients routinely underwent general anesthesia with endotracheal intubation followed by the placement of a uterine manipulator in a dorsal lithotomy position. Cefazedone sodium (1 g) was injected intravenously 30 min before the induction of anesthesia. After lifting the anterior abdominal wall, a 5-mm port was directly inserted at the infraumbilicus with a vertical skin incision. Carbon dioxide was insufflated through the port sleeve to create a pneumoperitoneum, and the intra-abdominal pressure was maintained at 15 mmHg. The intra-abdominal cavity was inspected with a 5-mm telescope. Transillumination was used to locate the superior and inferior epigastric vessels, and direct visualization was used to insert a secondary ancillary 5-mm port into the left upper quadrant. The 5-mm infraumbilical port was replaced with a 12-mm port (Fig. 1). If adhesiolysis was necessary, bipolar grasping forceps and endoscissors were inserted sequentially into the left upper quadrant port site. The 5-mm telescope was shifted to the left upper quadrant 5-mm port, and an endoscopic stapler (Endoscopic Linear Cutter®, Ethicon Endo-surgery, Cincinnati, OH, USA) was inserted into the umbilical 12-mm port. An assistant moved the uterus using the uterine manipulator on tension to one side. At the same time, the ovarian ligament, the salpinx, and the round ligament were simultaneously transected by the endoscopic stapler. This procedure was repeated on the contralateral side. A bladder flap was created by dissecting the broad ligament in front of the uterine artery with the endoscissors. If necessary, the ovary was removed by simultaneously transecting the infundibulopelvic ligament and the round ligament with the endoscopic stapler. When the laparoscopic step was completed, the carbon dioxide gas was removed, and vaginal portion of the procedure was performed in the usual fashion. The vaginal vault was sutured after insertion of a Foley catheter. Once again, the abdomen was insufflated, a survey was performed to ensure hemostasis, and we have confirmed any possible ureteric injuries in all operations by observing and identifying the

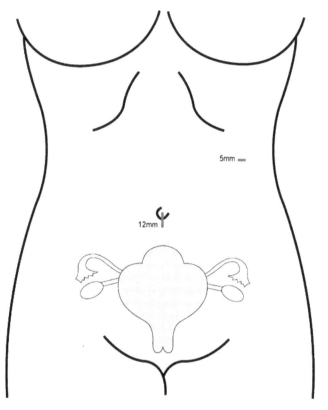

Fig. 1 Port-placement system for LAVH with the two-port method. The 5-mm telescope was located on the left upper quadrant 5-mm port site and an endoscopic stapler in the umbilical 12-mm port site

peristalsis, the absence of dilation of the both ureters after surgery, and by tracing its direction to the bladder (Fig. 2). A drainage tube was inserted into the left upper quadrant through the 5-mm port in some patients when persistent oozing was present or adhesiolysis had been performed.

The SAS program (version 9.1; SAS Institute Inc., Cary, NC, USA) was used for all statistical analyses.

Findings

During the study period, 176 women underwent LAVH with the two-port method. Table 1 presents the demographic and operative characteristics of the patients. Forty-two women (23.9%) had previous abdominal operative history, most commonly cesarean section (25 out of 176, 14.2%). The most common surgical indication was menorrhagia (102 out of 176, 58.0%), and the most frequent histopathological diagnosis was leiomyoma (118 out of 176, 67.0%). The median weight of the resected uterus was 230 g (range, 60–660 g). The median operating time was 58 min (range, 30–150 min). The median change in the hemoglobin level from before surgery to postoperative day 1 was 1.7 g/dL (range, 0.1–3.8 g/dL). The median hospital stay was 3 days (range, 2–7 days). None of the cases required an additional

Fig. 2 Sequential images of LAVH with the two-port method. **a** Laparoscopic view of uterus with multiple myomas. **b** Transection of the left ovarian ligament, salpinx, and round ligament with an endoscopic stapler through the umbilical 12-mm port site. **c** Transection of the right ovarian ligament, salpinx, and round ligament using the same method. **d** Immediate postoperative view

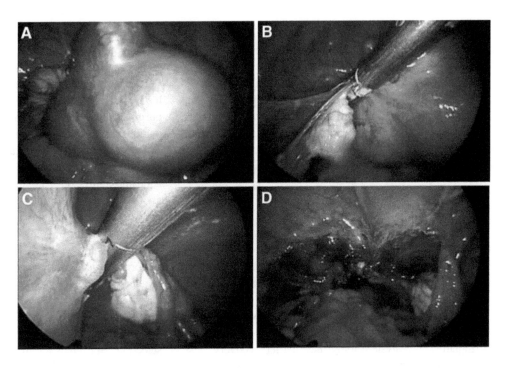

Table 1 Patients' characteristics and operative outcome for the two-port method

Characteristics	Median (range), number (%)
Age (years)	46 (33–60)
Parity	2 (0–5)
Body mass index (kg/m^2)	23.4 (17.6–29.6)
Operating time (min)	58 (30–150)
Uterine weight of removed specimen (g)	230 (60–660)
Hospital stay (day)	3 (2–7)
Estimated blood loss (mL)	200 (45–800)
Hemoglobin change (g/dL)	1.7 (0.1–3.8)
Complications (%)	1 (0.006)
Conversion to laparotomy (%)	0 (0)
Indications for LAVH	Number of subjects ($n=176$; %)
Menorrhagia	102 (58.0)
Lower abdominal pain	41 (23.3)
Carcinoma in situ of the uterine cervix	17 (9.7)
Dysmenorrhea	14 (8.0)
Microinvasive SCC of the uterine cervix	2 (1.1)
Previous abdominal surgery	Number of subjects ($n=42$; %)
Cesarean section	25 (14.2)
Appendectomy	7 (4.0)
Adnexectomy	6 (3.4)
Myomectomy	4 (2.3)
Histopathological diagnosis	Number of subjects ($n=176$; %)
Leiomyoma	118 (67.0)
Adenomyosis	39 (23.3)
Carcinoma in situ of the uterine cervix	17 (9.7)
Microinvasive SCC of the uterine cervix	2 (1.1)

SCC squamous cell carcinoma

port placement. There was no conversion to laparotomy in any cases. Eleven patients (6.3%) with anemia caused by menorrhagia received transfusion before or during the operation. No other intraoperative complications were noted. One case was complicated with an ileus postoperatively, but it was resolved with conservative treatment. All patients visited at 7 days, 2 months, and 12 months after two-port LAVH. There were no surgery-related complications.

Discussion

Since LAVH was first introduced in 1989 by Reich et al., various forms of laparoscopic hysterectomy such as laparoscopic supracervical hysterectomy or classic intra-fascial supracervical hysterectomy, LAVH, and total lapa-roscopic hysterectomy have been developed and modified [5–9]. LAVH has remained the widely performed method and the frequent type of laparoscopic hysterectomy.

Laparoscopic hysterectomy has earlier recovery, less postoperative pain, and cosmetic advantage when compared to conventional abdominal hysterectomy [10]. The number and size of ports used during laparoscopic surgery have been reported to be correlated with pain and analgesic use postoperatively [11–13]. Moreover, multiple skin incisions can lessen the patient's satisfaction postoperatively.

A study of two-port and four-port laparoscopic chole-cystectomy showed higher patient satisfaction scores on the scar in two-port than four-port group [14], and Al-Azawi et al. have demonstrated increased pain with increasing numbers of ports, especially more than four [15].

One of the unique techniques we used in this study is placement of the ports at the umbilicus and left upper quadrant. The vesicouterine peritoneum was easily accessed through the left upper quadrant port and, subsequently, the umbilical port. Instrument handling was convenient, and visibility was equally adequate using both the umbilical and left upper quadrant port sites. In a comparable study using two ports, a 2-mm minilaparoscope is fixed in the right lower quadrant, and the use of a laparoscopic instrument was possible only through the umbilical port [16]. Therefore, dissecting the vesicouterine peritoneum is not possible using this laparoscopic approach; thus, visualiza-tion and identification of the peritoneum are instead performed using a light-endorsed transvaginal section in the vaginal phase. Also, there has been a study on two-port LAVH using supraumbilical multichannel port and an ancillary port, but this method needed a 15-mm incision in the supraumbilical area for insertion of multichannel port. On the other hand, we used one 12-mm trocar and one 5-mm trocar [5].

Port insertion in the LUQ can decrease the risk of ilioinguinal or iliohypogastric nerve injury and nerve

entrapment syndrome [2]. Therefore, this two-port method seems to offer cosmetic satisfaction to the patients, less pain, fast recovery, and less port-associated complications. We used the endoscopic stapler device for dissecting and hemostasis in this study. It is widely used for these purposes, and its safety and utility have already been demonstrated in laparoscopic hysterectomy [17, 18].

However, if necessary, additional placement of ports should be performed to complete the procedure: severe adhesions, adnexal pathology, and large fibroids. Future areas of interest should include a direct comparison between LAVH using two-port method and conventional three- or four-port method.

LAVH using two ports, including a 5-mm telescope, was performed successfully for various benign uterine diseases in adequate operation times, without serious complications and increased surgical morbidity. LAVH with the two-port method is feasible and efficient with proper port placement, available laparoscopic instruments, and a suitable patient selection. But this is a retrospective study, so a randomized or comparative study will be required to determine the difference of pain and recovery between conventional and two-port LAVH.

Conflicts of interest The authors report no conflicts of interest. The authors alone are responsible for the content and writing of the paper.

References

1. Shen CC, Wu MP, Lu CH, Huang EY, Chang HW, Huang FJ, Hsu TY, Chang SY (2003) Short- and long-term clinical results of laparoscopic-assisted vaginal hysterectomy and total abdominal hysterectomy. J Am Assoc Gynecol Laparosc 10:49–54
2. Choi JS, Kyung YS, Kim KH, Lee KW, Han JS (2006) The four-trocar method for performing laparoscopically-assisted vaginal hysterectomy on large uteri. J Minim Invasive Gynecol 13:276–280
3. Ferrari MM, Berlanda N, Mezzopane R, Ragusa G, Cavallo M, Pardi G (2000) Identifying the indications for laparoscopically assisted vaginal hysterectomy: a prospective, randomised com-parison with abdominal hysterectomy in patients with symptom-atic uterine fibroids. BJOG 107:620–625
4. Darai E, Soriano D, Kimata P, Laplace C, Lecuru F (2001) Vaginal hysterectomy for enlarged uteri, with or without laparo-scopic assistance: randomized study. Obstet Gynecol 97:712–716
5. Yi SW, Park HM, Lee SS, Park SM, Lee HM, Sohn WS (2009) Two-port total laparoscopic hysterectomy with a multichannel port. J Laparoendosc Adv Surg Tech A 19:223–228
6. Reich H, DeCaprio J, McGlynn F (1989) Laparoscopy hysterec-tomy. J Gynecol Surg 5:213
7. Reich H, McGlynn F, Sekel L (1993) Total laparoscopic hysterectomy. Gynecol Endosc 2:59–63
8. Jenkins TR (2004) Laparoscopic supracervical hysterectomy. Am J Obstet Gynecol 191:1875–1884
9. Johnson N, Barlow D, Lethaby A, Tavender E, Curr E, Garry R (2006) Surgical approach to hysterectomy for benign gynaeco-logical disease. Cochrane Database Syst Rev (2):CD003677
10. Nieboer TE, Johnson N, Lethaby A, Tavender E, Curr E, Garry R, van Voorst S, Mol BWJ, Kluivers KB (2009) Surgical approach to

hysterectomy for benign gynaecological disease. Cochrane Database Syst Rev (3):CD003677. doi:10.1002/14651858.CD003677.pub4

11. Gagner M, Garcia-Ruiz A (1998) Technical aspects of minimally invasive abdominal surgery performed with needlescopic instruments. Surg Laparosc Endosc 8:171–179

12. Bisgaard T, Klarskov B, Trap R, Kehlet H, Rosenberg J (2000) Pain after microlaparoscopic cholecystectomy. A randomized double-blind controlled study. Surg Endosc 14:340–344

13. Leggett PL, Churchman-Winn R, Miller G (2000) Minimizing ports to improve laparoscopic cholecystectomy. Surg Endosc 14:32–36

14. Poon CM, Chan KW, Lee DW, Chan KC, Ko CW, Cheung HY, Lee KW (2003) Two-port versus four-port laparoscopic cholecystectomy. Surg Endosc 17:1624–1627

15. Al-Azawi D, Houssein N, Rayis AB, McMahon D, Hehir DJ (2007) Three-port versus four-port laparoscopic cholecystectomy in acute and chronic cholecystitis. BMC Surg 7:8

16. Tsai EM, Chen HS, Long CY, Yang CH, Hsu SC, Wu CH, Lee JN (2003) Laparoscopically assisted vaginal hysterectomy versus total abdominal hysterectomy: a study of 100 cases on light-endorsed transvaginal section. Gynecol Obstet Investig 55:105–109

17. Lee CL, Soong YK (1993) Laparoscopic hysterectomy with the Endo GIA 30 stapler. J Reprod Med 38:582–586

18. McMaster-Fay R (2004) Endoscopic stapling of large uterine vessels at laparoscopic hysterectomy for uterine fibroid masses of 500 g or more: a pilot study. Gynecol Surg 1:195–197. doi:10.1007/s10397-004-0046-8

Total laparoscopic hysterectomy for endometrial neoplasia

Mark Roberts · Carlota Rosales · Poornima Ranka

Abstract Total laparoscopic hysterectomy and bilateral salpingo-oophorectomy (TLH) offers an alternative and potentially more favourable procedure for women with early endometrial neoplasia. This cohort review presents the first 66 consecutive cases of TLH for endometrial neoplasia from one surgical team in a large teaching hospital. Data were collected for all women undergoing hysterectomy for suspected endometrial cancer, grade 1–2 adenocarcinoma, carcinoma in situ or severe atypical hyperplasia over 4 years using a prospectively kept theatre database. A total of 95 hysterectomies were identified, 66 (69%) underwent TLH, 18 (19%) underwent laparoscopically assisted vaginal hysterectomy (LAVH) and 11 (12%) had total abdominal hysterectomy (TAH) procedures. The mean age and body mass index of the patients in each group were similar, and average blood loss was lower in the TLH group (129 ml) compared to LAVH (185 ml) or TAH (247 ml). Total theatre time for TLH (113 min) was similar to LAVH (112 min) and less than the TAH group (127 min). Conversion rate from TLH to TAH was 0%. There were no major complications in the TLH group. These data report our early experience with a TLH and demonstrate a satisfactory record during its introduction. This new procedure offers a safe alternative to TAH for many women with no increased morbidity in agreement with recent literature. Although this paper reports a non-randomised series, we hope that it will serve to show that these techniques can be adopted safely by a new unit.

Keywords Total laparoscopic hysterectomy · Endometrial cancer · Neoplasia · Surgical route outcome · Severe atypia · Atypical hyperplasia · Treatment

Background

In 2009, one of the largest studies of the surgical approach to treat endometrial cancer was published [1]. The conclusions did not support routine systemic pelvis lymphadenectomy outside of clinical trials. Discussion highlighted the morbidity consequences of this radical approach without proven benefit; however, no suggestion is made on how to improve surgical outcome. It is worth noting that 93% of women underwent open hysterectomy, with the default approach being a mid-line incision, and the remaining 7% underwent laparoscopic hysterectomy.

Laparoscopic assisted vaginal hysterectomy with bilateral salpingo-oophorectomy (LAVH) has been described as an alternative to open hysterectomy with bilateral salpingo-oophorectomy (TAH) for suspected stage 1 endometrial cancer [2–4]. When compared, LAVH is associated with longer operating times and similar blood loss but less pain and shorter hospital stay. In deciding on the route of surgery, surgeons may consider findings such as obesity, which can compromise recovery because of the large abdominal incision required for TAH, or adequate vaginal access and cervical descent which would aid safe removal of the uterus with the main vaginal approach of LAVH. Such clinical findings are often seen in women with endometrial cancer, as common risk factors for the disease include obesity, nulliparity and increased age.

Total laparoscopic hysterectomy and bilateral salpingo-oophorectomy (TLH) offers an alternative and potentially more favourable procedure for these women. It has been shown in specialist centres to be an acceptable alternative to

M. Roberts (✉) · C. Rosales · P. Ranka
Women's Services, Royal Victoria Infirmary,
Newcastle upon Tyne NE1 4LP, UK
e-mail: mroberts.home@sky.com

TAH to treat women with endometrial pathology with no evidence of increased recurrence or impact on survival [5, 6]. Its benefits have included reduced hospital stay, shorter recovery time, fewer complications and less blood loss [7, 8]. The feasibility of a total laparoscopic approach for low grade endometrial cancer has improved since the ASTEC trial [1] has shown that routine pelvic lymphadenectomy is not necessary for grade 1 and 2 endometrial cancer. GOG-LAP2, a randomised controlled trial of more than 2,600 patients with early endometrial cancer comparing laparos-copy with laparotomy, also reported shorter hospital stay and fewer complications with a laparoscopic approach [9]. However, this study involved surgical staging and lympha-denectomy which is not supported by the ASTEC study [1]. In this large multi-centred study, there is limited surgeon or procedure quality control. These factors may explain the high laparoscopy conversion to laparotomy rate seen at 14.6%, reasons being mentioned including poor exposure, excessive bleeding and equipment failure.

We were obliged as part of local clinical governance protocol to confirm that the benefits described by others were achievable and realistic when TLH was introduced into our unit.

This cohort review presents the first 66 consecutive cases of TLH for endometrial neoplasia from one surgical team in a large teaching hospital. Cancers that are grade 1–2 endometrial malignancies and severe atypical hyperplasia are treated in this unit, whilst higher grades of cancer and endometrial sarcoma are referred to the local cancer centre. In the first year following introduction of TLH, a number of women were still offered LAVH or TAH, but by the fourth year of study, nearly all cases were treated with TLH. The study was primarily to look at the safety of the introduction of a new surgical method, and oncologic considerations were not the primary outcome of the study.

Methods

Data were collected from all women undergoing hysterec-tomy for endometrial cancer or severe endometrial atypia from January 2005, when TLH was first introduced to the unit, until December 2008. All surgery was undertaken or supervised by one gynaecological surgeon who had a caseload of 150–200 hysterectomies/year, which included other indications such as advanced endometriosis, ovarian masses and fibroids/menstrual disorders. All three surgical routes discussed in this paper were regularly used.

Diagnosis of severe atypical hyperplasia or grade 1–2 adenocarcinoma prior to surgery had been confirmed by Pipelle® endometrial biopsy or local anaesthetic hystero-scopy and direct biopsy. Severe atypia was taken as architectural and cytological atypia equivalent to carcinoma

in situ, and guideline management was the same as for low grade endometrial invasive cancer. Diagnostic and treat-ment methods were in line with the North of England Cancer Network Gynaeoncology Guidelines 2009. All cases were clinically FIGO stage I pre-operatively pending post-hysterectomy final staging. Any pre-operative FIGO stage II–IV and grade 3 malignancies were referred to the cancer centre for treatment and therefore are not included. A total of 95 hysterectomy and salpingo-oophorectomies were identified from a prospectively collected 'in theatre' database. Outcomes were further checked by retrospective review of all case notes and theatre records.

Surgical methods

All surgery was performed under general anaesthetic, and all patients received prophylactic antibiotics, low molecular weight heparin and TED® support stockings as standard.

TLH refers to hysterectomies performed entirely through laparoscopic ports but with vaginal removal of the specimen. A 10-mm trans-umbilical port is sited through which the laparoscope is inserted. In the right iliac fossa, a 5-mm port is placed for use by an assistant using a grasper. In the left iliac fossa, two 5-mm ports are placed as far apart as possible for use by the surgeon. Placement of the two ports in this position is to aid the surgical approach for suturing of the vaginal vault. At the start of the procedure, the cervix is inspected and peritoneal washings taken for cytology. Bipolar diathermy and incision are used to divide the infundibulo-pelvic ligaments and ovarian blood supply (Fig. 1), the round and the broad ligaments. The bladder is reflected from the anterior surface of the cervix using monopolar scissors until the outline of the vaginal probe (McCartney Tube® or VCare®) is delineated (Fig. 2). This identifies the cervico-vaginal margin and distal extent of dissection required to complete the hysterectomy. The uterine vessels are cauterised with bipolar diathermy (Fig. 3), and the vagina is opened with a monopolar hook by circumcising the cervix using the vaginal probe as a guide (Fig. 4). The uterus is removed via the vagina and the vaginal vault is closed using 2/0 PDS sutures which also re-align the uterosacral ligaments (Fig. 5). The procedure is completed after a careful check of haemostasis (Fig. 6).

Early on in the series, a McCartney Tube® was used as the vaginal probe. This is a hollow tube pushed up into the vagina to delineate the vaginal fornices and maintain pneumoperitoneum after the vagina is opened. Latterly, the VCare® uterine manipulator was used. This appeared to define the vaginal fornices much better for laparoscopic dissection. The tip of the VCare® is held in position by a small inflated balloon placed in the lower uterine cavity. Initially, we were concerned about uterine instrumentation with such a device, but after initial assessment in cases

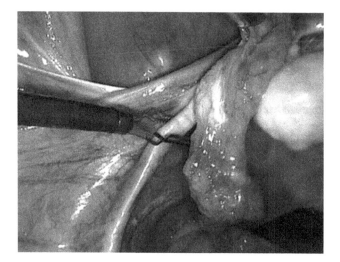

Fig. 1 Division of the left infundibulo-pelvic ligament

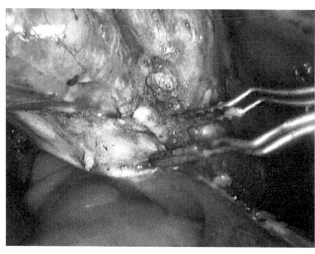

Fig. 3 Division of right uterine artery

without malignancy and subsequently with, we confirmed that histopathological assessment of the cervix/uterus was not impaired, there were no uterine perforations and none of the 66 cases had vaginal vault recurrence during the 1–5-year follow-up. We also did not experience tumour spillage into the vagina during surgery which is sometimes a problem when the uterus is manipulated during a TAH with difficult access.

By comparison, LAVH is maybe defined as a hysterectomy whereby a laparoscopic approach is used to mobilise the ovaries and obtain peritoneal washings and the rest performed vaginally. In this study, TAH is defined as an abdominal hysterectomy via a transverse suprapubic incision. Lymphadenectomy was not performed.

Data collected included age, body mass index (BMI), parity, procedure undertaken and hospital stay. Blood loss was determined by measurement of surgical swab weight after use and any aspirated blood. Theatre time was obtained from theatre records and was defined as time into

theatre to time out of theatre and as such includes time taken to transfer the patient to the operative table, positioning and preparation of the patient, cleaning at the end of the procedure and waking up from the anaesthetic. Hospital stay is defined as the number of post-operative nights spent in the hospital.

Findings

Of the 95 hysterectomies for endometrial neoplasia identified since the introduction of this new approach in 2005, a total of 66 (69%) underwent TLH, 18 (19%) underwent LAVH and 11 (12%) had TAH procedures. The surgical approach was decided on an individual patient basis following examination and discussion; however, the number of LAVH and TAH procedures declined each year with experience (Fig. 7). A higher proportion of TAH cases were nulliparous compared with TLH and LAVH. The chosen

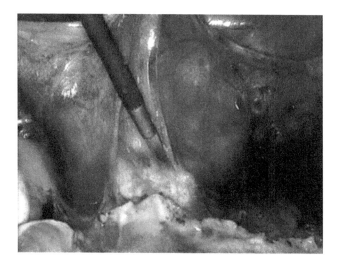

Fig. 2 Reflection of bladder

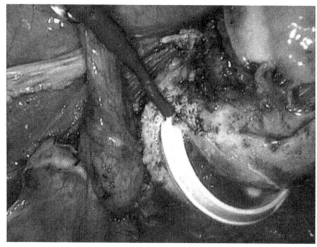

Fig. 4 Vaginal vault opened

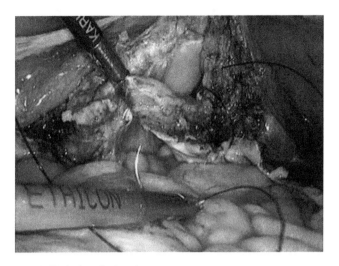

Fig. 5 Vaginal vault closed

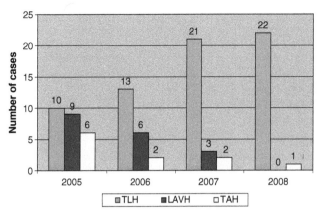

Fig. 7 Route of surgery in the years 2005–2008

surgical route was influenced by the presence (size and number) of fibroids, which were more common in nulliparous women. An abdominal approach would be chosen for a uterus over 12-week size to ensure that the uterus could be removed intact for histopathological examination. All TLH procedures were completed as intended; however, early in the series, one LAVH was converted to laparotomy after laparoscopic assessment identified a large subserosal fibroid that had not been considered prior to surgery.

The following data were initially collected without randomisation as the intent was to audit safe introduction of TLH, so the comparison of outcomes between the different surgical approaches is limited (Table 1). Nevertheless, it can be noted that mean age and BMI of the patients in each group were similar, and with this in mind, it

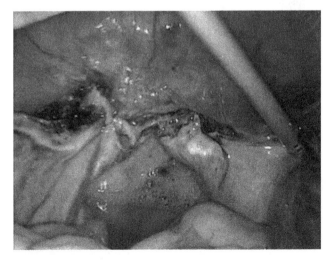

Fig. 6 Haemostasis check

is reassuring that measured blood loss and major haemorrhage (here taken as >1,000 ml) was actually lower in the TLH group (129 ml) compared to LAVH (185 ml) or TAH (247 ml).

Theatre times were obtained from theatre records and as such were recorded as time into theatre and time out of theatre. This would reflect total theatre usage rather than just operative time alone. Total theatre time for TLH (113 min) was similar to LAVH (112 min) and less than the TAH group (127 min).

Considering major complications, one of the LAVH patients had a small bowel injury repaired laparoscopically, and there were no other recorded cases of visceral injury in any of the groups. In the LAVH group, one patient also required intravenous antibiotics for an infected pelvic collection, which went on to require vaginal evacuation under anaesthetic 8 days post-operatively and the patient was given a 3-unit blood transfusion. Another of the LAVH cases had a BMI of 63 and was transferred post-operatively to HDU followed by a medical ward for treatment, including CPAP, antibiotics and physiotherapy. There were no cases of venous thrombosis or incisional hernia in any group.

The minor complications were noted as follows. Of the TLH cases, one developed a 3-cm chronic haematoma identified on CT scan 5 months post-operatively, which resolved spontaneously. Another was discharged home with oral antibiotics for persistent low grade pyrexia of unknown origin, 7 days post-operatively. One of the TLH cases required some superficial skin sutures under local anaesthetic on the ward for a dehiscence of the umbilical port site day 1 post-operatively. Of the LAVH cases, one was readmitted 3 weeks post-operatively for 4 days with a vault infection. There was no evidence of collection on scan and she was successfully treated with oral antibiotics. Following a difficult procedure due to a BMI of 55, a large uterus and abdominal adhesions, one of the TAH patients developed a wound infection and was discharged home on

Table 1 Summary of results comparing TLH, LAVH and TAH

	TLH	LAVH	TAH
Number	66	18	11
Mean age in years (SD)	63 (11.6)	60 (9.5)	61 (7.9)
Mean BMI (SD)	32.9 (8.24)	30.7 (10.7)	32.7 (9.33)
Nulliparous (%)	16 (24%)	1 (6%)	4 (36%)
Mean theatre time in minutes (SD)	113 (23.7)	112 (28.5)	127 (25.4)
Mean estimated blood loss (SD)	129 ml (395)	185 ml (187)	270 ml (247)
Major haemorrhage, >1,000 ml (%)	2 (3%)	0 (0%)	1 (9%)
Mean hospital stay in days (SD)	2.27 (1.6)	4.11 (2.7)	5.91 (3.0)
Major complications—injury to other organs, return to theatre or admission to HDU (%)	0 (0%)	3 (17%)	0 (0%)
Minor complications, infection or other complication managed conservatively (%)	3 (5%)	1 (6%)	1 (9%)

oral antibiotics. She represented 23 days post-operatively with a complete superficial wound dehiscence which required further antibiotics, a vacuum suction dressing and added hospital stay of 20 days.

In all cases, hysterectomy was performed following pre-operative diagnosis of severe atypical hyperplasia or grade 1–2 adenocarcinoma on endometrial biopsy. Post-operative histology on the whole uterus confirmed this in the majority of cases. The following cases were upstaged or upgraded: Of the TLH group, there were four cases with stage 3a endometrial adenocarcinoma diagnosed post-operatively. There was also one case of stage 3a carcinosarcoma. Two of the TAH cases had carcinosarcomas diagnosed at stages 3c and 1b. All cases are discussed at a weekly multidisciplinary team meeting and those requiring adjuvant therapy are referred to the local cancer centre. None of the cases underwent further surgical staging.

Conclusions

These data report our early experience with a TLH and demonstrate a satisfactory record during its introduction to a new unit. This new procedure offers a safe alternative to TAH for many women with no increased morbidity in agreement with recent literature [2, 9]. There is an excepted bias in the reported cases as the route chosen was not randomised; however, since introducing TLH, it has become the default procedure for endometrial pathology, reserving TAH as the default procedure for a grossly enlarged uterus.

We report a TLH to TAH conversion rate of 0% compared to 14% seen in the GOG-LAP2 study [9] probably in part due to the fact that pelvic lymphadenectomy was not performed in our series. The LACE trial, a randomised multi-centre trial comparing the laparoscopic with the open approach in early stage endometrial cancer,

has been started in Australia; however, this too involves lymphadenectomy. Given that lymphadenectomy is not supported by the ASTEC trial [1], our study better reflects current practice in Europe.

TLH is seen not only as a good alternative to TAH in terms of reduced blood loss and quicker recovery, but may also be advantageous over LAVH. It has been described that avoidance of the vaginal approach may reduce the risk of subsequent urinary incontinence and vault prolapse both of which are seen more often following vaginal rather than open hysterectomies [10–12]. Certainly, we found that routine post-operative indwelling bladder catheterisation is not required after TLH, perhaps because bladder dissection is minimised through use of the vaginal probe. This allows earlier mobilisation and more recently discharge home often on the first day following surgery.

Despite the fact that laparoscopy is usually associated with longer theatre times due to technical set up, our TAH theatre times were on average longer than the laparoscopic routes. This may reflect a more challenging case type, enlarged uterus, adhesions, high BMI and many co-morbidities.

Finally, it must be noted that the unit and surgical team investigated in this study is recognised for laparoscopic surgery, with these cases representing a small proportion of major and advanced laparoscopic procedures undertaken. In addition to this surgical expertise, it is likely that the cautious approach taken in establishing this new procedure may in part explain the satisfactory outcome data. Although this paper reports a non-randomised series, we hope that it will serve to show that these techniques can be adopted safely by a new unit. We demonstrate the ability to perform the majority of hysterectomies for endometrial cancer and severe atypical hyperplasia at a relatively low volume oncology unit. We await the results of the randomised multi-centred trial which is underway in the Netherlands [13], which is designed to include criteria for surgeons and is more applicable to practice in Europe.

References

1. ASTEC Study Group (2009) Efficacy of systematic pelvic lymphadenectomy in endometrial cancer (MRC ASTEC trial): a randomised study. Lancet 373(9658):125–136

2. Childers JM, Brzechffa PR, Hatch KD, Surwit EA (1993) Laparoscopically assisted surgical staging (LASS) of endometrial cancer. Gynecol Oncol 51(1):33–38

3. Eltabbakh GH, Shamonki MI, Moody JM, Garafano LL (2001) Laparoscopy as the primary modality for the treatment of women with endometrial carcinoma. Cancer 91(2):378–387

4. Hur M, Kim M, Kim JH, Moon JS, Lee JC, Seo DW (1995) Laparoscopically assisted vaginal hysterectomy. J Reprod Med 40 (12):829–833

5. Seracchioli R, Venturoli S, Ceccarin M, Cantarelli M, Ceccaroni M, Pignotti E et al (2005) Is total laparoscopic surgery for endometrial carcinoma at risk of local recurrence? A long-term survival. Anticancer Research 25(3c):2423–2428

6. Obermair A, Manolitsas TP, Leung Y, Hammond IG, McCartney AJ (2004) Total laparoscopic hysterectomy for endometrial cancer: patterns of recurrence and survival. Gynecol Oncol 92(3):789–793

7. O'Hanlan KA, Huang GS, Garnier AC, Dibble SL, Reuland ML, Lopez L et al (2005) Total laparoscopic hysterectomy versus total abdominal hysterectomy: cohort review of patients with uterine neoplasia. J Soc Laparoendosc Surg 9(3):277–286

8. Malzoni M, Tinelli R, Cosentino F, Perone C, Rasile M, Iuzzolino D et al (2009) Total laparoscopic hysterectomy versus abdominal hysterectomy with lymphadenectomy for early-stage endometrial cancer: a prospective randomized study. Gynecol Oncol 112(1):126–133

9. Walker JL, Piedmonte MR, Spirtos NM, Eisenkop JB, Barakat R (2009) Laparoscopy compared with laparotomy for comprehensive staging of uterine cancer: gynaecologic oncology group study LAP2. J Clin Oncol 27(32):5331–5336

10. Roovers JP, van der Bom JG, van der Vaart C Huub, Fousert DM, Heintz AP (2001) Does mode of hysterectomy influence micturition and defecation? Acta Obstet Gynecol Scand 80(10):945–951

11. Barrington JW, Edwards G (2000) Posthysterectomy vault prolapse. Int Urogynecol J Pelvic Floor Dysfunct 11(4):241–245

12. Zivkovic F, Tamussino K, Ralph G, Schied G, Auer-Grumbach M (1996) Long term effects of vaginal dissection on the innervation of the striated urethral sphincter. Obstet Gynecol 87(2):257–260

13. Bijen CBM, Briët JM, Bock GH, Arts HJG, Bergsma-Kadijk JA (2009) Total laparoscopic hysterectomy versus abdominal hysterectomy in the treatment of patients with early stage endometrial cancer: a randomized multi center study. BMC Cancer 9:23

23

Cardiac and gingival metastasis after total abdominal hysterectomy with bilateral salpingo-oophorectomy for primary uterine epithelioid angiosarcoma

Olivier Donnez · Etienne Marbaix ·
Patrick Van Ruyssevelt · Sarah Mitri · Jacques Donnez

Abstract Uterine epithelioid angiosarcomas are extremely rare; only 24 cases have been documented worldwide. We present a unique case of cardiac and gingival metastases developing 4 years after total abdominal hysterectomy with bilateral salpingo-oophorectomy for primary uterine epithelial angiosarcoma. Initial treatment remains total abdominal hysterectomy with bilateral salpingo-oophorectomy. Limited distant metastases may be surgically resected in selected cases in order to improve quality of life or to prevent sudden death in untreated patients. Optimal chemotherapy regimens must be determined.

Keywords Primary uterine angiosarcoma · Cardiac metastasis · Gingival metastasis

O. Donnez
Department of Gynecology,
Cliniques Universitaires de Mont-Godinne,
5530 Yvoir, Belgium

E. Marbaix
Department of Anatomopathology,
Université Catholique de Louvain,
1200 Brussels, Belgium

P. Van Ruyssevelt
Cardiovascular Department,
Centre Hospitalier de Jolimont-Lobbes,
7160 Haine-Saint-Paul, Belgium

S. Mitri · J. Donnez (✉)
Department of Gynecology, Université Catholique de Louvain,
Cliniques Universitaires St Luc,
Avenue Hippocrate 10,
1200 Brussels, Belgium
e-mail: jacques.donnez@uclouvain.be

Introduction

Epithelioid angiosarcoma was first described in 1864 by Klob [1]. It can arise from any blood or lymph vessels and most commonly occurs on the face and scalp and is linked to chronic lymphedema and previous irradiation [2]. It accounts for less than 2% of all sarcomas [3]. In the uterus, epithelioid angiosarcomas are extremely rare; only 24 cases have been documented worldwide [4, 5].

Metastases of uterine epithelioid angiosarcomas are poorly described in the literature. Here, we report the first case of cardiac metastasis arising from epithelioid angiosarcoma of the uterus 4 years after total abdominal hysterectomy with bilateral salpingo-oophorectomy. Successful resection of gingival metastasis is also reported.

Case report

The patient's oncological history dates back to a very early age. At just 2.5 years of age, she underwent surgical resection of a liposarcoma from the hip. Local recurrence was observed 1.5 years later, and surgical resection was followed by external radiotherapy. No metastatic lesions were identified. Unfortunately, no information is available on the timing or administered doses.

The patient then had an unremarkable medical history until the age of 58, when she presented with chronic cystitis and progressive abdominal discomfort. A large uterine tumor was diagnosed. Because of the considerable volume of the initial tumor, she underwent total abdominal hysterectomy and bilateral salpingo-oophorectomy. The uterine weight was 2,500 g. Histological examination of the uterus revealed a normal endometrium and normal adnexa on both sides. The uterine corpus was the site of the primary tumor. Histology, shown in Fig. 1a (low power magnification) and b (high power magnification), revealed irregular anastomotic vascular channels. Neoplastic cells had a pleomorphic vesicular nucleus with a prominent nucleolus and showed mitotic activity. The lesion was identified as an epithelioid angiosarcoma of the uterus. CD31 (Fig. 1c) was strongly immunolabeled in all neoplastic cells and CD34 (Fig. 1d) in most neoplastic

cells, while von Willebrand factor (Fig. 1e) was only faintly detected in some neoplastic cells. Cytokeratin (Fig. 1f) was immunolabeled in many neoplastic cells using the AE1–AE3 antibody mixture.

Bone metastasis in L2 and pulmonary lesions were also detected, and the patient underwent palliative adjuvant chemotherapy based on ifosfamide and doxorubicin (four regimens) associated with zoledronic acid. After two regimens, she presented with periodontal ulceration of the

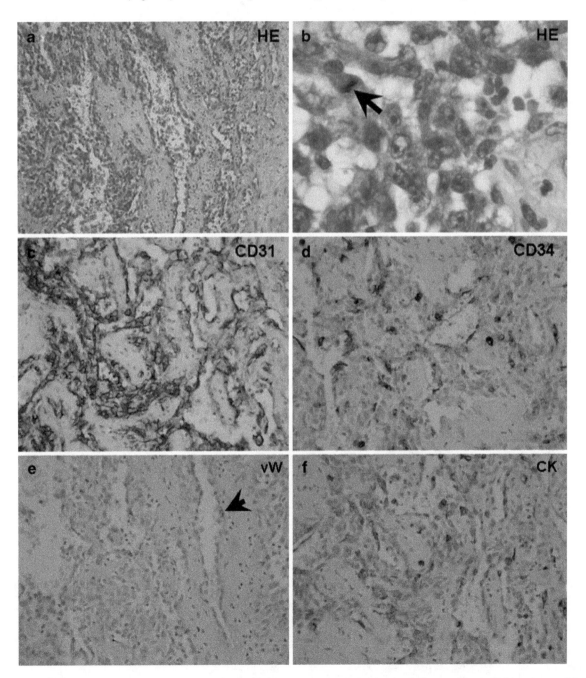

Fig. 1 **a** Low and **b** high power magnifications of the primary tumor in the uterine corpus reveal irregular anastomotic vascular channels. Neoplastic cells have a pleomorphic vesicular nucleus with a prominent nucleolus and show mitotic activity (*black arrow*). **c** CD31 is strongly immunolabeled in all neoplastic cells. **d** CD34 is immunolabeled in most neoplastic cells. **e** von Willebrand factor is faintly detected in some neoplastic cells (*black arrow*). **f** Cytokeratin is immunolabeled in many neoplastic cells using the AE1–AE3 antibody mixture

upper maxilla. Upon completion of the chemotherapy, the bone and pulmonary metastases were found to have regressed, but not the upper maxillary ulceration. The patient, therefore, underwent surgical resection of the maxilla, and histopathological examination (Fig. 2) revealed an angiosarcomatous growth beneath the squamous epithelium at the edge of the ulcer. One and a half years after the end of chemotherapy, chest and abdominal tomography confirmed the absence of recurrence. Bone scintigraphy showed stability of the lumbar spine, particularly L2, over a period of 4 years.

At the age of 62, the patient presented with hyperthermic syndrome associated with hyperleukocytosis (22,000/μl). A positron emission tomography scan revealed hyperfixation at the level of the superior pole of the left kidney and right cardiac ventricle. Cardiac echography was normal, and left adrenalectomy was performed. Histopathological examination did not evidence any neoplastic lesions, so immunohistochemical analysis was not carried out. The patient then received corticotherapy, and close follow-up was proposed. Two weeks later, she presented with dyspnea and distal cyanosis, and pulmonary scintigraphy showed bilateral embolism. Thoracic tomography revealed a mass inside the right atrium. Cardiac echography confirmed the presence of a 45-mm mass growing from the right atrial wall and obtruding the superior vena cava.

Because of the persistence of normal cardiac function and rapid development of the lesion, excisional surgery was proposed. After open heart surgery, a necrotic mass measuring 45 mm was observed issuing from the right wall of the right auricle (Fig. 3). En bloc excision and complete reconstruction of the right atrium using equine pericardium were performed. Histopathological findings (Fig. 4) showed endocardial aggregates of proliferating

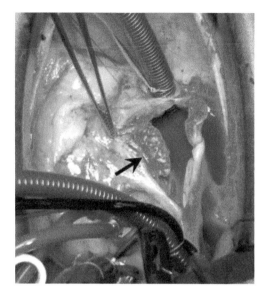

Fig. 3 Open heart surgery reveals a 4.5-cm mass in the right atrial wall (*black arrow*)

pleomorphic cells with central necrosis and confirmed the presence of cardiac metastasis of angiosarcomatous origin.

Unfortunately, during close postoperative follow-up, the patient developed acute severe right cardiac failure, complicated by refractory venous stasis and liver and kidney failures, and subsequently died. A recurrent pulmonary embolism was suspected.

Discussion

The 5-year relative survival rate for all uterine sarcomas is 43.5% (95% confidence intervals: 42.0–44.9) [6]. Uterine sarcomas other than leiomyosarcomas and endometrial

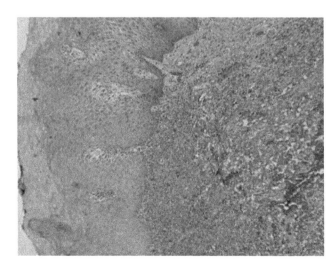

Fig. 2 Palatal metastasis shows an angiosarcomatous growth beneath the squamous epithelium at the edge of the ulcer

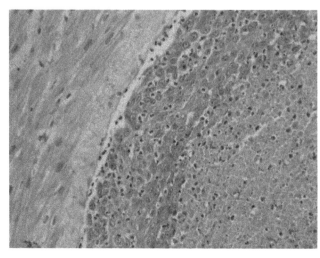

Fig. 4 Cardiac metastasis comprises endocardial aggregates of proliferating pleomorphic cells with central necrosis

stromal sarcomas are exceedingly rare. According to Olawaiye et al. [4] and Cardinale et al. [5], only 24 cases of uterine angiosarcoma have ever been published in the English-speaking literature. Since routine immunohisto-chemical investigation was introduced in the early 1980s, only 15 cases [4, 5, 7–15] have been documented using this technique in addition to morphological analysis. In the case we describe, angiosarcoma was microscopically identified by the freely anastomosing vascular channels, but also by positive immunohistochemical staining for endothelial cell antigens such as CD31, CD34, and von Willebrand factor. The same observations were made of both the gingival and cardiac metastases.

In Table 1, we present the last 16 cases of primary uterine angiosarcoma diagnosed by morphology and immunohisto-chemistry. We deliberately did not take into account cases reported before the early 1980s because of the absence of routine immunohistochemistry [7]. Ninety-three percent ($n=15/16$) of patients were peri- or postmenopausal at the time of diagnosis. One patient was only 35 years of age [5], but no data are available on her evolution after surgery. In this case, the prognosis was very poor due to the reported

presence of malignant cells in omental nodules and cytology fluid smears from pelvic irrigation and pleural effusions.

According to the literature, the prognosis of uterine angiosarcomas is very poor, with a median survival of just 13.5 months (Table 1). Small tumors [9, 12] appear to have a better prognosis. This view is upheld by Schammel and Tavassoli [12], who strongly believe that the endocavitary growth pattern might be considered a favorable prognostic factor. They previously reported a case of a patient still alive more than 3 years after a diagnosis of angiosarcoma, which is the only case of uterine angiosarcoma exhibiting an exophytic polyp rather than diffuse neoplastic infiltration of the myometrium. This is not supported by our findings, however. Our patient presented with diffuse myometrial infiltration of a 2,500-g uterus, and she survived for more than 4 years. Since we have no further information about the evolution of the cases described by Quinonez et al. [9] (>47 months' survival at the time of the case report) and Schammel et al. [12] (>36 months' survival at the time of the case report), our patient, having survived for 53 months, shows the longest overall survival observed after treatment of primary uterine angiosarcoma to date. This may have

Table 1 Sixteen cases of primary uterine angiosarcoma diagnosed by morphology and immunohistochemistry

Year	Age	Macroscopic features	Surgery	Adjuvant chemotherapy	Adjuvant irradiation	PFS months	OS months	Metastasis
1987	71	Massive enlargement of uterus	TAH, BSO	None	Yes	3	3	NA
1990	76	Massive enlargement of uterus	TAH, BSO	None	None	6	6	NA
1991	65	4.7-cm hemorr mass+bulky uterus	TAH, BSO LN	Cisplatin+adriamycin	Yes	47	47	NA
1993	56	Multiple hemorr myoma	TAH, BSO LN	Ifosfamide+adriamycin	Yes	2	7	NA
1993	61	10-cm uterine mass	TAH, BSO	None	None	1	1	NA
1994	58	12-cm mass	TAH, BSO	Unspecified type	Yes	2	2	NA
1998	49	6.3-kg uterine mass	TAH, BSO	None	None	3	3	NA
	58	12-cm uterine mass	TAH, BSO	Unspecified type	Yes	2	2	NA
	70	5-cm polypoid lesion, half myoma	TAH, BSO	None	None	36	36	NA
	75	6.3-cm lower uterus	TAH, BSO	None	None	7	7	NA
1999	59	12-week size uterus	TAH, BSO LN	None	None	0.4	2.5	Vaginal, lung, brain
2001	67	25x21-cm uterus	TAH, BSO	None	None	0	15	Gingival, lung, brain
2008	81	200-g uterus	TAH, BSO	None	None	0	6	Peritoneal spread
	35	2.400-g uterus	TAH, BSO	NA	NA	0	NA	Peritoneal+pleural spread
2008	54	11-cm bulky uterus	TAH, BSO	Gemcitabine+taxotere / Bevacizumab	None	3	12	Peritoneal+pleural spread
2009	58	2.500-g uterus	TAH, BSO	Ifosfamide+adriamycin	None	3	53	Bone, lung, gingival, heart

TAH total abdominal hysterectomy, *BSO* bilateral salpingo-oophorectomy, *LN* pelvic lymphadenectomy, *NA* not applicable

been due to the chemotherapy administered, but no other data are available in the literature on the impact of four regimens of ifosfamide and doxorubicin.

Complete surgical resection is generally accepted as the primary treatment in the literature. Olawaiye et al. [4] recommend total abdominal hysterectomy with bilateral salpingo-oophorectomy, as well as surgical excision of all macroscopic lesions observed in the peritoneal cavity. There are no data supporting routine pelvic or para-aortic lymphadectomy at the time of surgery. Indeed, no lymph node involvement has ever been reported, even in case of extensive peritoneal spread [9, 10, 14]. This is corroborated by histological findings, which show a strong tendency toward proliferation by hematogenous metastasis.

Olawaiye et al. [4] report that adjuvant chemotherapy may be of benefit in case of uterine angiosarcoma. Of patients (Table 1) who received adjuvant chemotherapy, 50% (n=3/6) were still alive more than 12 months after treatment (Table 1). Of those who did not receive chemotherapy, only 11% (n=1/9) survived after treatment. Moreover, the surviving patient was reported to have an angiosarcoma in a 5-cm intrauterine polyp, without transmural myometrial invasion [12]. These authors [4] were the only ones to use antiangiogenic agents associated with chemotherapy and, at the time of the publication, had achieved more than 12 months' survival in one of their patients. However, due to the disparity of chemotherapeutic regimens utilized, drug choice must be individually tailored.

On the subject of pelvic irradiation, the literature remains inconclusive. In Table 1, it is shown that 40% (n=2/5) of patients with pelvic irradiation were still alive 6 months after publication of the case report, compared to 70% (n=10) of those without irradiation. Based on these data, pelvic irradiation does not appear to offer any benefits.

Metastases of uterine angiosarcomas are poorly described. Mendez et al. [14] and Medina et al. [15] have both reported lung and brain metastases, and one case of gingival metastasis was recorded by Medina et al. [15]. In their opinion, surgical excision was necessary to improve the patient's quality of life. In our case, the appearance of gingival and pulmonary metastases during chemotherapy could have worsened the prognosis, but the patient survived more than 4 years after treatment. Again, this may have been due to the chemotherapeutic regimen, but further studies are required to confirm this.

Cardiac metastasis from primary uterine angiosarcoma has never before been reported. In the case we describe here, development of the lesion suggested an aggressive neoplasm, but this was not borne out by the 53 months of progression-free survival at the time of cardiac surgery. Surgery was decided upon because of the 4-year survival of the patient in an attempt to prevent fatal heart failure or sudden death by pulmonary embolization or acute valvular obstruction. In the literature, four cases of successful excision of intracavitary extension to the heart from recurrent low-grade endometrial stromal sarcomas have been documented [16–19], and the authors considered the surgical approach to be a viable option. Unfortunately, in our case, the patient died postoperatively of acute right-sided cardiac failure. This risk has to be weighed against the risk of sudden death in untreated cases.

Conclusion

Here, we present the longest progression-free survival of primary uterine sarcoma treated by total abdominal hysterectomy with bilateral salpingo-oophorectomy achieved to date. Adjuvant chemotherapy seems to offer some benefit in terms of overall survival, but further studies are needed to determine the optimal regimen. Pelvic radiotherapy does not appear to improve overall survival. Limited distant metastases may be surgically resected in selected cases in order to improve quality of life or to prevent sudden death in untreated patients [19].

Conflict of interest There is no actual or potential conflict of interest in relation to this article.

References

1. Klob: Cited by Horgan E (1930) Hemangioma of uterus. Surg Gynecol Obstet 50:990
2. Rao J, Dekoven JG, Beatty JD, Jones G (2003) Cutaneous angiosarcoma as a delayed complication of radiation therapy for carcinoma of the breast. J Am Acad Dermatol 49:532–538
3. Abrahamson TG, Stone MS, Piette WW (2001) Cutaneous angiosarcoma. Adv Dermatol 17:279–299
4. Olawaiye AB, Morgan JA, Goodman A, Fuller AF, Penson RT (2008) Epithelioid angiosarcoma of the uterus: a review of management. Arch Gynecol Obstet 278:401–404
5. Cardinale L, Mirra M, Galli C, Goldblem JR, Pizzolito S, Falconeri G (2008) Angiosarcoma of the uterus: report of 2 new cases with deviant clinicopathologic features and review of the literature. Ann Diagn Pathol 12:217–221
6. Gatta G, Ciccolallo L, Kunkler I, Capocaccia R, Berrino F, Coleman M, De Angelis R, Faivre J, Lutz JM, Martinez C, Möller T, Sankila R, the EUROCARE Working Group (2006) Survival from rare cancer in adults: a population-based study. Lancet Oncol 7:132–140
7. Witkin GB, Askin FB, Geratz JD, Reddick RL (1987) Angiosarcoma of the uterus: a light microscopic, immunohistochemical, and ultrastructural study. Int J Gynecol Pathol 6:176–184
8. Milne DS, Hinshaw K, Malcolm AJ, Hilton P (1990) Primary angiosarcoma of the uterus: a case report. Histopathology 16:203–205
9. Quinonez GE, Paraskevas MP, Diocee MS, Lorimer SM (1991) Angiosarcomas of the uterus: a case report. Am J Obstet Gynecol 164:90–92

10. Tallini G, Price FV, Carcangiu ML (1993) Epithelioid angiosarcoma arising in uterine leiomyomas. Am J Obstet Gynecol 100:514–518

11. Morrel B, Mulder AF, Chadha S, Tjokrowardojo AJ, Wijnen JA (1993) Angiosarcoma of the uterus following radiotherapy for squamous cell carcinoma of the cervix. Eur J Obstet Gynecol Reprod Biol 49:194–197

12. Schammel DP, Tavassoli FA (1998) Uterine angiosarcomas: a morphologic and immunohistochemical study of four cases. Am J Surgic Pathol 22:246–250

13. Darchenberg CB, Faust FJ, Borkowski A, Papadimitriuo JC (1994) Epithelioid angiosarcoma of the uterus arising in a leiomyoma with associated ovarian and tubal angiomatosis. Am J Clin Pathol 102:338–339

14. Mendez LE, Joy S, Angioli R, Estape R, Penalver M (1999) Primary uterine angiosarcoma. Gynecol Oncol 75:272–276

15. Medina BR, Barba EM, Torres AV, Trujillo SM (2001) Gingival metastasis as first sign of a primary uterine angiosarcoma. J Oral Maxillofac Surg 59:476–481

16. Vargas-Narron J, Keirn C, Barragan-Garcia R, Beltran-Ortega A, Rotberg T, Santana-Gonzalez A et al (1990) Intracardia extension of malignant uterine tumors. J Thorac Cardiovasc Surg 99:1099–1103

17. Mikami Y, Demopoulos RI, Boctor F, Febre EF, Harris M, Kronzen I et al (1999) Low-grade endometrial stromal sarcoma with intracardiac extension. Pathol Res Pract 195:501–508

18. Val-Bernarl JF, Hernandez-Nieto E (1999) Symptomatic intracavitary (non-invasive) cardiac metastasis from low-grade endometrial stromal sarcoma of the uterus. Pathol Res Pract 195:717–722

19. Yokoyama Y, OnoY ST, Fukuda I, Mizunuma H (2004) Asymptomatic intracardiac metastasis from a low-grade endometrial stromal sarcoma with successful surgical resection. Gynecol Oncol 92:999–1001

24

Use of vaginal mesh for pelvic organ prolapse repair

Virginie Bot-Robin · Jean-Philippe Lucot ·
Géraldine Giraudet · Chrystèle Rubod · Michel Cosson

Abstract The use of mesh for pelvic organ prolapse repair through the vaginal route has increased during this last decade. The objective is to improve anatomical results (sacropexy with mesh seeming better than traditional surgery) and keep still the advantage of vaginal route. Numbers of cohort series and randomized control trials have been recently published. These works increase our knowledge of advantages and risks of mesh. It has been shown that the use of mesh to treat cystocoele through vaginal route improves anatomical results when compared to traditional surgery. The rate of complications, especially de novo dyspareunia, remains equivalent between the two techniques.

Keywords Pelvic organ prolapse · Gynaecologic surgical procedure · Vaginal surgery · Female · Mesh · Review

Background

Recommendations and reviews were recently published in the USA and in France about the surgical treatment of pelvic organ prolapse (POP) in women. In 2010, a Cochrane review gathered all randomized studies published until February 2009 [1]. Authors concluded that prosthetic reinforcement when treating cystocoele by vaginal route seems to lessen the risk of anatomic recurrence, but better satisfaction, better quality of life and decrease of re-interventions could not be demonstrated. There were not enough data to prove the impact of mesh when treating prolapse in the posterior compartment through the vaginal route [1].

Mucowski warned surgeons on the increased number of patients complaining after treatment of POP with prosthetic reinforcement mesh [2]. Over 1,000 undesirable effects were reported between 2005 and 2010 to the US Food and Drug Administration (FDA). A report listed the most frequent due to the technique (vaginal erosion, infection, pelvic pain, urinary problems and recurrence of prolapse). The FDA also encouraged surgeons to declare all adverse effects they could consider linked to the mesh, even those that come under a non-mandatory declaration. Finally, to improve (1) knowledge of surgeons about the possible complications of this procedure and (2) informed counselling provided to concerned women, the International Urogynecological Association and the International Continence Society recently proposed a classification of the complications related directly to the insertion of prostheses in this indication [3].

Since then, several randomized trials and many cohorts were published. Our aim is to collect and analyze them all.

V. Bot-Robin (✉) · J.-P. Lucot · G. Giraudet · C. Rubod ·
M. Cosson
Department of Gynaecologic Surgery, Jeanne de Flandre Hospital,
Centre Hospitalier Régional et Universitaire,
59000 Lille, France
e-mail: virginiebotrobin@gmail.com

C. Rubod · M. Cosson
Faculty of Medicine, University of 'Lille Nord de France',
59000 Lille, France

Method

A computerized bibliographic enquiry on Pubmed used the keywords: "pelvic organ prolapse", "mesh", "graft", "vaginal surgery", with limits: "randomized control trial" and "clinical trial". We added to the review of Savary [4] all randomized trials published in English or French until

December 2010. To study the adverse effects, we also included prospective or retrospective works. We excluded fundamental studies (using or not animals) and anatomic studies. All included articles were analyzed by two reviewers.

For each randomized study, data were collected on a standardized file which noted: the objectives of the study (main and secondary) with their criteria of judgement (standardized scales), the approval of an ethical committee and the written consent of the patients, the length of inclusion, the calculation of the number of included patients, inclusion and exclusion criteria, the blind definition, the method of randomization, the anatomic level treated, the material used and surgical technique, the method used to homogenize the techniques, surgeons and centres, the statistical method used, the number of patients included and lost to follow-up, the duration of the study and follow-up, the anatomic and functional results, the complications and adverse effects and the conclusions of the authors.

In other studies, we used similar reading files without the items specific to randomized studies.

Findings

Sixteen randomized trials matching our inclusion criteria were published: one in 2006 [5], two in 2007 [6, 7], four in 2008 [8–11], four in 2009 [12–15] and five in 2010 [16–20]. We added two publications of Nieminen, reporting long-term results of the randomized trial initially written by Hiltunen in 2007 [6, 21, 22]. Table 1 sums up for each study the number of patients included, the anatomic level involved, the surgical technique and mesh used and the main and secondary criteria of evaluation. The work of Allahdin was dismissed because of the lack of precision about the conception and the description of surgery [8].

Thirteen of these randomized trials mainly compared traditional surgery and use of mesh on anatomic results [5–7, 10–14, 17–20, 22]. Twelve studied non-absorbable synthetic (NAS) polypropylene implants [6, 8–12, 14, 16, 19–22] and six absorbable biomesh (AB) [5, 7, 13, 15, 17, 18]. Anatomic results are summed up in Table 2.

Improvement of symptoms and quality of life were the main objectives of two studies: Nieminen in 2008 (polypropylene NAS mesh versus colporrhaphy) and Guerette in 2009 (bovine pericardium graft versus colporrhaphy) [13, 21]. They were secondary objectives in the other 15 studies. Among studied symptoms, nine authors took interest in the impact of the mesh reinforcement on sexuality. Nieminen used an original questionnaire as no validated one existed in a Finnish translation. Authors studied not only sexuality but also symptoms and quality of life [21]. For Guerette,

sexuality was the main objective: they used the validated questionnaire "Pelvic Organ Prolapse/Urinary Incontinence Sexual Questionnaire" (PISQ-12) [13], also used by Nguyen [10]. Some authors only reported existence or not of a sexual activity and/or pre- and post-surgical dyspareunia. Functional results are summed up in Table 3.

Since December 2010, six randomized studies have been published [23–28]: two studies comparing the anatomical outcomes after 12 months between conventional vaginal prolapse surgery and polypropylene mesh insertion (respectively, $n=189$ versus $n=200$ and $n=97$ versus $n=93$) [23, 28], one study comparing the improvement of symptoms and quality of life 2 years after a 2×2 factorial design first described by Allahdin (Vicryl mesh $n=32$ or not $n=34$ and PDS $n=33$ or Vicryl suture $n=33$) [8, 25], one study comparing the anatomical outcomes after 36 months between sacrospinous ligament fixation (SSLF, $n=8$) and posterior intravaginal slingplasty (IVS, $n=14$) for uterovaginal or vaginal vault prolapse [24], one study comparing the anatomical outcomes after 24 months between laparoscopic sacropexy ($n=53$) and vaginal mesh (Prolift Kit, $n=55$) for the treatment of post hysterectomy vault prolapse [26], and one study comparing the sexual function at 12 months after either a vaginal surgical repair with native tissue or a trocar-guided mesh insertion in patients with recurrent POP [27]. The work of Madhuvrata was also dismissed because of the lack of precision about the conception, the description of surgery and the complication rates for different groups (no mesh versus mesh).

For Maher, the rate of anatomic success (all compartments, state 0 or 1) is significantly higher after sacropexy (77% versus 43%) with a higher rate of re-intervention in the Prolift group (79% versus 87%). But the number of symptomatic prolapse is similar [26]. Altman and Withagen showed a number of anatomic failures (state 2 or higher) observed after a tension-free vaginal mesh insertion significantly less important than after a conventional vaginal repair after 12 months (respectively, 65.5% versus 39.2% and 45.2 versus 9.6%) [23, 28]. Heinonen showed a similar rate of anatomic recurrence between the two apical support operations (21% in the IVS group and 13% in the SSLF group) with only one symptomatic patient in each group and no re-intervention [24]. Surgery is significantly shorter for vaginal route when comparing with laparoscopic sacropexy [26], but longer when comparing with conventional vaginal repair [23]. All these studies showed an improvement of quality of life and symptoms of POP in both groups, most often with no significant difference between the two surgical techniques [23, 26–28]. Complications in these recent randomized studies are described in the paragraphs below.

Finally, during the study period, we collected 108 nonrandomized trial (NRT) which studied the surgical treat-

Table 1 Randomized trials summary

Trial	Number	Level of prolapse	Graft type and technique compared	Main objective(s)/Criterion(a) Secondary objective(s)/Criterion(a)
Hiltunen 2007 [6]	202	ANT	Polypropylene mesh fixed by 4 lateral arms NAS (Parietene®) versus Colporrhaphy	Anatomic results/POP-Q<2 at 2 et 12 months POP symptoms improvement, per and post-surgical complications, and postvoidal urine residual volume at 2 and 12 months/non-validated questionnaire, clinical examination
Allahdin 2008 [8]	66	–	1° Polyglactin mesh AS versus Colporrhaphy 2° Polydiaxone suture AS versus Polyglactin suture AS	QoL and POP symptoms improvement / POPPY (Bugge et al. 2005)
Nguyen 2008 [10]	76	ANT	Polypropylene mesh fixed by 4 lateral arms NAS (IntePro® + Perigee System®) versus Colporrhaphy	Anatomic results/POP-Q<2 at 1 year (intermediate analysis) Sexual functional results and QoL improvement/validated questionnaire
Nieminen 2008 [21]	202	ANT	Polypropylene mesh fixed by 4 lateral arms NAS (Parietene®) versus Colporrhaphy	POP symptoms improvement and sexual functional results/non-validated questionnaire
Sivasliolgu 2008 [11]	90	ANT	Polypropylene mesh fixed by 4 lateral arms NAS (Parietene®) versus Colporrhaphy	Anatomic results/POP-Q: Ba<−1 at 1 year QoL improvement, dyspareunia, cicatrisation and complications/validated questionnaire, clinical examination
Carey 2009 [12]	139	ANT + POST	Free Polypropylene mesh NAS (Gynemesh®) versus Colporrhaphy	Anatomic results/POP-Q<2 at 12 years POP symptoms, QoL and satisfaction improvement/validated questionnaire
Lunardelli 2009 [14]	32	ANT	Polypropylene mesh fixed by 4 lateral arms NAS (Nazca TC®) versus Site-specific surgical anterior vaginal prolapse repair: reinsertion of the pubocervical fascia into the tendinous arch	Anatomic results/POP-QI with a difference of Ba point of 1 cm between the 2 groups
Ek 2010 [16]	50	ANT	Polypropylene mesh fixed by 4 lateral arms NAS (Prolift®) versus Colporrhaphy	Urodynamic examination/MUCP<40 cmH2O
Iglesia 2010 [19]	65	ANT + / - POST	Hysterectomy and: Polypropylene mesh NAS anterior or total (Prolift®) versus Uterosacral ligament suspension as Schull described or Sacrospinofixation of vaginal dome as Richter described	Anatomic results/POP-Q<2 at 3 and 12 months POP symptoms and QoL improvement, complications/validated questionnaire, clinical examination
Nieminen 2010 [22]	202	ANT	Polypropylene mesh fixed by 4 lateral arms NAS (Parietene®) versus Colporrhaphy	Anatomic results/POP-Q<2 at 3 years POP symptoms improvement and complications/non-validated questionnaire, clinical examination
Meschia 2007 [7]	206	ANT	Porcine skin collagen implant with lateral fixation AB (Pelvicol®) versus Plication of the pubocervical fascia	Anatomic results / POP-Q<2 at 3, 6 and 12 months, then once a year Complications/clinical examination at 3, 6 and 12 months, then once a year
Guerette 2009 [13]	94	ANT	Bovine pericardium collagen matrix implant with 2×2 lateral fixation AB versus Colporrhaphy	Anatomic results, POP symptoms improvement, sexual functional results, cicatrisation and complications/validated questionnaire, clinical examination, POP-Q at 3, 6, 12 and 24 months
Natale 2009 [15]	190	ANT	Porcine skin collagen implant AB (Pelvicol®) versus Polypropylene mesh NAS (Gynemesh®)	Incidence of erosions/decrease of 15% POP symptoms and QoL improvement, sexual functional results/validated questionnaire
Feldner 2010 [17]	56	ANT	Porcine collagen implant (submucosa of small intestine) with 3×2 lateral fixation AB versus Colporrhaphy	Anatomic results / POP-Q<2 (Ba point) at 1 year POP symptoms and QoL improvement, complications/validated questionnaire, clinical examination

Table 1 (continued)

Trial	Number	Level of prolapse	Graft type and technique compared	Main objective(s)/Criterion(a) Secondary objective(s)/Criterion(a)
Hviid 2010 [18]	61	ANT	Porcine skin collagen implant with lateral fixation AB (Pelvicol®) versus Plication of the fascia + colpectomy	Anatomic results/POP-Q: Ba<−1 at 1 year QoL improvement/validated questionnaire
De Tayrac 2008 [9]	49	MOY	Polypropylene mesh with lateral fixation NAS (IVS®) versus Sacrospinofixation	Pain the first day post-surgery/VAS Operating time, pre- and post-surgical complications, length of stay, satisfaction, QoL improvement, sexual activity, anatomic results, erosion, surgical procedure facility
Paraiso 2006 [5]	106	POST	Porcine skin implant with central and lateral fixation (Fortagen®) versus Plication of the fascia or Site-specific surgical repair	Anatomic results/POP-Q: Bp<or=−2 at 1 year POP symptoms and QoL improvement, sexual functional results/validated questionnaire
Lopes 2010 [20]	32	POST	Hysterectomy and: Polypropylene mesh fixed by 4 lateral arms NAS (Nazca TC®) versus Sacrospinofixation +/- pubocervical fascia repair if indicated	Anatomic results/POP-Q and POP-Q-I at 1 year POP symptoms and QoL improvement, complications/validated questionnaire, clinical examination

POP pelvic organ prolapse, *QoL* quality of life, *AS* absorbable and synthetic, *NAS* non-absorbable and synthetic, *AB* absorbable and biologic, *MUCP* maximum urethral closure pression

ment of POP with reinforcement mesh, mainly NAS meshes (92/108 studies). Complications are described in Tables 4 and 5. It seemed important to distinguish complications due to the dissection or the suspension of the mesh through trans-obturator or trans-levator and the complications due to the mesh itself (vaginal exposition, mesh shrinkage, dyspareunia, infection...).

Bleeding

In randomized studies, there was no significant difference between the two techniques (traditional surgery or using graft) when comparing "average blood loss" (596 patients in seven studies) [5, 7, 13, 14, 18–20] or "important blood loss" (446 patients in four studies) [6, 9, 12, 17]. A superior blood loss in the group with prosthetic reinforcement was found by Hiltunen and Altman [6, 23]. Heinonen reported one transfusion in the IVS group [24]. Sixty-seven non-randomized studies reported their per-surgical bleeding or post surgical haematomas. However, definition of bleeding varied from one study to another: most often the subjective impression of the surgeon, sometimes a more precise quantification (>200, 300, 400, 500 or 1,000 ml), or the need of blood transfusion. Other causes of bleeding have been reported as a vascular lesion in concomitant surgery (such as a hysterectomy) [29]. The precise time of onset of important bleeding due to the mesh set up (opening of pararectal or paravesical fossa, passage through trans-obturator or trans-levator) was never reported. No death due to

haemorrhage occurred in these series. Post-surgical haematomas were seen in 2.15% out of 6,034 patients (41 NRT). Their localization and their management were different according to the teams (vaginal mesh, surgical draining, simple clinical monitoring...) and not always explained. Only three studies reported infection of haematoma (three cases out of 368 patients, 0.8%); all were seen after using a NAS mesh [30–32]. In the recent randomized studies published, Heinonen reported one haematoma in the IVS group [24], Withagen observed significantly more haematomas in the group with mesh reinforcement [28], and Altman found no difference between the two groups (mesh versus not) [23].

Visceral injury

Non-randomized studies showed, respectively, 1.94%, 1.6% and 1.55% of bladder, urethral or ureteral injuries, while in randomized studies, these complications were reported, respectively, in three studies for bladder injury (meaning four patients out of 160) [6, 9, 19], one study for urethral injury (one patient out of 29) [17] and one study for ureteral injury (one patient out of 31) [5]. No rectal injury was reported in randomized studies, versus 0.58% out of 5,877 patients in cohorts (47 NRT). Two non-randomized studies have mentioned vaginal perforations (4.35% of 99 patients) [33, 34]. Randomized studies showed no difference with or without mesh reinforcement regarding to these complications, and recently Altman confirmed this result [23].

Table 2 Anatomic results (graft surgery versus traditional surgery)

Trial	Number	Number of patients studied (graft surgery versus traditional surgery)	Results (graft surgery versus traditional surgery)
Hiltunen[a] 2007 [6]	202	2 months: 201 (104 versus 97) 12 months: 200 (104 versus 96)	One-year recurrence rate in favour of graft reinforcement (7% versus 38%)
Nguyen[a] 2008 [10]	76	75 (37 versus 38)	One-year recurrence rate in favour of graft reinforcement (11% versus 45%)
Sivasliolgu[a] 2008 [11]	90	85 (43 versus 42)	One-year recurrence rate in favour of graft reinforcement (9% versus 28%)
			POP-Q difference for points Aa, Ba and C in favour of graft reinforcement
Carey[a] 2009 [12]	139	124 (63 versus 61)	No significant POP-Q difference<2 at 1 year (81% versus 65.6%)
Lunardelli 2009 [14]	32	32 (16 versus 16)	POP-Q difference for points Aa and Ba in favour of graft reinforcement (mean follow-up=8.5 months)
Iglesia 2010 [19]	65	65 (32 versus 33)	No significant difference for recurrence rate with mean follow-up=9.7 months (59% versus 72%)
			Point Ba higher in the group with graft reinforcement
Nieminen 2010 [22]	202	182 (97 versus 85)	Two-year recurrence rate in favour of graft reinforcement (12% versus 41%)
Meschia 2007 [7]	206	201 (98 versus 103)	One-year recurrence rate in favour of graft reinforcement for point Ba (7% versus 19%)
			No significant difference for recurrence rate on the posterior wall
Guerette 2009 [13]	94	1 year: 72 (35 versus 37) 2 years: 44 (17 versus 27)	No significant difference for recurrence rate (15% versus 22% after 1 year, 23.5% versus 37% after 2 years)
Feldner 2010 [17]	56	56 (29 versus 27)	One-year recurrence rate in favour of graft reinforcement (13.8% versus 40.7%)
			POP-Q difference for point Ba in favour of graft reinforcement
Hviid 2010 [18]	61	3 months: 50 (27 versus 23) 12 months: 54 (28 versus 26)	No significant difference for recurrence rate after 3 and 12 months (15% versus 7%)
Paraiso 2006 [5]	106	81 (26 graft reinforcements versus 27 plication of the fascia versus 28 site-specific surgical repair)	One-year recurrence rate (meaning Bp point>−2) higher and earlier in the group with graft reinforcement (46% versus 22% versus 14%)
			No significant difference for recurrence rate between these 3 groups if recurrence is defined by Bp>0
Lopes 2010 [20]	32	30 (14 versus 16)	No significant difference for recurrence rate after 12 months whatever level treated
De Tayrac[b] 2008 [9]	49	45 (21 versus 24)	No significant difference for recurrence rate whatever level treated (anterior 4.8% versus 25%, apex 4.8% versus0%, posterior 0% versus 4.2%) with mean follow-up=16.8 months
Natale[b] 2009 [15]	190	190 (96 Gynemesh® versus 94 Pelvicol®)	No significant difference for recurrence rate after 24 months (28.1% versus 43.6%)

[a] From these trials: number of patients with 1-year follow-up: 247 anterior graft reinforcement NRS versus 236 anterior traditional surgery. Mean recurrence rate after 1 year: with graft reinforcement surgery=11.5%, without graft reinforcement surgery=36.35%

[b] In this study, anatomic results are secondary criteria

Mesh exposition

The rate of graft exposition, whatever its type (NAS or AB) was 7.6% on average. In randomized studies, it was higher with NAS meshes (most studies): 44 patients out of 398 in nine trials [6, 9–12, 14, 15, 19, 20]. But it varied largely, from 0% to 35.7% of cases [13, 17, 20]. Mean frequency of exposition was lower for AB meshes (<1%), excepted in one study [35]. In the majority of randomized trials, mesh expositions were treated with local excision (most often under local anaesthesia) and/or vaginal oestrogen cream [6, 9–12, 14, 15, 20, 28]. A total removal of the mesh in this indication is exceptional. Milani showed that mesh exposure was independently associated with deterioration in sexual function [27].

Infection

Three randomized studies did not show a significant increase of local infection on surgical site [6] or urinary

Table 3 Functional results (graft surgery versus traditional surgery)

Trial	Number	Number of patients studied (graft surgery versus traditional surgery)	Results (graft surgery versus traditional surgery)
Nieminen[a] 2008 [21]	202	182 (97 versus 85)	Score for vaginal bulge significantly lower in the mesh group 2 years after surgery
			Scores for sexual function did not differ between the groups at baseline and 2 years after surgery
			Score for dyspareunia significantly lower in the mesh group
			Higher rate of patient reported their vagina to be too loose for intercourse in the mesh group
Guerette[a] 2009 [13]	94	1 year: 72 (35 versus 37)	Better UDI-6 score after surgery in both groups
		2 years: 59 (26 versus 33)	Scores for sexual function did not differ between the groups at baseline and after surgery
			Better rate of dyspareunia and PISQ-12 score after surgery in both groups
Hiltunen 2007 [6]	202	2 months: 201 (104 versus 97)	Majority of the symptoms resolved after surgery in both groups
		12 months: 200 (104 versus 96)	Symptomatic recurrence higher in mesh group 12 months after surgery (4% versus 15%)
			Stress urinary incontinence reported more frequently in the mesh group 12 months after surgery (23% versus 10%)
Nguyen 2008 [10]	76	75 (37 versus 38)	Better PFDI-20 and PFIQ-7 scores after surgery in both groups
			Lower POPDI-6 and UDI-6 scores, and higher CRADI-8 score in the mesh group
			Sexual function, PISQ-12 score and rate of dyspareunia did not differ between the groups at baseline and after surgery
Sivasliolgu 2008 [11]	90	85 (43 versus 42)	Better P-QOL score after surgery in both groups
Carey 2009 [12]	139	124 (63 versus 61)	Worsening PSI-QOL, SUDI, SIIQ and CCCS scores after surgery in both groups
			Rate of dyspareunia did not differ between the groups at baseline and after surgery
Lunardelli 2009 [14]	32	32 (16 versus 16)	Similar rate of de novo stress urinary incontinence between the groups after surgery (6.25%)
Ek 2010 [16]	50	47 (22 versus 25)	Higher rate of de novo stress urinary incontinence in mesh group after surgery (32% versus 8%)
			Lower MUCP in mesh group after surgery in overweight women
			Lower MUCP in mesh group after surgery in 65-years old or older patients
Iglesia 2010 [19]	65	65 (32 versus 33)	Better scores about symptoms, quality of life and dyspareunia after surgery in both groups
Nieminen 2010 [22]	202	182 (97 versus 85)	All symptoms of prolapse resolved after surgery in both groups
			Sexual function did not differ between the groups at baseline and 2 years after surgery
Meschia 2007 [7]	206	201 (98 versus 103)	Improvement of symptoms of prolapse after surgery in both groups
Natale 2009 [15]	190	190 (96 Gynemesh® versus 94 Pelvicol®)	Improvement of quality of life after surgery in Gynemesh® group in the domains: prolapse impact, social limitations, emotions, and severity measures.
			Improvement of quality of life after surgery in Pelvicol® group in all domains with the exclusion of physical limitations
			Comparing the postoperative quality of life in both groups: better impact of Pelvicol® in the domains: social limitations and emotions
			Better PISQ-12 score after surgery in Pelvicol® group
			Comparing the postoperative sexuality in both groups: better impact of Pelvicol®
Feldner 2010 [17]	56	56 (29 versus 27)	Better P-QOL score after surgery in both groups
Hviid 2010 [18]	61	3 months: 50 (27 versus 23) 12 months: 54 (28 versus 26)	Better P-QOL score after surgery in both groups

Table 3 (continued)

Trial	Number	Number of patients studied (graft surgery versus traditional surgery)	Results (graft surgery versus traditional surgery)
De Tayrac 2008 [9]	49	45 (21 versus 24)	Lower pain and buttock pain in IVS® group the first day after surgery
			No difference of "mean VAS" and "rate of patients with VAS>5" in both groups after long term follow-up (4.8 versus 12.5%)
			No difference of rate of patients "satisfy" and "very satisfy" in both groups after long term follow-up (85.7% versus 79.2%)
			Better UDI, POPDI, CRADI, UIQ, CRAIQ and POPIQ score after surgery in both groups
			Absence of improvement of PISQ-12 score after surgery in both groups
Paraiso 2006 [5]	106	81 (26 graft reinforcements versus 27 plication of the fascia versus 28 site-specific surgical repair)	Better PFDI-20 and PFIQ-7 scores after surgery in all groups
			Better quality of life after surgery in all groups
			Better PISQ-12 scores after surgery in all groups
			Absence of lower rate of dyspareunia after surgery in all groups
Lopes 2010 [20]	32	30 (14 versus 16)	Better quality of life (KHQ) 1 year after traditional surgery but without statistically significant difference

PISQ-12 Pelvic Organ Prolapse/Urinary Incontinence Sexual Questionnaire, *UDI-6* Urogenital Distress Inventory Questionnaire, *PFDI-20* Pelvic Floor Distress Inventory-Short Form Questionnaire, *PFIQ-7* Pelvic Floor Impact Questionnaire–Short Form Questionnaire, *POPDI-6* Pelvic Organ Prolapse Distress Inventory Questionnaire, *CRADI-8* Colorectal–Anal Distress Inventory Questionnaire, *P-QOL* Prolapse Quality Of Life Questionnaire, *MUCP* maximum urethral closure, *KHQ* King's Health Questionnaire

[a] In these studies, functional results and sexuality are the main criteria

infection [10, 17] in one or other technique. Paraiso was the only one to report a pelvic abscess after surgery [5]. In 11 non-randomized studies (623 patients), nine of which using NAS meshes, no post-surgical infection was detected [33, 36–45]. Six studies with NAS meshes reported post-surgical hyperthermia, meaning 3.15% out of 755 cases [46–51]. Other frequent infections were

urinary, low or high (13 studies, 1,899 patients, mean frequency 5.8%), and infection of the surgical site (nine studies, 1,287 patients, mean frequency 2%). These complications were mainly seen with NAS grafts (28 out of 32 studies). Deep infection (abscess, cellulites) or generalized infections were reported in 14 cases, four times of which with a prosthesis IVS.

Table 4 Pre- and post-surgery complications in mesh groups		Randomized trials	Non randomized trials
	Major bleeding	5.3%	1.23% (0–3.6)
		8 patients out of 152 in 4 trials (1.6% to 13.8%) [9, 12, 17, 18]	29 trials *n*=4164
	Blood transfusion	3.1%	2.05% (0–25)
		2 patients out of 63 in 2 trials (2.7% to 3.1%) [5, 19]	24 trials *n*=3379
	Haematoma	3%	2.15% (0–8.3)
		4 patients out of 131 in 2 trials (3.8% to 9.5%) [5, 7]	41 trials *n*=6034
	Bladder injury	2.5%	1.94% (0–8.3)
		4 patients out of 160 in 3 trials (0% to 9.6%) [6, 9, 19]	51 trials *n*=6827
	Ureteral injury	1 patients out of 31 in 1 trials [5]	1.55%
			2 trials *n*=359
	Urethral injury	1 patients out of 29 in 1 trials [17]	1.6%
			1 trial *n*=123
	Vaginal injury	0	4.35% (1.6–5.5)
			2 trials *n*=99
NAS non-absorbable and synthetic, *AS* absorbable and synthetic	Rectal injury	0	0.58%
			47 trials *n*=5877

Table 5 Pre- and post-surgery complications in mesh groups

Graft type	Randomized trials			Non randomized trials				
	All	NAS meshes	Biologic meshes	All	NAS meshes	AS meshes	Mixed meshes	Biologic meshes
Mesh Exposition	6.1% 45 patients out of 733 in 13 trials (0% to 35.7%)	11% 44 patients out of 398 in 9 trials (5% to 35.7%) [6, 9–12, 14, 15, 19, 20]	0.34% 1 patient out of 298 in 5 trials (0% to 3.6%) [7, 13, 15, 17, 18]	7.7% (0–34.1) 98 trials n=10076	7.9% (0–34.1) 84 trials n=8747	6.4% (0–12.9) 2 trials n=173	7.9% (0–30) 8 trials n=786	5.5% (0–16.7) 4 trials n=370
De novo urinary incontinence	6.3% 26 patients out of 415 in 8 trials (0% to 40%)	7.8% 25 patients out of 319 in 7 trials (0% to 40%) [6, 9, 11, 14–16, 20]	1 patient out of 96 in 1 trial [15]	7% (0–24%) 26 trials n=3078	6.6% (0%–24%) 24 trials n=2941	0	5.6% 1 trial n=36	16.8% 1 trial n=101
De novo Dyspareunia	5.3% 9 patients out of 170 in 4 trials (0% to 27.8%)	6.7% 9 patients out of 135 in 3 trials (4.6% to 27.8%) [10–12]	None out of 35 patients in 1 trial [13]	9.2% (0–69) 42 trials n=3444	9.2% (0–69) 35 trials n=3008	3% 1 trial n=90	14.9% (4.5–27) 3 trials n=115	4.9% (0.9–10) 3 trials n=231

NAS non-absorbable and synthetic, *AS* absorbable and synthetic

Pain

Mesh shrinkage was reported in 6.8% of cases but none in randomized studies. Frequency was higher with NAS prosthesis (7.9%). Chronic pelvic pain was observed in 5.6% of patients with mesh. In randomized studies, three chronic pains were described, all in the prosthetic reinforcement group: in the buttock (Lopes, two cases out of 14 patients) [20] or in the leg (Nguyen one case out of 37 patients) [10]. Altman and Withagen did not find a significant difference between both groups for this postoperative symptom [23, 28].

Most studies did not specify the type of dyspareunia (de novo or not) or the rate of sexually active patients before and after surgery. Mean rate of dyspareunia in non-randomized studies is 9.2%. In the majority of randomized studies, the rate of postoperative dyspareunia does not differ significantly with or without graft (nine patients out of 170 in four trials) [10–13, 26, 28].

General complications

Less frequently, these are reported in Table 6. Two studies on AB meshes compared the rate of general complications between the two groups: Guerette did not find any significant difference [13], and Feldner found a higher rate in the group with prosthetic reinforcement [17]. Among non-randomized studies, three authors claimed absence of post-surgical complications (for 186 treated patients) [43, 52–54].

De novo stress urinary incontinence

Concerning stress urinary incontinence (SUI), there is a great disparity in definition and assessment between studies: the rates varied from 0% to 24%. Some authors only included patients without SUI before surgery. Distinction between SUI and urgenturia was not systematic. Five randomized studies evaluated the post-surgical rate of SUI, but only Ek and Altman showed a higher frequency of de novo SUI after prosthetic reinforcement [16, 23]. When de novo SUI is clearly defined, it was reported in 26 cases out of 415 patients in eight trials [6, 9, 11, 14–16, 20].

Discussion

Number of studies

This literature review shows that many studies have been recently published on cure of prolapse with mesh inserted through the vaginal route. The number of controlled randomized trials and the use of standard questionnaires

Table 6 Long-term complications in non randomized trials

Graft type	All kind of meshes	NAS meshes	Biologic meshes
Chronic pain (buttock, groin, perinea)	5.6% (0–24.4)	5.8% (0–24.4)	0.9%
	25 trials $n=3307$	24 trials $n=3206$	1 trial $n=101$
Vesicovaginal or rectovaginal fistula	1.5% (0.3–5)	1.6% (0.3–5)	0.9%
	9 trials $n=1576$	8 trials $n=1475$	1 trial $n=101$
Shrinkage	6.8% (1.3–17)	7.9% (1.3–17)	1.5
	6 trials $n=1530$	5 trials $n=1398$	1 trial $n=132$
Vaginal adhesion	3.1% (0.9–6.9%)	3.1% (0.9–6.9%)	0
	5 trials $n=835$	5 trials $n=835$	
Granuloma	4.7% (0.8–13)	4.7% (0.8–13)	0
	5 trials $n=533$	5 trials $n=533$	
Leukorrhea	5.6% (0–4)	5.6% (0–4)	0
	4 trials $n=447$	4 trials $n=447$	

show the will of real objective evaluation of these techniques. Few surgical techniques have undergone such an assessment, both on anatomic and functional results. But some questionnaires seem unsuited to the specificity of prolapse surgery: for example, they are not very pertinent on sexuality and dyspareunia. Works actually try to adapt them more precisely. Moreover, surgical standards are not always respected: hysterectomy is systematic for Iglesia, though it is classically a risk factor for mesh exposition [19]. Lopes also inserts the synthetic mesh between vagina and fascia, which is not recommended and could explain the rate of vaginal mesh exposition in this study: 35% [20].

Anatomic results

For the treatment of cystocoele, five randomized trials on the seven published show that the risk of anatomic recurrence is reduced with NAS mesh. The global rate of relapse at 1 year is estimated around 37% after traditional surgery (87 patients out of 237) and at 11% with NAS mesh (27 patients out of 247) [6, 10–12]. We must remain careful: our review does not represent a meta-analysis, and many biases may exist. But NAS meshes seem to bring an anatomic benefit when treating cystocoele. One of these studies demonstrates after a 3-year follow-up the anatomic benefit of NAS meshes (12% of recurrence after 104 grafts versus 41% after 96 traditional surgery) [22]. Carey did not find any benefit with a sub-vesical mesh, but in his surgical description, it was the only observation where prosthesis was left free without any suspension [12]. This technical variation seems to be important: in all other studies, sub-vesical mesh is suspended by its four arms. Carey changed his technique, using a vaginal support device after intervention and during 1 month [55]. Clinical results are not yet enough to conclude, and no comparative study has been published. The second trial showing no benefit of NAS prostheses was stopped after an unacceptable rate of

meshes expositions (five patients out of 32, 15%) [19]. Hysterectomy was also systematic during the cure of cystocoele. The high number of failures at 1 year (59% and 72%), the concomitant hysterectomy and also the surgeon skills were questioned [56].

Two studies tried to assess the benefit of treating rectocele with a trans-vaginal mesh [5, 20]. For Paraiso, anatomic failures were more important with a biological prosthesis [5]. Lopes did not either find any anatomic benefit in this indication with a synthetic graft [20]. Pre-rectal mesh cannot be recommended with the actual data. But it seems surprising that a prosthetic surgery more efficient than traditional surgery in the anterior compartment might not be equally in the posterior one. We might need to collect a more important number of cases to show its benefit. Lopes also did not calculate the number of subjects enquired to include.

Treatment of apex is one of the actual discussions in 2011. Suspension to the sacrospinous ligament (SSL) seems the reference technique for the vaginal route. When the four arms of a sub-vesical prosthesis are bound to the tendinous arch of pelvic fascia, apex remains free. Classically SSL is reached by colpotomy and rectal dissection. When there is no rectocele, anterior route by paravesical fossa may be tempted. Prolapse of apex and bladder will be cured in the same surgical time. The sub-vesical prosthesis having several arms: two will be bound to the SSL. Traditional techniques of fixing cannot be used. Two recent systems seem interesting: harpoon or threading (Capio™). De Tayrac published a series of 48 patients whose sub-vesical prostheses were fixed with Capio™ to the SSL by anterior route and also to the tendinous arch of pelvic fascia [57]. The rate of anatomic success was 96% for cystocoele and 98% for apex after 8 months follow-up. The cure of apical prolapse cannot only be realised by a sub-vesical obturating prosthesis. Suspension to SSL must be completed by a Richter's traditional method, a posterior prosthesis or an anterior one with anterior access of SSL. No technique seems better than the other.

Infracoccygeal sacropexy is described in several publications. The rate of mesh exposition was high, probably due to the multifilament grafts used. Data are scarce, and compilation and analysis of results are difficult as studied populations are heterogeneous (with or without hysterectomy) [58].

Question of moderate and long-term recurrence has recently find answers in several cohorts with longer follow-up. In 2010, Jacquetin showed a stability of anatomic results in the cohort TVM with a three-level surgery after 3 years follow-up [59]. Letouzey reports a rate of failures growing from 11% at 3 years to 24% after 5 years follow-up, in the treated compartment (cystocoele) [34]. But in the technical surgery description, authors let the graft free, without suspension. An anatomic failure does not always mean re-intervention: in the TVM cohort, re-intervention for anatomic failure was 3% at 3 years. And Letouzey reports no re-intervention for anatomic failure at 5 years. In January 2011, Maher demonstrates better anatomic results of sacropexy compared to Prolift kit without any difference in functional terms. The rate of anatomic failures after Prolift seems very important (57%) at 2 years, largely more than literature data and also the rate of re-interventions (22% for all indications, 5% for pelvic organ prolapse) at 2 years. Such major discrepancies compared to the general results questions the specific skills of the particular teams using this vaginal route [26].

Use of AB meshes does not seem useful: two randomized studies on four published did not show a reduced rate of recurrence when compared to traditional surgery [13, 18].

Functional results

They were evaluated most often by standardized and validated questionnaires. Seven randomized studies evaluated the treatment of cystocoele by meshes. Improvement of urinary symptoms is significant but is equivalent without prosthetic reinforcement. The contradiction between anatomic and functional results leads to question the modalities of evaluation and the criteria used. How can it be explained that symptom scores do get better after traditional surgery though anatomic relapse will reach 37%?

De novo urinary incontinence is found in 11% of women after prosthetic surgery and 7% after traditional surgery. Only considering sub-vesical NAS prostheses, the rate is 16% versus 8.5% in the surgery without mesh. It is difficult to conclude as indications to treat urinary incontinence vary largely from one study to another. Management of urinary symptoms remains a complex chapter we will not open here.

In the two studies of Paraiso and Lopes about vaginal surgery with graft reinforcement in posterior prolapse, functional results were identical when comparing results with or without mesh [5, 20].

Complications

The main complication of prosthetic surgery by vaginal route is mesh exposition. Frequency varies largely from 0% to 35.7% [13, 17, 20]. Our increasing knowledge of this particular risk leads to a standardization of surgical technique: no systematic hysterectomy, no inverted-T colpotomy when dissecting cystocoele, infiltration, dissection and positioning of the mesh while keeping the fascia on the vaginal wall, absence of colpectomy, meticulous check-up so there is no transfixion of prosthetic arms in lateral vaginal cul-de-sac. Surgical experience is also linked to the complication rate, with a learning curve evoked by Dwyer [60]. Moreover, management of this complication seems simple enough for most authors. It should not be considered as a major complication.

Infection has become exceptional with the use of polypropylene.

The most dreaded problem is the mesh shrinkage, sometimes with pain and dyspareunia. Its definition is not clear, and the frequency is difficult to evaluate. In cohort studies, the rate of dyspareunia could not be homogenized: the pre- and post-surgical sexual activity figures and inclusion criteria vary (some teams only suggest mesh surgery at time of relapse). There may be sometimes association to other surgery (colpectomy, myorraphy...). Letouzey finds no de novo dyspareunia at 5 years, but the rate is 9% (3/33) in the TVM series [34, 59]. Randomized studies on sexuality and dyspareunia show no significant difference between vaginal surgery with mesh and traditional surgery [5, 9, 10, 12, 13, 21, 22]. De novo dyspareunia reaches 10% in average. This rate seems superior than after sacropexy but data vary largely with this technique: Handa reports 14.5% after sacropexy by laparotomy [61]. There may be improvement of pre-surgical dyspareunia after vaginal prosthetic surgery [13, 21, 59, 62]. In a prospective cohort on 96 patients who underwent placing of a mesh by vaginal route, Hoda found a significant increasing of sexuality with a 2-year follow-up [63]. He signals a transient deterioration during the first 3 months after surgery, which might correspond to healing. But the questionnaires used are not suitable for the evaluation of dyspareunia and sexuality in the post-operative period.

New trends

To reduce surgical risk and post-surgical pain after the trans-obturator or trans-levator passage of the arms, it might be changed for suspension to the tendinous arch of pelvic fascia and also SSL by harpoon, Capio™ suture capture device, clip or vaginal device. These techniques are being evaluated. Suspension of a posterior prosthesis by harpoon (Elevate™) has been reviewed in 139 patients [64]. Authors report one rectal injury during dissection, two haematomas and two buttock pains. On 48 suspensions with Capio™, de Tayrac reports: one bladder injury during dissection, two embedded needles, three paravesical haematomas, two ureteral kinking, two major sciatic neuralgias and 54% of patients had buttock pain during around 8 days (2 to 70 days) [57]. Carey suggests a post-surgical intra-vaginal device but has complications due to dissection: one rectal injury and one paravesical haematoma needing re-intervention [55]. In a multicentre study with the same technique ($n=136$), authors also report two bladder injuries [62]. Intra-vaginal device was lost six times; two devices had to be taken away for infection and two for discomfort. Premature ablation of the device may generate more anatomic failures.

Severe complications were seen with trocars, but they remain exceptional [65]. The complication rate in studies with or without trocars does not seem very different: they most often happened during dissection. Some are specific of the techniques without trocar (kinking, sciatic neuralgia) with no benefit on post-surgical pain. These are preliminary studies and more important series are needed to conclude. Special care must be given to tension when positioning the mesh: when excessive, it becomes a contributing factor to chronic pain, shrinkage, rectal compression [66]. Surgeons must be especially careful when they use a graft without tension adjustment device.

The weight of the non-absorbable material and the elasticity of the mesh seem to favour prosthetic shrinkage. Prostheses used in prolapse surgery stem from hernia surgery and their mechanic properties may be unsuited to vaginal tissues. No author reported anatomic relapse due to the "breaking" of the prosthesis: they may be too robust and rigid. We might wait for meshes specifically developed for genital prolapse. Semi-absorbable mesh with a special knitting and different transversal and longitudinal elasticity was used and published after 1 year of experimentation [31]. Authors report 2% of de novo dyspareunia but cure of pre-surgical dyspareunia in 76% of cases and 4% of de novo pelvic pains. These results may seem encouraging though there are 22% of anatomic failures in the treated compartment with only 1-year follow-up. Long-term survey is necessary to be sure the benefit for pain is not obtained to the detriment of anatomic results.

Conclusion

Literature is every day growing, and the use of mesh by vaginal route is now coming to maturity with certain indications and middle-term data. Compared to traditional vaginal surgery, use of a non-absorbable synthetic sub-vesical mesh to treat cystocoele gives an anatomic benefit. All skilled surgeons have identical functional results and rate of complications, when technical surgical rules are respected. New techniques might give further improvements, but we have yet no sufficient data to conclude. Meshes specifically designed for vaginal surgery might allow even more ameliorations. Comparison with sacropexy by skilled teams (knowing both techniques) might also be interesting.

Declaration of interest Dr. Lucot Jean-Philippe: teaching sessions with Prolift® (Johnson &Johnson), IPSEN and Endofast® (IBI)

Pr. Cosson Michel: teaching sessions with Prolift® (Johnson &Johnson), IPSEN, funding for fundamental research Ethicon®, patents in progress with Ethicon®, Cousin Biotech®

References

1. Maher C, Feiner B, Baessler K, Adams EJ, Hagen S, Glazener CM (2010) Surgical management of pelvic organ prolapse in women. Cochrane Database Syst Rev 4:CD004014
2. Mucowski SJ, Jurnalov C, Phelps JY (2010) Use of vaginal mesh in the face of recent FDA warnings and litigation. Am J Obstet Gynecol 203(2):103, e1–4
3. Haylen BT, Freeman RM, Swift SE, Cosson M, Davila GW, Deprest J et al (2011) An International Urogynecological Association (IUGA)/International Continence Society (ICS) joint terminology and classification of the complications related directly to the insertion of prostheses (meshes, implants, tapes) and grafts in female pelvic floor surgery. Neurourol Urodyn 30 (1):2–12
4. Savary D, Fatton B, Velemir L, Amblard J, Jacquetin B (2009) What about transvaginal mesh repair of pelvic organ prolapse? Review of the literature since the HAS (French Health Authorities) report. J Gynecol Obstet Biol Reprod (Paris) 38 (1):11–41
5. Paraiso MF, Barber MD, Muir TW, Walters MD (2006) Rectocele repair: a randomized trial of three surgical techniques including graft augmentation. Am J Obstet Gynecol 195(6):1762–1771
6. Hiltunen R, Nieminen K, Takala T, Heiskanen E, Merikari M, Niemi K et al (2007) Low-weight polypropylene mesh for anterior vaginal wall prolapse: a randomized controlled trial. Obstet Gynecol 110(2 Pt 2):455–462
7. Meschia M, Pifarotti P, Bernasconi F, Magatti F, Riva D, Kocjancic E (2007) Porcine skin collagen implants to prevent anterior vaginal wall prolapse recurrence: a multicenter, randomized study. J Urol 177(1):192–195
8. Allahdin S, Glazener C, Bain C (2008) A randomized controlled trial evaluating the use of polyglactin mesh, polydioxanone and polyglactin sutures for pelvic organ prolapse surgery. J Obstet Gynaecol 28(4):427–431
9. de Tayrac R, Mathe ML, Bader G, Deffieux X, Fazel A, Fernandez H (2008) Infracoccygeal sacropexy or sacrospinous suspension for uterine or vaginal vault prolapse. Int J Gynaecol Obstet 100(2):154–159
10. Nguyen JN, Burchette RJ (2008) Outcome after anterior vaginal prolapse repair: a randomized controlled trial. Obstet Gynecol 111 (4):891–898

11. Sivaslioglu AA, Unlubilgin E, Dolen I (2008) A randomized comparison of polypropylene mesh surgery with site-specific surgery in the treatment of cystocoele. Int Urogynecol J Pelvic Floor Dysfunct 19(4):467–471

12. Carey M, Higgs P, Goh J, Lim J, Leong A, Krause H et al (2009) Vaginal repair with mesh versus colporrhaphy for prolapse: a randomized controlled trial. BJOG 116(10):1380–1386

13. Guerette NL, Peterson TV, Aguirre OA, Vandrie DM, Biller DH, Davila GW (2009) Anterior repair with or without collagen matrix reinforcement: a randomized controlled trial. Obstet Gynecol 114 (1):59–65

14. Lunardelli JL, Auge AP, Lemos NL, Carramao Sda S, de Oliveira AL, Duarte E et al (2009) Polypropylene mesh vs. site-specific repair in the treatment of anterior vaginal wall prolapse: preliminary results of a randomized clinical trial. Rev Col Bras Cir 36(3):210–216

15. Natale F, La Penna C, Padoa A, Agostini M, De Simone E, Cervigni M (2009) A prospective, randomized, controlled study comparing Gynemesh, a synthetic mesh, and Pelvicol, a biologic graft, in the surgical treatment of recurrent cystocoele. Int Urogynecol J Pelvic Floor Dysfunct 20(1):75–81

16. Ek M, Tegerstedt G, Falconer C, Kjaeldgaard A, Rezapour M, Rudnicki M et al (2010) Urodynamic assessment of anterior vaginal wall surgery: a randomized comparison between colporraphy and transvaginal mesh. Neurourol Urodyn 29(4):527–531

17. Feldner PC Jr, Castro RA, Cipolotti LA, Delroy CA, Sartori MG, Girao MJ (2010) Anterior vaginal wall prolapse: a randomized controlled trial of SIS graft versus traditional colporrhaphy. Int Urogynecol J Pelvic Floor Dysfunct 21(9):1057–1063

18. Hviid U, Hviid TV, Rudnicki M (2010) Porcine skin collagen implants for anterior vaginal wall prolapse: a randomized prospective controlled study. Int Urogynecol J Pelvic Floor Dysfunct 21(5):529–534

19. Iglesia CB, Sokol AI, Sokol ER, Kudish BI, Gutman RE, Peterson JL et al (2010) Vaginal mesh for prolapse: a randomized controlled trial. Obstet Gynecol 116(2 Pt 1):293–303

20. Lopes ED, Lemos NL, Carramao Sda S, Lunardelli JL, Ruano JM, Aoki T et al (2010) Transvaginal polypropylene mesh versus sacrospinous ligament fixation for the treatment of uterine prolapse: 1-year follow-up of a randomized controlled trial. Int Urogynecol J Pelvic Floor Dysfunct 21(4):389–394

21. Nieminen K, Hiltunen R, Heiskanen E, Takala T, Niemi K, Merikari M et al (2008) Symptom resolution and sexual function after anterior vaginal wall repair with or without polypropylene mesh. Int Urogynecol J Pelvic Floor Dysfunct 19(12):1611–1616

22. Nieminen K, Hiltunen R, Takala T, Heiskanen E, Merikari M, Niemi K et al (2010) Outcomes after anterior vaginal wall repair with mesh: a randomized, controlled trial with a 3 year follow-up. Am J Obstet Gynecol 203(3):235, e1–8

23. Altman D, Vayrynen T, Engh ME, Axelsen S, Falconer C (2011) Anterior colporrhaphy versus transvaginal mesh for pelvic-organ prolapse. N Engl J Med 364(19):1826–1836

24. Heinonen PK, Nieminen K (2011) Combined anterior vaginal wall mesh with sacrospinous ligament fixation or with posterior intravaginal slingplasty for uterovaginal or vaginal vault prolapse. Eur J Obstet Gynecol Reprod Biol 157(2):230–233

25. Madhuvrata P, Glazener C, Boachie C, Allahdin S, Bain C (2011) A randomized controlled trial evaluating the use of polyglactin (Vicryl) mesh, polydioxanone (PDS) or polyglactin (Vicryl) sutures for pelvic organ prolapse surgery: outcomes at 2 years. J Obstet Gynaecol 31(5):429–435

26. Maher CF, Feiner B, DeCuyper EM, Nichlos CJ, Hickey KV, O'Rourke P (2011) Laparoscopic sacral colpopexy versus total vaginal mesh for vaginal vault prolapse: a randomized trial. Am J Obstet Gynecol 204(4):360, e1–7

27. Milani AL, Withagen MI, The HS, Nedelcu-van der Wijk I, Vierhout ME (2011) Sexual function following trocar-guided mesh or vaginal native tissue repair in recurrent prolapse: a randomized controlled trial. J Sex Med. doi:10.1111/j.1743-6109.2011.02392.x

28. Withagen MI, Milani AL, den Boon J, Vervest HA, Vierhout ME (2011) Trocar-guided mesh compared with conventional vaginal repair in recurrent prolapse: a randomized controlled trial. Obstet Gynecol 117(2 Pt 1):242–250

29. Apfelbaum D, David-Montefiore E, Darai E (2009) Mid-term results of the grade 3–4 genital prolapse cure by vaginal route using a total hammock of porcine skin implant associated with bilateral sacro-spinofixation. J Gynecol Obstet Biol Reprod (Paris) 38(2):125–132

30. de Tayrac R, Devoldere G, Renaudie J, Villard P, Guilbaud O, Eglin G (2007) Prolapse repair by vaginal route using a new protected low-weight polypropylene mesh: 1-year functional and anatomical outcome in a prospective multicentre study. Int Urogynecol J Pelvic Floor Dysfunct 18(3):251–256

31. Milani AL, Hinoul P, Gauld JM, Sikirica V, van Drie D, Cosson M (2011) Trocar-guided mesh repair of vaginal prolapse using partially absorbable mesh: 1 year outcomes. Am J Obstet Gynecol 204(1):74, e1–8

32. Sergent F, Sentilhes L, Resch B, Diguet A, Verspyck E, Marpeau L (2007) Prosthetic repair of genito-urinary prolapses by the transobturateur infracoccygeal hammock technique: medium-term results. J Gynecol Obstet Biol Reprod (Paris) 36(5):459–467

33. Araco F, Gravante G, Overton J, Araco P, Dati S (2009) Transvaginal cystocoele correction: Midterm results with a trans-obturator tension-free technique using a combined bovine pericardium/polypropylene mesh. J Obstet Gynaecol Res 35(5):953–960

34. Letouzey V, Deffieux X, Gervaise A, Mercier G, Fernandez H, de Tayrac R (2010) Trans-vaginal cystocoele repair using a tension-free polypropylene mesh: more than 5 years of follow-up. Eur J Obstet Gynecol Reprod Biol 151(1):101–105

35. Simsiman AJ, Luber KM, Menefee SA (2006) Vaginal para-vaginal repair with porcine dermal reinforcement: correction of advanced anterior vaginal prolapse. Am J Obstet Gynecol 195(6):1832–1836

36. Balakrishnan S, Lim YN, Barry C, Corstians A, Kannan K, Rane A (2008) Prospective evaluation of the safety and efficacy of the Apogee system for treatment of vault prolapse. J Obstet Gynaecol 28(6):618–620

37. Lee YS, Han DH, Lim SH, Kim TH, Choo MS, Seo JT et al (2010) Efficacy and Safety of "Tension-free" Placement of Gynemesh PS for the Treatment of Anterior Vaginal Wall Prolapse. Int Neurourol J 14(1):34–42

38. Lin TY, Su TH, Huang WC (2010) Polypropylene mesh used for adjuvant reconstructive surgical treatment of advanced pelvic organ prolapse. J Obstet Gynaecol Res 36(5):1059–1063

39. Mahdy A, Elmissiry M, Ghoniem G (2008) The outcome of transobturator cystocoele repair using biocompatible porcine dermis graft: our experience with 32 cases. Int Urogynecol J Pelvic Floor Dysfunct 19(12):1647–1652

40. Moore RD, Miklos JR (2009) Vaginal repair of cystocoele with anterior wall mesh via transobturator route: efficacy and complications with up to 3-year followup. Adv Urol 2009:743831

41. Okui N, Okui M, Horie S (2009) Improvements in overactive bladder syndrome after polypropylene mesh surgery for cystocoele. Aust N Z J Obstet Gynaecol 49(2):226–231

42. Rane A, Kannan K, Barry C, Balakrishnan S, Lim Y, Corstiaans A (2008) Prospective study of the Perigee system for the management of cystocoeles—medium-term follow up. Aust N Z J Obstet Gynaecol 48(4):427–432

43. Sentilhes L, Sergent F, Resch B, Berthier A, Verspyck E, Marpeau L (2006) Prolapsus isolé de l'étage postérieur posthystérectomie: résultats préliminaires d'une technique utilisant les voies vaginales et transobturatrice basse. Ann Chir 131:533–539

44. van Raalte HM, Lucente VR, Molden SM, Haff R, Murphy M (2008) One-year anatomic and quality-of-life outcomes after the Prolift procedure for treatment of posthysterectomy prolapse. Am J Obstet Gynecol 199(6):694, e1–6

45. Withagen MI, Vierhout ME, Milani AL (2010) Does trocar-guided tension-free vaginal mesh (Prolift) repair provoke prolapse of the unaffected compartments? Int Urogynecol J Pelvic Floor Dysfunct 21(3):271–278

46. Abdel-Fattah M, Ramsay I (2008) Retrospective multicentre study of the new minimally invasive mesh repair devices for pelvic organ prolapse. BJOG 115(1):22–30

47. Eboue C, Marcus-Braun N, von Theobald P (2010) Cystocele repair by transobturator four arms mesh: monocentric experience of first 123 patients. Int Urogynecol J Pelvic Floor Dysfunct 21(1):85–93

48. Fatton B, Amblard J, Debodinance P, Cosson M, Jacquetin B (2007) Transvaginal repair of genital prolapse: preliminary results of a new tension-free vaginal mesh (Prolift technique)—a case series multicentric study. Int Urogynecol J Pelvic Floor Dysfunct 18(7):743–752

49. Gagnon LO, Tu LM (2010) Mid-term results of pelvic organ prolapse repair using a transvaginal mesh: the experience in Sherbrooke, Quebec. Can Urol Assoc J 4(3):188–191

50. Ganj FA, Ibeanu OA, Bedestani A, Nolan TE, Chesson RR (2009) Complications of transvaginal monofilament polypropylene mesh in pelvic organ prolapse repair. Int Urogynecol J Pelvic Floor Dysfunct 20(8):919–925

51. Wetta LA, Gerten KA, Wheeler TL 2nd, Holley RL, Varner RE, Richter HE (2009) Synthetic graft use in vaginal prolapse surgery: objective and subjective outcomes. Int Urogynecol J Pelvic Floor Dysfunct 20(11):1307–1312

52. Migliari R, De Angelis M, Madeddu G, Verdacchi T (2000) Tension-free vaginal mesh repair for anterior vaginal wall prolapse. Eur Urol 38(2):151–155

53. Migliari R, Usai E (1999) Treatment results using a mixed fiber mesh in patients with grade IV cystocoele. J Urol 161(4):1255–1258

54. Sand PK, Koduri S, Lobel RW, Winkler HA, Tomezsko J, Culligan PJ et al (2001) Prospective randomized trial of polyglactin 910 mesh to prevent recurrence of cystocoeles and rectoceles. Am J Obstet Gynecol 184(7):1357–1362, discussion 62–4

55. Carey M, Slack M, Higgs P, Wynn-Williams M, Cornish A (2008) Vaginal surgery for pelvic organ prolapse using mesh and a vaginal support device. BJOG 115(3):391–397

56. Jacquetin B, Cosson M, Debodinance P, Hinoul P (2010) Vaginal mesh for prolapse: a randomized controlled trial. Obstet Gynecol 116(6):1457–1458, author reply 8

57. de Tayrac R, Boileau L, Fara JF, Monneins F, Raini C, Costa P (2010) Bilateral anterior sacrospinous ligament suspension associated with a paravaginal repair with mesh: short-term clinical results of a pilot study. Int Urogynecol J Pelvic Floor Dysfunct 21(3):293–298

58. Jia X, Glazener C, Mowatt G, Jenkinson D, Fraser C, Bain C et al (2010) Systematic review of the efficacy and safety of using mesh in surgery for uterine or vaginal vault prolapse. Int Urogynecol J Pelvic Floor Dysfunct 21(11):1413–1431

59. Jacquetin B, Fatton B, Rosenthal C, Clave H, Debodinance P, Hinoul P et al (2010) Total transvaginal mesh (TVM) technique for treatment of pelvic organ prolapse: a 3-year prospective follow-up study. Int Urogynecol J Pelvic Floor Dysfunct 21(12):1455–1462

60. Dwyer P, O'Reilly B (2004) Transvaginal repair of anterior and posterior compartment prolapse with Atrium polypropylene mesh. BJOG 111(8):831–836

61. Handa V, Zyczynski HM, Brubaker L, Nygaard I, Janz N, Richter HE et al (2007) Sexual function before and after sacrocolpopexy for pelvic organ prolapse. Am J Obstet Gynecol 197(6):629.e1–629.e6

62. Zyczynski HM, Carey MP, Smith AR, Gauld JM, Robinson D, Sikirica V et al (2010) One-year clinical outcomes after prolapse surgery with nonanchored mesh and vaginal support device. Am J Obstet Gynecol 203(6):587, e1–8

63. Hoda MR, Wagner S, Greco F, Heynemann H, Fornara P (2010) Prospective follow-up of female sexual function after vaginal surgery for pelvic organ prolapse using transobturator mesh implants. J Sex Med 8(3):914–922

64. Lukban J, Roovers J, Moore RD, Patel M, Courtieu C, Mayne C (2010) A prospective multicenter study evaluating Elevate TM apical and posterior for treatment of posterior and/or apical vaginal wall prolapse: 12 month follow-up. Int Urogynecol J Pelvic Floor Dysfunct 21(suppl 1):s405–s406

65. Touboul C, Nizard J, Fauconnier A, Bader G (2008) Major venous hemorrhagic complication during transvaginal cystocoele repair using the transobturator approach. Obstet Gynecol 111(2 Pt 2):492–495

66. Emmanuelli E, Rubod C, Poncelet E, Lucot J-P, Quinton J-F, Cosson M (2010) Cure de rectocèle par prothèse type Transvaginal Mesh et compression rectale: à propos de trois cas. Pelvi-périnéologie 5(4):243–246

25

Sentinel lymph node in endometrial cancer

Elisabete Gonçalves · Odete Figueiredo · Fernanda Costa

Abstract The role of complete pelvic and para-aortic lymphadenectomy in early endometrial cancer remains controversial in gynecologic oncology. Sentinel lymph node detection is an alternative to assess lymphatic spread in several solid tumors. The authors review the literature related to the detection of sentinel lymph node in endometrial cancer, the techniques employed, and its results and feasibility. The authors review reported case series of endometrial cancer in which the sentinel lymph node biopsy was performed. A systematic literature review was conducted using the PubMed database. Different techniques were used considering lymphatic imaging mapping (colorimetric, isotopic, and fluorescence procedures) and injection site (subserous, hysteroscopic, and cervical). Detection rates of sentinel lymph node were heterogeneous, varying between 44 and 100 % with false-negative rates between 0 and 33 %. Although technically demanding, hysteroscopy approach was associated with the highest detection rate. The largest trials showed a good detection rate with cervical injection, a more reproducible procedure. The laparoscopic route improved the results. Immunohistochemistry staining improved the micrometastasis detection in sentinel lymph node. Cost-effectiveness of systematic lymphadenectomy compared with sentinel lymph node procedure and its value on adjuvant therapies as well as a standardized reproducible and reliable technique must be assessed.

Keywords Sentinel lymph node · Endometrial cancer · Lymph node mapping · Ultrastaging

E. Gonçalves (✉) · O. Figueiredo · F. Costa
Division of Gynecology Oncology, Department of Gynecology and Obstetrics of Centro Hospitalar Tâmega e Sousa, Lugar do Tapadinho, Guilhufe,
4564-007 Penafiel, Portugal
e-mail: elisabetegoncalvesms@yahoo.com

Background

Endometrial cancer (EC) represents the most frequent malignancy of the female genital tract in developed countries. In 2011, 46,470 new cases of EC were diagnosed and 8,120 EC-related deaths occurred in the USA [1]. Seventy percent are diagnosed at an early stage [2] and are treatable by surgical intervention.

EC is surgically staged using the 2009 International Federation of Gynecology and Obstetrics (FIGO) staging system. Surgical treatment consists of peritoneal washing, total hysterectomy, bilateral salpingo-oophorectomy, and pelvic and para-aortic (PA) lymphadenectomy [2].

The risk of metastatic involvement of lymph nodes is dependent on histological type, grade, depth of myometrial invasion, and lymphovascular invasion [3, 19]. Nevertheless, the risk of metastatic disease to pelvic lymph nodes at initial stages (IA grade 1–2) is 0–7 % associated to a low risk of recurrence (3–6 %) [3]. On the other hand, advanced stages and grade 3 endometrial cancer are associated with a lymph node metastatic involvement as high as 20 % [3]. When pelvic nodes are positive, PA nodal involvement occurs approximately in 50 %, and in up to 6 % of patients, it may occur isolated [4]. Therefore, in 80–90 % of early stage endometrial cancer, pelvic and PA lymphadenectomy is useless, incurring morbidity [3].

Survival impact of systematic lymphadenectomy in patients with EC is widely discussed. The ASTEC trial shows no evidence of benefit for systematic lymphadenectomy for early EC in terms of overall and recurrence-free survival [5].

The sentinel lymph node (SLN), by definition, is the first node to receive metastasizing cancer cells, as first described in 1960 by Gold et al. for parotid cancer [6]. In 1996, Burke et al. reported the SLN first application in EC [7].

Nowadays, lymphatic mapping is an accepted alternative to assess lymphatic spread in several solid tumors. EC lymphatic mapping has not gained the same popularity. The uterus has a complex lymphatic drainage due to lymphatic channels in the broad and infundibulo-pelvic ligaments [7]; therefore, the lymphatic spread is through external iliac and obturator (mainly) and PA area, respectively (Fig. 1), and the best technique to detect SLN is yet unestablished [7].

First studies of SLN in EC included small-size samples and various injections sites revealing heterogeneous results. In 2008, a consensus panel stated that SLN in EC was worthy of further investigation [8]. Prospective investigation is reviving SLN in EC.

EC patients are usually obese and aged [9]. The primary goal of SLN in EC consists in reducing the morbidity of a full lymphadenectomy (by decreasing surgical time), as well as early (need of blood transfusion, fever, wound infection, thromboembolism [10]) and late complications (lymphocysts formation, leg lymphedema, transient neuralgias [3, 6, 8–14]). Besides, SLN allows an accurate exploration of all drainage routes as well as those considered aberrant or not routinely examined [12]. It is suggested that SLN could have a value in isolated PA metastatic node detection. PA metastasis is a

known adverse prognostic factor in EC [15], and there is no reliable way to predict its involvement [16]. SLN detection could select patients that beneficiate from PA lymphadenectomy that would be performed in presence of a positive SLN. For this purpose, the most accurate technique involves hysteroscopic injection [17]. Moreover, the use of more sensitive techniques for SLN detection could better identify pelvic nodes and probably reduce the reported incidence of isolated infra-renal metastasis [8]. The secondary goal is to improve detection of micrometastasis, which is associated with a recurrence risk [13], with resource to ultra-sectioning and immunohistochemistry (IHC) protocols [3, 6, 8–13]. Therefore, the risk of recurrence related to positive lymph nodes missing despite a full lymphadenectomy could be reduced [12], and SLN could improve selection of patients for adjuvant therapy. Despite the controversy concerning therapeutic benefit of lymphadenectomy, some experts argue that lymph node staging is necessary to guide appropriate adjuvant therapy [18]. Adjuvant therapies based only on uterine factors may result in over or under treatment [12, 32]. Identification of microscopic disease outside the uterus can help to determine the need of adjuvant therapy. SLN application in EC is more accurate than MRI and intra-operative frozen section analysis in assessing lymph node status [1, 8] and SLNs are three times more likely to harbor disease than non-SLNs [34]. SLN in EC, incorporating ultrastaging, may improve selection of women at high risk and could potentially avoid 80 % full unnecessary lymphadenectomy [6]. The authors review the concerning techniques employed and their results and feasibilities to detect SLN node in EC.

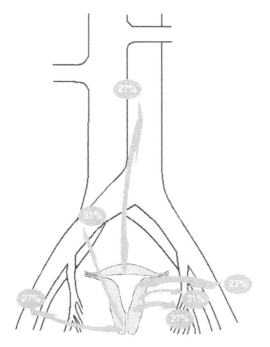

Fig. 1 Main routes of lymphatic drainage and relative distribution of lymphatic nodes in EC. The concept of SLN depends on the uterus's lymphatic drainage. There are two main interconnected routes through broad and infundibulo-pelvic ligaments, these last ones considered the secondary routes. The cervix and the lower uterine segment drain mainly through parametria to external iliac and common iliac nodes. The uterine corpus drains primarily to the external iliac nodes; other pathways include the inter iliac, common iliac, and obturator area. Uterine fundal drainage is relatively consistent through the ovarian vessels to the infra-renal PA area

Material and methods

The authors performed a comprehensive and systematic search on the PubMed database for published studies with keywords "sentinel lymph nodes," "endometrial cancer," "lymphadenectomy," and "ultrastaging". We selected studies evaluating techniques to detect SLN including original articles, meta-analysis, reviews, and opinion articles published up to October 2012.

Authors analyzed lymphatic mapping methodology, injection site, surgical route, and detection of micrometastasis, of which advantages and disadvantages, rates of detection of SLN, and negative prognostic values were correlated.

Findings

Twenty-three publications with at least 15 cases were included. Eighteen studies were prospective, and one was a meta-analysis involving 26 studies. Four studies analyzed subserosal injection, five hysteroscopic injection, and one peri-tumoral ultrasound guided injection. Eleven analyzed cervical injection. One evaluated cervical and subserosal injections simultaneously. The meta-analysis intended to assess the diagnostic performance of SLN through univariate regression analysis. The characteristics of these studies are summarized in Table 1.

SLN detection varies depending on the lymphatic mapping procedure, injection site, and surgical route [9]. Other factors include surgeon experience, delay between injection and detection, and previous pelvic radiotherapy or surgery.

Lymphatic mapping procedure

The detection of SLN is performed using colorimetric imaging of blue dyes (isosulfan blue, patent blue, and methylene blue), isotopic mapping with Technetium-99 (Tc-99), or both, through injection in a defined location [3, 8, 9]. Half-life is relatively long to allow a deferred identification of SLN, and both have a safety profile [9]. Blue dye imaging is injected before surgery, after induction of anesthesia [11]. Isotopic imaging implies an injection, ideally 18 h before surgery, with control scintigraphic images obtained with a gamma camera.

During surgery, pelvic and lower PA regions are inspected for colored lymph node channels and dye uptake. Radioactive pelvic and PA lymph nodes are localized using a gamma probe (usually before opening the retroperitoneum). Dissection of pelvic lymph nodes with or without PA management is performed and followed by hysterectomy with bilateral salpingo-oophorectomy.

Dual detection (colorimetric and isotopic) was associated with the highest detection rate and lowest false-negative rate, independent of injection site [9, 22], with detection rates ranging from 46 to 87 % [3]. Ballester et al. demonstrated a SLN detection rate of 57 % with simple colorimetric imaging against 94 % in double detection, using cervical injection [23]. Later, Ballester et al. found low correlation between day-before lymphoscintigraphy and surgical SLN mapping querying its usefulness and cost-effectiveness in routine practice [24].

Solima et al. found a high detection rate of SLN when performed by hysteroscopic injection of radiolabeled albumin colloids and suggested that this result may be explained by the low interval between hysteroscopic injection and sentinel node detection, not exceeding 6 h [21]. Kang et al. found no statistical difference in a meta-analysis when comparing dye, isotope, or both [20].

Other medical dyes, such as Indocyanine green (ICG) with near-infrared fluorescence, have recently been reported for use in mapping [8, 22]. Roy et al. applied robotically assisted fluorescence imaging with ICG for lymphatic mapping in early stage cervical and endometrial cancer reporting

a 7.8 % increase in SLN detection [8, 22]. Holloway et al. compared, in a prospective study with 35 women with EC, colorimetric and fluorescence imaging. Bilateral SLNs were detected in 97 % using the robotic near-infrared imaging system and in 77 % patients by colorimetric analysis [8]. Holloway et al. found this technique easy to perform and complimentary to traditional calorimetric imaging. If these findings are corroborated in the future with larger multicentric trials, Holloway et al. argue that gynecologist oncologists will be more confident omitting lymphadenectomy for low-risk EC by performing less morbid SLN biopsies and will improve the precision of staging for high-risk EC [8].

Injection site

Considering the complexity of uterus lymphatic drainage [7, 9], the injection site is the most evaluated issue for SLN detection. Despite being a major determinant [3], the optimal site remains unclear [14]. Different injection sites were experimented, and combined techniques were also proposed [3, 9, 14].

Subserosal/myometrial injection

This was the first procedure used for SLN detection in EC, as published by Burke et al. The 15 patients involved underwent laparotomy, and after obtaining peritoneal washings, the uterus was exposed and the fallopian tubes were occluded; blue dye was injected into subserosal myometrium at three midline places (empirical-midline injections were used to maximize the probability of observing bilateral lymphatic drainage). The colored lymphatic channels were dissected in pelvic and PA regions followed by standard surgical staging [7]. They reported a SLN detection rate of 67 % with a false-negative rate of 50 % [3, 7, 9, 25]. Other seven articles describe this technique (Table 1). Detection rate ranges considerably between 0 and 92 % with sensibilities spanning 50–100 %. False-negative range is 0–50 %, and the negative predictive value is 75–100 %. Altgassen et al. reported the highest detection rate (92 %), which was related with the higher number of myometrial injections performed (eight) [25]. Moreover, adding to the safety and feasibility, this technique has a good accuracy to detect PA lymph nodes with a rate of detection of 31–34 %. Disadvantages attributed to this technique include surgical planning difficulties and required dissection of all anatomical areas of lymphatic drainage [25].

Peri-tumoral/hysteroscopic injection

The hysteroscopic injection is technically the most difficult, mainly because of direct access to the injection site [3, 9, 14, 27]. Success rate is reported as high as 64–100 % [9]. Disadvantages include eventual local anesthesia or sedation for good tolerance and the complex logistics of performing

Table 1 Characteristics of studies evaluating SLN in EC, grouped according to the injection site

Authors, year	Injection site	Study type	N	FIGO staging[a] (%)	Method	Surgical route	PA nodes	Median N lymph nodes	Bilateral SLN detection (%)	Detection rate (%)	Sensibility (%)	NPV	FN rate (%)	Pathology assessment
Pericervical/cervical injection or combined/comparison with cervical injection														
How et al. [28], 2012	PC	Pros	100	I-86.0; II-1.0; III-13.0	B + Tc 99	Rob	HR	2	72	92	89	99	1	HE/IHC
Barlin et al. [14], 2012	PC PC + SS (34)	Pros	498	I-79.0, I-2.0 III-17.0, IV-2.0	B B + Tc 99 (75)	Rob/Lap Lapar	Yes	3.0	51	81	98.1	99.8	1.9	HE/IHC
Holloway et al. [7], 2012	PC	Pros	35	NA	F + C C F	Rob	Yes	At least 1	100	100 77 97	90	96	NA	HE/IHC
Ballester et al. [9], 2011	PC	Pros	125	I-94.0 II-6.0	B + Tc 99	Lap/ Lapar	No	1.5	69	89	84	97	16	HE/IHC
Khoury-Collado et al. [13], 2011	PC PC + SS	Pros	266	I-78.0, II-2.0, III-19.0, IV-1.0	B B+Tc 99	Lap/ Lapar/ Rob	No	3.0	67	84	NA	NA	NA	HE/IHC
Mais et al. [5], 2010	PC	Pros	34	I-91.2, II-2.9, III-5.9	B	Lap	No	1–4	NA	62 82 42	100	NA	50	HE/IHC
Abu-Rustum et al. [34], 2009	PC PC+SS	Pros	21 21	I-84.0, II-2.0, III-14.0, IV-2.0	B+Tc 99	Lapar Lap/ Lapar	Yes	3	NA	86 81 90	100	100	0	HE/IHC
Barranger et al. [35], 2009	PC	Pros	33	I-90.9, II-9.1	B+Tc 99	Lap	No	2.5	54.5	81.8	NA	NA	0	HE/IHC
Ballester et al. [21], 2008	PC	Pros	46	NA	B+Tc 99	Lap/ Lapar	No	2.6	62.5	87	100	NA	0	HE/IHC
Bats et al. [29], 2008	PC	Pros	43	I-60.5, II-14.0, III-25.5	B+Tc 99	Lap/ Lapar	No	2.9	53.3	69.8	100	NA	0	HE/IHC
Perone et al. [9], 2008	PC HYS	Pros	23 17	NA	Tc 99	Lap	No	1.7 1.4	38 27	70 65	100	100	0	HE/IHC
Holub et al. [27], 2004	PC+SS	NA	25	I	B	Lap	NA	2.1	81	84	100	100	0	HE
Peri-tumoral: hysteroscopic or intra-myometrial guided transvaginal ultrasound injection														
Torné et al. [23], 2012	IM	Pros	74	I-66.1, II-21.6, III-10.9, IV-1.4	Tc 99	Lap	Yes	2.8	29.2	82.1	92.3	97.7	NA	HE/IHC
Solima et al. [18], 2012	HYS	Pros	59	I-72.9, II-5.1, III-20.3, IV-1.7	Tc 99	Lapar/ Lap	HR	2.6	NA	95	90	98	1.7	IHC
Delaloye et al.[36], 2007	HYS	Pros	60	I-64.0, II-11.0, III-25.0	B+Tc 99	Lapar/ Lap	Yes	3.7	44.8	82	89	97	11	HE/IHC
Maccauro et al. [25], 2005	HYS	Unk	26	I-83.0, III-27.0	B+Tc 99	Lapar	No	2.5	18	100	100	100	0	HE/IHC
Raspagliesi et al. [26], 2004	HYS	Pros	18	I-72.2, III-27.8	B+Tc 99	Lapar	HR	3	55.6	94	NA	NA	0	HE
Niikura et al. [32], 2004	HYS	Pros	28	I-78.6, II-10.7, III-10.7	Tc 99	Lapar	Yes	3.1	NA	82	100	100	0	HE/IHC

Table 1 (continued)

Authors, year	Injection site	N	FIGO staging[a] (%)	Method	Surgical route	PA nodes	Median N lymph nodes	Bilateral SLN detection (%)	Detection rate (%)	Sensibility (%)	NPV	FN rate (%)	Pathology assessment
Subserosal or comparison with subserosal injection													
Robova et al. [33], 2009	SS HYS	67 24	I-83.5, II-11.0, III-5.5	B+Tc 99	Lapar	Yes	2.2	67.2	73.1 50	74 50	NA NA	NA NA	IHC
Lopes et al. [11], 2007	SS	40	NA	B	Lapar	Yes	NA	NA	77.5	83	98	4	HE/ICH
Altgassen et al. [22], 2007	SS	23	I-64.0, II-36.0	B	Lapar	Yes	3	NA	92	62.5	92.5	5	HE/IHC
Burke et al. [6], 1996	SS	15	NA HR	B	Lapar	Yes	3.1	NA	67	67	NA	33	H
Combined													
Kang et al. [16], 2011	PC HYS SS PC+SS Other	1101	NA	B Tc 99 B+Tc 99	Lap/ Lapar	NA	2.6	61	78	93	NA	NA	NA

Blue D B Blue dye, *C* Colorimetric, *F* Fluorescence Indo Cyanine Green, *HR* high-risk endometrial cancer, *HYS* hysteroscopy, *IM* intra-myometrial cancer, *Lap* laparoscopy, *Lapar* laparotomy, *N* number of cases, *NA* not available/applicable, *NPV* negative predictive value, *PC* pericervical/cervical, *Pros* prospective, *Rob* robotic assisted laparoscopy, *SS* subserosal, *Unk* unknown

[a] FIGO Staging 1998, except for Torné et al. (FIGO 2009 staging)

the injection per-operatively, considering that the use of radioactive agents is not allowed in the conventional operating theater [9, 27]. Another issue raised concerns with the repeated hysteroscopy that could favor the dissemination of tumor cells through the fallopian tubes to the peritoneal cavity [3, 9, 27]. Maccauro et al. and Raspagliesi et al. reported one case of positive peritoneal cytology [28, 29]. However, the dissemination risk is low if less than 70 mmHg is used to distend uterine cavity [28]. Gien et al. evaluate peritoneal washings after hysteroscopy and found no positive cytology for malignancy [14].

Niikura et al. suggested that with hysteroscopic guidance and the possibility to determine the injection point into the endometrium, the isotope pathway will mimic the natural lymphatic drainage of cancer cells [28]. It is associated with the highest reported SLN detection rates [28], ranging between 40 and 100 %, and it detects PA lymph nodes with rates as high as 57 % [3, 9, 19, 28].

Raspgaliesi et al. and Maccauro et al., in their series with 18 and 26 patients, respectively, injected a radioactive tracer and blue dye by hysteroscopy and performed surgery 3–4 h after. They found a 100 % SLN detection, and all metastatic nodes were identified as SLN [14, 28, 29].

Solima et al. published in 2012 the largest serial with 80 patients using office hysteroscopic technetium injection (office hysteroscopy was performed without cervical dilation or local/general anesthesia, with maximum intracavitary pressure of 40 mmHg). Radiolabeled albumin 99 Tc was injected peritumoral at 3, 6, 9, and 12 h subendometrially; if the entire cavity was involved, technetium was injected at four uterine surfaces and the fundus. Gamma camera images were obtained starting 15 min after injection, every 5 min in 1 h. Pelvic and PA lymphadenectomies were performed systematically in EC serous or clear cell histological types, and for endometrioid type when intraoperative staging was equal or higher than IB G2. They reported at least one SLN in 76 of the 80 patients. Ten of these patients (17 %) had node metastases. Thirty-three patients (56 %) had SLN in the PA region. Negative predictive value (NPV) was 98 % (95 % CI 89.4–100) and sensitivity 90 % (55.5–99.8). Solima et al. related the SLN detection rate with the low interval between hysteroscopic injection and surgery, up to 6 h [21].

Lately, a new approach for SLN detection in EC was proposed by Torné et al.: transvaginal ultrasound-guided myometrial injection of radiotracer (TUMIR) consists in a myometrial injection of radiotracer guided by trans-vaginal ultrasound resembling the embryo transfer procedure. The protocol procedure described by Torné et al. used a Tc 99 injection in the anterior and posterior myometrium wall, guided by ultrasound and performed under local anesthesia, 18–24 h before surgery. Identification of SLN was performed with lymphoscintigraphy preoperatively. Patients underwent laparoscopy, and radioactive pelvic and PA SLNs were identified with a gamma probe and subsequently removed; PA and pelvic lymphadenectomies, hysterectomy, and bilateral salpingo-oophorectomy followed. TUMIR was feasible in 90.5 % of patients and showed a SLN identification in 55 patients (74.3 %). The sensitivity and NPV of SLN detected were, respectively, 92.3 and 97.7 %. No complications were registered. The advantages of TUMIR pointed by the authors are visualization of the exact injection site and puncture at the myometrial layer of the uterus; in this location, lymphatics are more significant compared to the subendometrial layer, allowing adequate information of the lymph node drainage of the endometrium. Disadvantages pointed are related with SLN detection failure associated with higher tumor size and technical skill requirements [26].

Cervical injection

Larger trials for SLN detection used cervical injection. Usually, a radioactive tracer is injected at two or four cardinal points in the cervix, the day preceding the surgery. Lymphoscintigraphy is then obtained. Immediately prior to surgery, a dye is injected at the same cervical sites.

The rate of detection ranges between 70 and 97 % [3, 8, 27]. This is the most reproducible technique since the cervix is an accessible and easy site to perform the injection [16, 27]. It is also well tolerated by patients [24]. A potential concern with cervical injection is that it could represent more cervical drainage instead of corporal drainage [3, 9, 14]. SLNs are more often localized at the pelvis (93.1–100 %) [9]; the SLN detection of PA is lower than through hysteroscopic and myometrial injection, around 3 % [9]. However, deep cervical injection at 3 and 9-o'clock positions prior to total hysterectomy may demonstrate good blue dye spread to the lower uterine segment and to the cornua of the uterus [14]. Besides, it is considered a good technique that shows a high bilateral pelvic detection rate [9], and cervical injection detects, on average, 63 % of bilateral pelvic SLN against to 48 and 35 % peritumoral and myometrial injections [9]. Holub et al. used a combined cervical and myometrial injection of blue dye and reported a SLN detection rate of 80 % [31].

A French multicentric prospective trial published by Ballester et al. (SENTI-ENDO), involving 125 patients, used cervical dual labeling injection. Pelvic SLNs were detected in 89 % of the patients (31 % unilateral and 69 % bilateral). They explained this low detection rate with the long interval between radiocolloid injection and SLN procedure, with a median time of 22 h [11]. SLN in the PA region was detected in 5 % of patients. For each hemipelvis as a unit, the presence of SLN was correctly identified in 100 % of patients; however, at the patient level analysis, three patients with a type 2 EC had false-positive results, giving a sensitivity of 84 % and a NPV of 97 % [11].

In 2012, Barlin et al. published the largest prospective cohort, using a blue dye cervical injection. The surgical algorithm consisted in peritoneal washings and retroperitoneal evaluation with excision of all mapped SLN and suspicious nodes; in the absence of mapping, a side specific pelvis node dissection was performed. The overall SLN detection rate was 81 % with optimal bilateral mapping in 51 %. There were seven false negatives, leading to a sensitivity of 85.1 %, a false-negative rate of 14.9 %, and NPV of 98.1 %; after algorithm application, the false-negative rate dropped to 2 % [18].

Recently, How et al. published the first prospective data of 100 patients with EC undergoing SLN mapping. How et al. assessed SLN through a dual injection of Tc 99 and patent blue dye administrated during surgery, superficially in cervical submucosa and deeply in the cervix stroma. The surgical route was robot assisted, with a median time between incision and first blue node detection of 60.3 min. SLN detection rate was 92 %, with a pelvic bilateral detection rate of 72 % and PA level of 15 %. There was one false negative, leading to a sensitivity of 89 % and a NPV of 99 %. During one procedure, How et al. noted in the infundibulo-pelvic ligament blue lymphatics, demonstrating that cervical injection could drain through this pathway [32]. Few studies evaluated directly the injection site with tumor localization and site of SLN identification.

Raspagliesi and Delaloye et al. in their series with hysteroscopic injection found no correlation between the site of SLN and site of the tumor [29, 37], stating that metastatic spread may not follow a stepwise progressive drainage [37]. According to Maccauro et al. and Niikura et al., the PA basin is frequently involved in drainage from the uterus corpus, and therefore, peri-tumoural injection allows a more complete detection of the corpus drainage [10] and becomes mandatory for assessing the PA area [28]. Also, subserosal injection could improve PA lymph node detection, considering its fundal drainage [33].

Only 16 % of EC cancer is located in the lower part of the uterus [25], and cervical injection may miss higher pelvic or PA sentinel node identification [10]. That is why Holloway et al. recommended that should SLN not be identified with cervical injection, para-rectal and the pre-sacral space should be inspected, which may lead to identification of the common iliac or PA SLN [8]. Distribution of SLN and positive nodes according to the studies evaluating SLN in EC is found in Table 2.

Surgical route

The laparoscopic route seems to allow a higher SLN identification than laparotomy [6]. Mais et al. evaluated 34 patients in a prospective cohort with the purpose of comparing SLN detection in laparoscopy vs laparotomy. Cervical injection with blue dye was performed. Median time between injection and

Table 2 Distribution of SLN and positive nodes according the studies evaluating SLN in EC

Anatomic location of nodes (%) — Authors; site of injection	How et al. [30]: PC	Barlin et al. [14]: PC (PC+SS)	Holloway et al. [7]: PC	Ballester et al. [9]: PC	Khoury-Collado et al. [13]: PC	Mais et al. [5]: PC	Abu-Rustum et al. [35]: PC	Barranger et al. [36]: PC	Ballester et al. [21]: PC	Bats et al. [31]: PC	Perone et al. [9]: PC/HYS	Holub et al. [29]: PC+SS	Torné et al. [24]: IM	Solima et al. [18]: HYS	Delaloye et al. [37]: HYS	Maccauro et al. [26]: HYS	Raspagliesi et al. [27]: HYS	Niikura et al. [28]: HYS	Robova et al. [34]: SS/HYS	Lopes et al. [11]: SS	Altgassen et al. [23]: SS	Burke et al. [6]: SS
Obturator	NA	NA	NA	NA	NA				NA	NA		NA		NA							NA	
SLN detection						1	24	6			0,6/0,6	NA	25		20	14	15	20	15	17		13
Positive SLN						NA	NA	1			0/1	4	NA		0	0	NA	0	NA	NA		NA
C. iliac	NA	NA	NA	NA	NA	NA					NA										NA	
SLN detection							8	3	6	10		18	20	18	17	18	19	6	10	3		19
Positive SLN							NA	NA	NA	0		NA	NA	NA	NA	0,5	1,5	NA	0	NA		NA
Ext. iliac	NA	NA	NA	NA	NA	NA				NA	NA										NA	NA
SLN detection							30	68	78			26	27	30	31	25	25	25	59	25		
Positive SLN							NA	11	NA			NA	NA	NA	0	3	NA	1	NA	NA		
Int. iliac	NA	NA	NA	NA	NA	NA			NA	NA	NA	NA		NA					NA		NA	
SLN detection							36	0					1		18	3	4	6		19		3
Positive SLN							NA	0					NA		3	0	NA	0		NA		NA
Interiliac	NA	NA	NA	NA	NA	NA						NA			NA	NA	NA	NA	NA	NA	NA	
SLN detection							0	20	16	83	94/94		15	31								7
Positive SLN							0	6	NA	9	1/4/1		NA	NA								NA
Parametrium	NA	NA	NA	NA	NA	NA					0			NA			NA	NA			NA	
SLN detection							0	0	0	0		0	0		0	0			6			0
Positive SLN							0	0	0	0		0	0		0	0			NA			0
Presacral	NA	NA	NA	NA	NA	NA		NA	NA			NA		NA			NA	NA				NA
SLN detection							0			7	0		0		0	0			1	2	2	
Positive SLN							0			0	NA		0		0	0			0	NA	0	
Pelvic		NA	NA			NA	NA	NA		NA	NA					NA	NA	NA	NA			
SLN detection	91			95	94				100			100	70	77	86					65	94	42
Positive SLN	9			16					25			4	7	4						1,6	4	NA
PA		NA	NA			NA																
SLN detection	9			5	6		4	0	0	0	0/18	0	30	21	14	21	27	20	8	35	6	39
Positive SLN	1			0			NA	0	0	0	NA	0	1	2	0,5	1,5	1	0	NA	6	0	NA

C-.Common; Ext.-External; HYS-Hysteroscopy; IM-Intra-myometrial guided transvaginal ultrasound; Int.-Internal; NA-Not available/applicable; PA-Para-aortic; PC-Peri-cervical/Cervical

pelvic lymph nodes dissection was 20–30 min with laparoscopic approach and 40–50 under laparotomy. SLN detection rate was 82 % with laparoscopy, significantly higher than with laparotomy which was 42 %. Levenback et al. found, while mapping the cervix, that blue SLN was identifiable in the pelvis 5–16 min after injection and so remained for 9–30 min [7].

Globally, detection rates of SLN range between 44 and 100 % [3, 9, 21]. Achieving an acceptably low false-negative rate is crucial for lymphatic mapping as an alternative to standard protocols [8, 14]. False-negative rates range between 0 and 33 %. SLN detection ranges from 0 to 92 % with colorimetric techniques, 0 to 82 % with isotopic, and 46 to 87 % with dual techniques. In relation to the injection site, hysteroscopy has a detection rate of 50–100 %, cervical of 69–94 %, and myometrial of 67–92 % [9]. A meta-analysis showed a SLN detection rate of 78 %, lower than for other solid tumors, with a sensitivity of 95 %. In this meta-analysis, cervical injection was correlated with an increase of the detection rate, hysteroscopic injection was associated with a decrease of detection rate and myometrial injections with a decrease of sensitivity [18]. PA node evaluation is less studied. Burke et al. found 31 SLN, and 12 of them were in the PA area. Niikura et al. detected SLN in 82 % of patients, with at least 1 PA SLN in 18 of 25 patients, and SLN located in the PA area in 3 of 23 patients [30]. Delpesh et al. reported a lower detection rate of SLN in the PA region using cervical injection alone compared with cervical combined with subserosal or peritumoral injections. Peritumoral or subserosal myometrial injection may enable detection of isolated PA node involvement. In cervical injection studies, PA nodes were not systematically sampled. SENTI-ENDO identified 5 in 111 with an associated SLN in the PA region. Detection of isolated PA node involvement would improve outcome prediction and may decrease the complications of postoperative whole pelvis radiotherapy by limiting the use of extended surgical staging [33].

Ultrastaging

Lymph node status is an important factor and a criterion for adjuvant therapy in EC [9]. Ultrastaging of lymph nodes is a main focus of the SLN concept and implies serial sectioning and IHC [11, 34]. The main limitation of these techniques is their time-consuming and costly nature, inappropriate for routine use [3, 34].

At the Philadelphia Consensus Conference, macrometastasis was defined as a single focus of metastatic disease per node measuring more than 2 mm, micrometastasis measuring between 0.2 and 2 mm and submicrometastasis measuring less than 0.02 mm, including the presence of a single noncohesive tumor cell [9, 34].

The relation between micrometastasis and risk of recurrence/prognosis has been demonstrated in an increasing number of malignancies suggesting that micrometastasis should be an indication for adjuvant therapy, including early EC [34]. Yabushita et al. analyzed the relation between disease recurrence and presence of pelvic nodes micrometastasis in early EC and found its presence was associated with recurrent disease [34].

The conventional examination of SLN with hemi-section and analysis under hematoxylin and eosin (HE) is not very effective for micrometastasis detection [9]. Ultrastaging protocols involve serial sectioning techniques (with intervals of 3 mm), and each of these sections will be analyzed into a panel of anti-cytokeratin antibodies [9, 34]. The signal amplification produced by IHC may improve sensitivity of micrometastasis detection [32]. The rate of detection of micrometastasis ranged from 0 to 15 % according to a review [34]. Niikura et al., using serial sectioning and IHC, noted that micrometastases were detected in 5 % negative SLN and only in 0.3 % of nonsentinel nodes [30]. Ballester et al. showed that ultrastaging detected metastasis underdiagnosed by conventional histology in 11 % and also showed that SLN biopsy upstaged 10 % of low-risk and 15 % of intermediate-risk EC patients [11]. Holloway et al. concluded that metastasis was solely identified by ultrastaging and IHC in 4/10 patients with node metastasis, which represents a 67 % increase in identification of node metastasis compared to routine HE [8]. Khoury-Collado et al. found metastasis only detected by ultrastaging protocols in 3 % of patients and that SLNs are more prone to be metastatic than non SLNs [35].

Conclusions

Patients with gynecological malignancies, particularly with small tumors of the vulva, have significantly profited from SLN mapping. Since its first application in 1996, SLN in EC is still debated. Considering the surgical risk of EC patients, the lower risk of metastasis in early stages and the controversial role of therapeutic lymphadenectomy in unselected patients, SLN biopsy, incorporating ultrastaging, could find its indication in low-and intermediate-risk women with EC: it brings the advantages of a conservative and more sensitive procedure and might select patients for adjuvant therapy. Moreover, SLN biopsy lends itself to laparoscopic surgery, which is an attractive alternative [10, 19].

The uterus has a complex lymphatic drainage due to its midline position, and therefore, the best technique for lymphatic ways highlighting remains in discussion. Data on

SLN in EC are very heterogeneous in methodology and studied population. Injection site is the most discussed issue. Subserosal myometrial injection has considerable variability in SLN detection and lower sensitivity; hysteroscopic injection has demonstrated the highest detection rates; however, it adds costs and is technically demanding; cervical injection is more reproducible, yet the least reliable in PA mapping. A meta-analysis estimated a detection rate of SLN in EC of 78 %, lower than for other solid tumors. Recent larger studies, with more consistent results and higher detection rates, point the SLN procedure as feasible, reliable, and easy to incorporate in surgical management.

In the future, cost-effectiveness of potential benefits from SLN procedure compared with adjuvant therapies should be evaluated in low- and intermediate-risk women with EC. Also, larger, prospective and controlled trials are needed to evaluate the most reproducible and effective standardized procedure to detect SLN in EC.

Acknowledgments We thank to João Santos, MD.

Statement of responsibility All authors gave substantial contributions to the article on reviewing recent literature and actively participating on its elaboration. The authors approved the final version of the manuscript.

Conflict of interest The authors declare that they have no competing interests.

References

1. Garg G, Gao F, Wright J (2013) The risk of lymph node metastasis with positive peritoneal cytology in endometrial cancer. Int J Gynecol Cancer 23:90–97. doi:10.1097/ICG.0b013e318275afd2
2. Dogan NU, Gungor T et al (2011) To what extent should para-aortic lymphadenectomy be carried out for surgically staged endometrial cancer? Int J Gynecol Cancer 22:607–610. doi:10.1097/IGC.0b013e3182434adb
3. Lecuru F, Bats S et al (2012) Technique et résultats du prélèvement du ganglion sentinelle dans le cancers du col et du corps de l'utérus. EMC. doi:10.1016/S1624-5857(12)57321-7
4. AlHilli MM, Mariani A (2013) The role of para-aortic lymphadenectomy in endometrial cancer. Int J Clin Oncol. doi:10.1007/s10147-013-0528-7, Article online
5. Amos C, Blake P et al (2009) Efficacy of systematic pelvic lymphadenectomy in endometrial cancer (MRC ASTEC trial): a randomised study. Lancet 373(9658):125–136. doi:10.1016/S0140-6736(08)61766-3
6. Mais V, Peiretti M et al (2010) Intraoperative sentinel lymph node detection by vital dye through laparoscopy or laparatomy in early endometrial cancer. J Surg Oncol 101:408–412. doi:10.1002/jso.21496
7. Burke TW, Levenbeck C et al (1996) Intraabdominal lymphatic mapping to direct selective pelvic and paraaortic lymphadenectomy in women with high-risk endometrial cancer: results of a pilot study. Gynecol Oncol 62:169–173
8. Holloway RW, Bravo RAM et al (2012) Detection of sentinel lymph nodes in patients with endometrial cancer undergoing robotic-

assisted staging: a comparison of colorimetric and fluorescence imaging. Gynecol Oncol Article in Press. doi:10.1016/j.ygyno.2012.04.009

9. Bonneau C, Bricou A, Barranger E (2011) Current position of the sentinel lymph node procedure in endometrial cancer. Bull Cancer 98(2):133–145. doi:10.1684/bdc.2011.1304

10. Perone AM, Casadio P et al (2008) Cervical and hysteroscopic injection for identification of sentinel lymph node in endometrial cancer. Gynecol Oncol 111:62–67. doi:10.1016/j.ygyno.2008.05.032

11. Ballester M, Dubernard G et al (2011) Detection rate and diagnostic accuracy of sentinel-node biopsy in early stage endometrial cancer: a prospective multicentric study (SENTI-ENDO). Lancet Oncology 12:469–476. doi:10.1016/S14702045(11)70070-5

12. Lopes LAF, Nicolau SM et al (2007) Sentinel lymph node in endometrial cancer. Int J Gynecol Cancer 17:1113–1117. doi:10.1111/j.1525-1438.2007.00909.x

13. Lelievre L, Camatte S et al (2004) Sentinel lymph node biopsy in cervix and corpus uteri cancers. Int J Gynecol Cancer 14:271–278

14. Khoury-Collado F, Abu-Rustum NR (2008) Lymphatic mapping in endometrial cancer: a literature review of current techniques and results. Int J Gynecol Cancer 18:1163–1168. doi:10.1111/j.1525-1438.2007.01188.x

15. Fujimoto T, Fukuda J, Tanaka T (2007) Role of complete para-aortic lymphadenectomy in endometrial cancer. Curr Opin Obstet Gynecol 21:10–14. doi:10.1097/GCO

16. Nasuh D, Gungor T et al (2012) To what extend should PA lymphadenectomy be carried out for surgically staged endometrial cancer. Int J Gynecol Cancer 22:607–610. doi:10.1097/IGC.0b013e3182434adb

17. Bouquier J, Bricou A, Delpech Y (2010) Y a-t-il un intérêt au curage lomboartique dans les cancers de l'endomètre opérables. Bulletin du Cancer 97(2):199–207. doi:10.1684/bdc.2009.0956

18. Barlin JN, Khoury-Collado F et al (2012) The importance of applying a sentinel lymph node mapping algorithm in endometrial cancer staging: beyond removal of blue nodes. Gynecol Oncol Article in Press. doi:10.1016/j.ygyno.2012.02.021

19. Kitchener HC (2011) Sentinel-node biopsy in endometrial cancer: a win-win scenario? Lancet Oncol 12:469–470. doi:10.1016/S14702045(11)70093-6

20. Kang S, Yoo HJ et al (2011) Sentinel lymph node biopsy in endometrial cancer: meta-analysis of 26 studies. Gynecol Oncol 123:522–527. doi:10.1016/j.ygyno.2011.08.034

21. Solima E, Martinelli F et al (2012) Diagnostic accuracy of sentinel node in endometrial cancer by using hysteroscopic injection of radiolabeled tracer. Gynecol Oncol 126:419–423. doi:10.1016/j.ygyno.2012.05.025

22. Rossi EC, Ivanova A, Boggess JF (2012) Robotically assisted fluorescence-guided lymph node mapping with ICG for gynecologic malignancies: a feasibility study. Gynecol Oncol 124(1):78–82. doi:10.1016/j.ygyno.2011.09.025

23. Ballester M, Dubernard G et al (2008) Use of the sentinel node procedure to stage endometrial cancer. Ann Surg Oncol 5:1523–1529. doi:10.1245/s10434-008-9841-1

24. Ballester M, Rouzier R et al (2009) Limits of lymphoscintigraphy for sentinel node biopsy in women with endometrial cancer. Gynecol Oncol 112(2):348–352. doi:10.1016/j.ygyno.2008.11.004

25. Altgassen C, Pagenstecher J et al (2007) A new approach to label sentinel nodes in endometrial cancer. Gynecol Oncol 105(2):457–461. doi:10.1016/j.ygyno.2007.01.021

26. Torné A, Pahisa J et al (2012) Transvaginal ultrasound-guided myometrial injection of radiotracer (TUMIR): a new method for sentinel lymph node detection in endometrial cancer. Gynecol Oncol. doi:10.1016/j.ygyno.2012.10.008

27. Dubernard G, Darai E, Ballester M (2012) Arguments in favour of sentinela lymph node dissection in endometrial cancer. Gynécologie Obstétrique & Fertilité 40:261–263. doi:10.1016/j.gyobfe.2012.02.005

28. Maccauro M, Lucignani G et al (2005) Sentinel lymph node detection following the hysterocopic peitumoral injection of 99 mTc-labelled albumin nanocolloid in endometrial cancer. Eur J Nucl Med Mol Imaging 32(5):569–574. doi:10.1007/s00259-004-1709-4

29. Raspagliesi F, Ditto A et al (2004) Hysteroscopic injection of tracers in sentinel node detection of endometrial cancer: a feasibility study. Am J Obstet Gynecol 191(2):435–439. doi:10.1016/j.ajog.2004.03.008

30. Niikura H, Okamura C et al (2004) Sentinel lymph node detection in patients with endometrial cancer. Gynecol Oncol Feb:92(2):669–674. doi:10.1016/j.ygyno.2003.10.039

31. Holub Z, Jabor A et al (2004) Laparoscopic detection of sentinel lymph nodes using blue dye in women with cervical and endometrial cancer. Med Sci Monit 10(10):CR587–CR591

32. How J, Lau S et al (2012) Accuracy of sentinel lymph node detection following intra-operative cervical. Gynecol Oncol 127(2012):332–337. doi:10.1016/j.ygyno.2012.08.018

33. Bats AS, Clement D et al (2008) Does sentinel node biopsy improve the management of endometrial cancer? Data from 43 patients. J Surg Oncol 97(2):141–145. doi:10.1002/jso.20857

34. Bézu C, Coutant C et al (2010) Ultrastaging of lymph node in uterine cancers. J Exp Clin Cancer Res 29(5):1–8

35. Khoury-Collado F, Murray MP et al (2011) Sentinel lymph node mapping for endometrial cancer improves the detection of metastatic disease to regional lymph nodes. Gynecol Oncol 122:251–254. doi:10.1016/j.ygyno.2011.04.030

36. Robova H, Charvat M et al (2009) Lymphatic mapping in endometrial cancer: comparison of hysteroscopic and subserosal injection and the distribution of sentinel lymph nodes. Int J Gynecol Cancer 19(3):91–394. doi:10.111/IGC.0b013e3181a1c0b1

37. Delaloye J-F, Pampallona S et al (2007) Intraoperative lymphatic mapping and sentinel node biopsy using hysteroscopy in patients with endometrial cancer. Gynecol Oncol 106:89–93. doi:10.1016/j.ygyno.2007.03.003

26

Trocar-guided polypropylene mesh for pelvic organ prolapse surgery—perioperative morbidity and short-term outcome of the first 100 patients

Pia Heinonen · Seija Ala-Nissilä · Riikka Aaltonen · Pentti Kiilholma

Abstract This study was conducted to assess the subjective outcome, complications and cure rates of prolapse surgery with a standardized trocar-quided polypropylene mesh in the first 100 patients. A follow-up visit was made after 2 months after the operation and the subjective outcome was assessed with a postal questionnaire 1 year postoperatively. An anterior mesh was used in 48, posterior mesh in 45, total mesh in five and combined anterior and posterior mesh in two patients. All patients had one or more subjective symptoms. Forty-seven percent of the patients had undergone prolapse surgery and 16% an anti-incontinence operation previously. Two patients had peroperative bleeding of more than 1,000 ml, antibiotic treatment was needed in 28 patients and two hematomas were evacuated. A total of 16 patients underwent an anti-incontinence operation for de novo stress urinary incontinence. Four patients needed cystocele repair after a posterior mesh and eight patients posterior repair after an anterior mesh. The mesh exposure was diagnosed in 14 patients. No serious complications occurred. Fifty-three (60%) patients reported all preoperative symptoms cured, 27 (30%) reported persistent symptoms and five patients were hesitant. Of the respondents, 63 (71%) were satisfied with the operation. We found that the mesh procedures were associated with a quite high amount of minor postoperative problems.

Keywords Pelvic organ prolapse · Polypropylene mesh · Prolift™ · Subjective outcome

P. Heinonen (✉) · S. Ala-Nissilä · R. Aaltonen · P. Kiilholma
Department of Obstetrics and Gynecology, University of Turku,
20520 Turku, Finland
e-mail: pia.heinonen@tyks.fi

Abbreviations

POP pelvic organ prolapse
SUI stress urinary incontinence
TVT tension-free vaginal tape
TOT transobturator tape

Introduction

Pelvic organ prolapse (POP) has a significant impact on the quality of life of women. Depending on the prolapsed compartment, symptoms may include urinary incontinence, voiding dysfunction, feeling of bulge, difficulty to defecate or fecal incontinence and sexual dysfunction [1]. Symptom relief is an obvious and important outcome measure for patients with pelvic organ dysfunction, but still most studies on POP surgery tend to report objective or anatomical cure as the primary outcome [1].

POP is the most common indication for benign gynecologic surgery and often occurs together with stress urinary incontinence (SUI). Patients' knowledge about urinary incontinence increased substantially over the last decade while knowledge about POP lags behind [1]. Many women treat their symptoms conservatively and only those who experience profound impairment seek surgical solutions. The real incidence of POP is, consequently, unknown but is estimated to vary between 38% and 41% of the female population [2, 3]. The lifetime risk for undergoing an operation for prolapse or urinary incontinence by age of 80 years is 11.1–11.8% [4, 5].

In traditional POP surgery using only native inherently weak or damaged supportive tissues in the pelvic floor, the recurrence rate is no less than 17–29% [4, 6]. The development of new surgical techniques with meshes and biomaterial implants to reinforce the vaginal wall support has improved results especially by patients undergoing anterior repair, where the failure rate after traditional repair is as high as 40% [7]. Reconstructions using meshes are efficient [8, 9] and overall anatomical cure rates of up to 79–86% 1 year after POP surgery have been reported [10].

New techniques must be evaluated for safety as well as effectiveness. The serious perioperative complication rates related to procedures using meshes in vaginal surgery have been low [11, 12]. However, postoperative mesh-related adverse events, e.g., mesh erosion, may affect the quality of life in the long-term follow-up.

In this study, we have evaluated the subjective outcome and patient satisfaction after pelvic prolapse repair with a standardized trocar-quided polypropylene mesh. The data includes the learning curves of four senior urogynecologists. Complications and any reoperations were reported during follow-up for 1 year. A specific aim was to examine the patient-related outcomes of this technique.

Materials and methods

This is a clinical follow-up study covering the first 100 patients operated on in the Turku University Central Hospital between June 2005 and April 2007 with the use of a transvaginal polypropylene mesh (Prolift™, Ethicon, Sommerville, NJ, USA). All operations were performed by four senior urogynecologists.

The data was collected from the hospital records from the preoperative visit to the follow-up visit 2 months after the operation. After an average of 1 year after the operation, a questionnaire was sent to all patients enquiring for the subjective outcome, pelvic floor symptoms and sexual function. The questionnaire was designed by the investigators, since there was no disease-specific, validated quality-of-life questionnaire on functional pelvic floor symptoms available in Finnish. The questionnaire included a detailed list of symptoms (Appendix). Formal, informed consent was obtained from all the patients.

The indication for using mesh was recurrent vaginal prolapse or large primary POP with a paravaginal tissue defect. Validated POP quantification was not used. Of the 100 patients, 49 used vaginal estrogen treatment and 30 had systemic hormone replacement therapy. All patients underwent a clinical examination to assess the site and degree of prolapse. In cases with a history of urinary incontinence a cough test was performed. With the patient in supine position a stress test with a 300-ml bladder volume was performed; a positive cough test was considered to indicate SUI. In these patients, an anti-incontinence operation was planned concomitantly. Urinary sampling was performed before and after the operation. Before the operation, a single dose of metronidazole (500 mg) and of cefuroxime (1.5 g) was given intravenously. There were eight patients who reported penicillin allergy and they received metronidazole (500 mg) and clindamycin (600 mg) intravenously. Prophylaxis against venous thrombosis was used during the hospital stay. If there was bacterial growth in the preoperative urine sample, an appropriate antimicrobial agent was administered. The criteria for wound infection were soreness, redness, exudation and swelling of the wound. Even a mild increase in the CRP level or fever was treated with antibiotics. Urinary retention was diagnosed if the postvoid residual urine volume was more than 150 ml.

A polypropylene mesh was used in all operations. The patients were in the lithotomy position during the procedure. Usually spinal anesthesia was used; nine patients required general anesthesia. Prilocaine with epinephrine was infiltrated in the operative site. The procedure was performed as previously described by Fatton and co-workers [13]. The vaginal mucosa was sutured with continuous or separate absorbable stitches. Finally vaginal packing and urinary catheter were inserted and they were removed in the next morning.

Statistical analysis was done with the SAS® System for Windows, version 8.2 (SAS Institute Inc., Cary, NC, USA). The study was approved by the ethics committee of the Hospital District of Southwest Finland.

Results

Of the 100 patients, an anterior mesh was used in 48, posterior mesh in 45, total mesh in five patients and combined anterior and posterior mesh in two patients. The baseline characteristics and preoperative symptoms are detailed in Table 1. Previous gynecological operations had

Table 1 Baseline characteristics of the 100 patients operated on using transvaginal mesh

Characteristics	
Age, mean (SD)	65 (10)
BMI, mean (SD)	27 (4)
Parity, mean (SD)	2.6 (1.3)
Preoperative symptoms, n^a	
• Feeling of pressure	56
• Difficulties in emptying the bladder	46
• Difficulties in defecation	30
• Urinary incontinence	29
• Urinary urgency	19
• Anal incontinence	7
• Dyspareunia	4

[a] Patients may have had one or more symptoms

been performed in 72 patients, 47 for POP and 16 for urinary incontinence (Table 2). The operation characteristics and concomitant surgery are presented in Table 3. Of the patients, 32% underwent some concomitant operation. Two patients who underwent anterior repair had blood loss exceeding 1,000 ml. Concomitant hysterectomy was performed in one of these procedures. No other serious intraoperative complications such as perforation of adjacent organs occurred.

Postoperatively, 28 patients were treated with antibiotics (Table 4). One haematoma was evacuated after posterior repair during hospital stay and one after anterior repair 3 weeks postoperatively. These hematomas were located under the vaginal mucosa and in both patients the mesh remained intact. Urinary retention ($n=5$) was treated with an indwelling catheter in three patients for 2 days, with a suprapubic catheter in one patient for 10 days and by observation alone for 2 days in one patient. Exposure of the mesh was reported in 14 patients at follow-up visit 2 months after the operation. In nine patients partial resection of the mesh, trimming and resuturation of the vaginal mucosa was performed. In five patients, exposure was treated by vaginal estrogen alone.

De novo SUI occurred in follow-up visit in 20 patients: in 18 patients after anterior repair and in two patients after posterior repair. This required anti-incontinence surgery for 16 patients (retropubic tape in ten and transobturator tape in six), which was performed at a mean period of 8 months after initial surgery. All of these patients became continent. The remaining four patients with de novo SUI were treated conservatively with pelvic floor muscle training. Six patients complained of urinary frequency and four had difficulties in emptying their bladder or rectum. Twelve reoperations due to POP were necessary during the follow-up of 1 year. In four cases with

Table 2 Previous surgery of the 100 patients operated on using transvaginal mesh

Number of patients with previous operations[a]	72
Previous operations for POP	47
• Anterior and/or posterior colporrhaphy	39
• Vaginal hysterectomy	29
• Sacrospinous ligament fixation	9
Anti-incontinence operations	16
• Burch colposuspension	8
• TVT	5
• Burch and TVT	1
• TOT	1
• Marshall–Marchetti–Kranz operation	1
Hysterectomy for other indications than POP	36

[a] Forty-three patients have had two or more previous gynecological procedures

Table 3 Operation characteristics and concomitant surgery in 100 patients operated on using transvaginal mesh

Characteristics	
Operation time, median (range)	72 min (27–160)
• Anterior mesh	88 min (27–160)
• Posterior mesh	60 min (30–83)
• Total mesh	110 min (72–160)
• Anterior and posterior mesh	113 min (110–125)
Blood loss, median (range)	100 ml (10–1100)
• Anterior mesh	180 ml (30–110)
• Posterior mesh	45 ml (10–500)
• Total mesh	150 ml (50–550)
• Anterior and posterior mesh	350 ml (250–450)
Hospital stay, median (range)	3 days (0–12)
Concomitant operations, n	32
• Traditional anterior or posterior colporrhaphy	14
• Sacrospinous fixation	12
• Anti-incontinence operation	6
• Vaginal hysterectomy	2

initial posterior mesh an anterior repair was done and in eight cases of anterior mesh a posterior repair was necessary.

A questionnaire after an average of 1 year was responded by 89 patients after one remainder. Fifty-three (60%) patients reported that all of their preoperative symptoms had been cured, 27 (30%) had persistent symptoms and five were uncertain as to the outcome. The most common persistent symptoms reported were urge incontinence ($n=12$), SUI ($n=8$) and urinary frequency ($n=6$). Forty-three patients (48%) complained of one or more de novo symptoms: 15 had pain or dyspareunia, nine had lower urinary tract symptoms, nine had bowel symptoms, seven had a feeling of tension and seven sensation of bulge and ten had urinary incontinence. Sixteen (42%) of the 38 sexually active patients reported dyspareunia postoperatively. In the majority of these

Table 4 Complications related to 100 operations using transvaginal mesh

Complication	
Bleeding >1,000 ml	2
Transient urinary retention	5
Hematoma	2
Mesh exposure	14
Patients with postoperative antibiotic treatment	28
• Bacteriuria	15
• Wound infection	6
• Elevated CRP and/or mild fever	7
De novo SUI	20

patients dyspareunia was infrequent. Four patients reported it frequently and two at every intercourse. Sixty-three (71%) patients were satisfied with the operation and 73 (82%) would recommend the procedure to a friend.

Discussion

This study reports the data on our first 100 patients with POP operated on using a polypropylene mesh. All complications and subjective symptoms or complaints were carefully registered and reported.

The exposure rate of the mesh was 14%; also small, nonsymptomatic exposures were recorded. In the literature, mesh exposure rates have varied between 7% and 17% [10, 14–16]. The erosion rate of vaginal meshes may to be related to surgeon's experience. According to a retrospective review [15] the erosion rate decreased from 19% to 4% during a mean follow-up time of 29 months. The fact that our study was conducted in the beginning of the learning curves of four doctors in a new surgical technique may thus have affected the rate of exposures.

We had two intraoperative bleeding complications of blood loss of more than 1,000 ml. The patients recovered uneventfully and they had no hematomas at operative site. The mean blood loss was fourfold in using anterior or total mesh compared to posterior mesh (Table 3). Other investigators have similar results. Elmer et al. [10] reported a twofold bleeding rate in patients who underwent anterior repair compared to posterior repair. The high rate of recurrence in the anterior compartment and scarring at the operative site after previous repair may complicate surgical preparation of the anterior compartment. Anterior vaginal dissection may also be associated with excessive bleeding due to injury to vascular structures in the paravesical space [11]. In addition, the passage of four supportive arms of the anterior mesh compared with two arms in the posterior procedure may contribute to a relatively greater blood loss related to anterior procedures.

In our study, one-fourth of the patients received antibiotic treatment postoperatively and no serious mesh-related infections occurred. Still, the overall rate of infections is quite high (28%, Table 4) compared to previous studies, where 8.7–13.6% of the patients were treated for infections [11, 13, 14]. This refers to our policy to treat also mild postoperative infections in our first mesh patients in order to prevent more serious adverse events. In addition, a routine postoperative urine sampling despite of missing urinary symptoms had led to a treatment of asymptomatic bacteriuria. It is a known fact that patients with asymptomatic bacteriuria should not be treated with antibiotics in order to prevent increasing antimicrobial resistance [17]. Nowadays, after achieving more experience in mesh surgery urinary samples after the operation are taken only of symptomatic patients.

Occult SUI occurs in 11–22% of patients after POP surgery [18]; in this study, de novo SUI rate was 20% and most of these patients needed surgery for SUI later on. Six patients underwent concomitantly an anti-incontinence operation (Table 3). The anterior repair with mesh raises the risk for postoperative SUI from 10% to 23% compared to traditional colporraphy [14]. Anti-incontinence operations in association with vaginal surgery are reportedly an efficient treatment of occult SUI [19], but the risk for urinary retention must be taken into consideration [20, 21]. Therefore, although routine preoperative stress test might be positive, one must consider carefully whether concomitant SUI surgery is essential. Sufficient preoperative information about occult SUI and the possibility to treat it later by surgery is important notions. However, subsequent surgery for stress incontinence should not be reported as a reoperation related to prolapse repair [1].

The rather high rate of de novo symptoms reported by our patients postoperatively (48% of the respondents) may partially be artificial, since we used a very detailed questionnaire enquiring subjective outcome. Additionally, questionnaires were filled in 1 year postoperatively which may affect the reliability of reporting preoperative symptoms. However, the prevalence of persistent subjective symptoms was comparable to a recent review where urinary symptoms were persistently reported by 22.7% patients and bowel symptoms by 4.3% after surgery using a non-absorbable mesh [22]. Presumably because of persistent or de novo subjective complaints, satisfaction with the operation was reported by 71% of the respondents. It is increasingly recognized that in POP surgery subjective outcome is a more appropriate measure of efficacy than objective measures [22].

Although the anatomy after the operation was restored at the follow-up visit 2 months after the operation, by the end of the first postoperative year 12 patients had undergone another procedure for POP. After initial anterior prolapse surgery another procedure was performed in the posterior compartment for eight patients. In the remaining four patients anterior prolapse occurred after a posterior mesh procedure. De novo prolapse rate in the non-mesh-treated site in 1 year follow-up is reported to be concerning high 23% and reoperation rate 4% [23]. In our study, reoperation rate for prolapse in another compartment was 12% during 1 year follow-up. The need for another operation for POP during a short-term follow-up might be possibly related to the previous POP surgery but a new procedure at a new site could also be recorded as "primary" surgery [1]. In our study, no validated method was used in pre- and postoperative examination but the follow-up was 1 year, which is considered as a minimum adequate period of time to assess the efficacy of prolapse repair [22]. There have been reports of anatomically high success rates when meshes are used [10–12, 16] and also significant improvements in the patients' quality of life have been reported [9]. Anatomical cure is naturally a remarkable indicator for outcome, especially when evaluating new surgical techniques for treating POP. However, it is also important to assess the patients' subjective outcome and symptoms and not just the objective outcome as indicator for good achievement. Paradoxically one may consider the anatomical result as a surrogate endpoint, while the real, meaningful endpoint is reflected by patient-related outcomes. Physicians have a tendency to underestimate the complaints of the patients [24, 25], and this makes it even more important that, when evaluating the success of any operation, especially in POP surgery, the patients' quality of life is considered.

In our study, 100 patients underwent POP repair for which a transvaginal polypropylene mesh was used. In our clinic indications for using mesh is a recurrent vaginal prolapse or large primary POP with a paravaginal tissue defect. In this non-controlled study a comparison with the traditional techniques was not possible. Although many patients experienced subjective complaints or some problems such as mesh exposure or minor infections after operation, there were no serious postoperative complications. The results for the very first 100 procedures performed in our hospital were only fair considering the quite high rate of de novo symptoms and prolapses.

Our study represents the situation where new skills are learned and prevailing practice has not yet been composed with a new procedure. Although all the surgeons have studied the mesh technique in theory and also in hands-on training, their inexperience in new surgery must have affected our complication and re-operation rates. Our preliminary results of the subsequent 100 patients operated on by the same procedure reveal a decrease in complication rates. A careful preparation and training before introducing new surgical techniques is essential to improve the results of the surgery. Consequently, it will be necessary to evaluate the objective long-term outcome as well as subjective outcome and satisfaction of the procedure using validated questionnaires.

Acknowledgements Dr Robert Paul reviewed the language of this manuscript.

Conflict of interest Pia Heinonen received a grant from the University of Turku (Finland). She also received money to support travel to the NUGA Congres Stockholm 2008 for the study or otherwhise from Astellas Pharma. Pia Heinonen's travel and accommodation expenses were covered or reimbursed by Bard (Mesh workshop in New York 2008).

References

1. Freeman RM (2010) Do we really know the outcomes of prolapse surgery? Maturitas 65:11–14
2. Hendrix SL, Clark A, Nygaard I, Aragaki A, Barnabei V, McTiernan A (2002) Pelvic organ prolapse in the Women's Health Initiative: gravity and gravidity. Am J Obstet Gynecol 186:1160–1166
3. Swift S, Woodman P, O'Boyle A, Kahn M, Valley M, Bland D, Wang W, Schaffer J (2005) Pelvic Organ Support Study (POSST): the distribution, clinical definition, and epidemiologic condition of pelvic organ support defects. Am J Obstet Gynecol 192:795–806
4. Olsen AL, Smith VJ, Bergstrom JO, Colling JC, Clark AL (1997) Epidemiology of surgically managed pelvic organ prolapse and urinary incontinence. Obstet Gynecol 1997;89:501–506
5. Fialkow MF, Newton KM, Lentz GM, Weiss NS (2008) Lifetime risk of surgical management for pelvic organ prolapse or urinary incontinence. Int Urogynecol J 19:437–440
6. Denman MA, Gregory WT, Boyles SH, Smith V, Edwards SR, Clark AL (2008) Reoperation 10 years after surgically managed pelvic organ prolapse and urinary incontinence. Am J Obstet Gynecol 198:555.e1–555.e5
7. Maher C, Baessler K (2006) Surgical management of anterior vaginal wall prolapse: an evidence based literature review. Int Urogynecol J 17:195–201
8. Sand PK, Koduri S, Lobel RW, Winkler HA, Tomezsko J, Culligan PJ, Goldberg R (2001) Prospective randomized trial of polyglactin 910 mesh to prevent recurrence of cystoceles and rectoceles. Am J Obstet Gynecol 184:1357–1362
9. de Tayrac R, Deffieux X, Gervaise A, Chauveaud-Lambling A, Fernandez H (2006) Long-term anatomical and functional assessment of trans-vaginal cystocele repair using a tension-free polypropylene mesh. Int Urogynecol J 17:483–488
10. Elmer C, Altman D, Ellström Eghn M, Axelsen S, Väyrynen T, Falconer C (2009) Trocar-guided transvaginal mesh repair of pelvic organ prolapse. Obstet Gynecol 113:117–126
11. Altman D, Falconer C, for the Nordic Transvaginal Mesh Group (2007) Perioperative morbidity using transvaginal mesh in pelvic organ prolapse repair. Obstet Gynecol 109:303–308
12. de Tayrac R, Devoldere G, Renaudie J, Villard P, Guilbaud O, Eglin G (2007) The French Ugytex Study Group. Prolapse repair by vaginal route using a new protected low-weight polypropylene mesh: 1-year functional and anatomical outcome in a prospective multicentre study. Int Urogynecol J 18:251–256
13. Fatton B, Amblard J, Debodinance P, Cosson M, Jacquetin B (2007) Transvaginal repair of genital prolapse: preliminary results of a new tension-free vaginal mesh (Prolift™ technique)—a case series multicentric study. Int Urogynecol J 18:743–752
14. Hiltunen R, Nieminen K, Takala T, Heiskanen E, Merikari M, Niemi K, Heinonen PK (2007) Low-weight polypropylene mesh for anterior vaginal wall prolapse: a randomised controlled trial. Obstet Gynecol 110:455–462
15. Dwyer PL, O'Reilly BA (2004) Transvaginal repair of anterior and posterior compartment prolapse with Atrium polypropylene mesh. BJOG 111:831–836
16. Milani R, Salvatore S, Soligo M, Pifarotti P, Meschia M, Cortese M (2005) Functional and anatomical outcome of anterior and posterior vaginal prolapse repair with prolene mesh. BJOG 112:107–111

17. Colgan R, Nicolle L, McGlone A, Hooton T (2006) Asymptomatic Bacteriuria in Adults. Am Fam Physician 74:985–990
18. Haessler AL, Lin LL, Ho MH, Betson LH, Bhatia NN (2005) Re-evaluating occult incontinence. Curr Opin Obstet Gynecol 17:535–540
19. Meltomaa S, Backman T, Haarala M (2004) Concomitant vaginal surgery did not affect outcome of the tension-free vaginal tape operation during a prospective 3-year follow-up study. J Urol 172:222–226
20. Fatton B (2009) Is there any evidence to advocate SUI prevention in continent women undergoing prolapse repair? An overview. Int Urogynecol J 20:235–245
21. Partoll LM. Efficacy of tension-free vaginal tape with other pelvic reconstructive surgery (2002) Am J Obstet Gynecol 186:1292–1295
22. Jia X, Glazener C, Mowatt G, MacLennan G, Bain C, Fraser C, Burr J (2008) Efficacy and safety of using mesh or grafts in surgery for anterior and/or posterior vaginal wall prolapse: systematic review and meta-analysis. BJOG 115:1350–1361
23. Withagen MIJ, Vierhout ME, Milani AL (2010) Does trocar-guided tension-free vaginal mesh (Prolift™) repair provoke prolapse of the unaffected compartments? Int Urogynecol J 21:271–278
24. de Boer TA, Gietelink DA, Vierhout ME (2008) Discrepancies between physician interview and a patient self-assessment questionnaire after surgery for pelvic organ prolapse. Int Urogynecol J 19:1349–1352
25. Srikrishna S, Robinson D, Cardozo L, Gonzalez J (2008) Is there a discrepancy between patient and physician quality of life assessment? Int Urogynecol J Pelvic Floor Dysfunct 19:517–520

Permissions

List of Contributors

Glenn E. Bigsby IV, Robert W. Holloway, Sarfraz Ahmad, George Ebra and Neil J. Finkler
Florida Hospital Gynecologic Oncology, Florida Hospital Cancer Institute, 2501 N. Orange Ave., Suite 800, Orlando, FL 32804, USA

Michael D. Sombeck
Radiation Oncology Program, Florida Hospital Cancer Institute, Orlando, FL 32804, USA

Kirsten B. Kluivers
Department of Obstetrics & Gynaecology, Radboud University Nijmegen Medical Centre, 6500 HB Nijmegen, The Netherlands

Florien A. Ten Cate Joan Melendez, Ravi Bhatia, Abiodun Fakokunde and Wai Yoong and Marlies Y. Bongers
Department of Obstetrics & Gynaecology, Máxima Medical Centre, De Run 4600, 5504 DB Veldhoven, The Netherlands

Hans A. M. Brölmann
Department of Obstetrics & Gynaecology, VU University Medical Centre, De Boelelaan 1117, 1081 HV Amsterdam, The Netherlands

Jan C. M. Hendriks
Department of Epidemiology and Biostatistics, Radboud University Nijmegen Medical Centre

Grigor Gortchev, Slavcho Tomov, Latchesar Tantchev, Angelika Velkova and Zdravka Radionova
Gynecologic Oncology Clinic, Medical University, 8A, Georgi Kochev Blvd, Pedro F. Escobar, Jason Knight, Matthew Kroh, Sricharan Chalikonda, Jihad Kaouk and Robert Stein Department of OB/GYN and Women's Health Institute, Cleveland Clinic, Desk A-81, 9500 Euclid Avenue, Cleveland, OH 44195, USA

Joan Melendez, Ravi Bhatia, Abiodun Fakokunde and Wai Yoong
Department of Obstetrics and Gynaecology, North Middlesex University Hospital, London N18 1QX, UK

Munawar Hussain
St. Michael's Hospital and Bristol Centre for Reproductive Medicine, Bristol, UK St. Michael's Hospital, University Hospitals Bristol NHS Trust, Bristol BS2 8EG, UK

Funlayo Odejinmi
Whipps Cross University Hospital NHS Trust, London E11 1NR, UK

Sivakami Rajamanoharan
Chelsea and Westminster Hospital, NHS Foundation Trust, 369 Fulham Road, London SW10 9NH, UK

Tim Duncan
Department of Gynaecological Oncology, Norfolk and Norwich University Hospitals, Colney Lane, Norwich NR4 7UY, UK

Jafaru Abu
Department of Obstetrics and Gynaecology, Nottingham University Hospitals, City Campus, Nottingham NG1 5PB, UK

M. D. Blikkendaal, A. R. H. Twijnstra, C. D. de Kroon and F. W. Jansen
Department of Gynaecology, Leiden University Medical Centre, RC Leiden, the Netherlands

S. C. L. Pacquee, J. P. T. Rhemrev and M. J. G. H. Smeets
Department of Gynaecology, Bronovo Hospital, JH The Hague, the Netherlands

D. Ghosh, P. Wipplinger and D. L. Byrne
Department of Gynaecology, Royal Cornwall Hospital

Danish S. Siddiqui
Department of Obstetrics and Gynecology, School of Medicine and Public Health, University of Wisconsin, 945 N 12th Street-1K,m Milwaukee, WI 53233, USA

Hussain Ali
St. John's Hospital, Lebanon, MO, USA

Kiley A. Bernhard
Aurora Health Care, Milwaukee, WI, USA

Vincenzo Berghella
Jefferson Medical College, Thomas Jefferson University, Philadelphia, PA, USA

Suneet P. Chauhan
Eastern Virginia Medical School, Norfolk, VA, USA

A. R. H Twijnstra and F. W. Jansen
Department of Gynecology, Leiden University Medical Center, 2300 RC Leiden, The Netherlands

A. Dahan
Department of Anesthesiology, Leiden University Medical Center, Leiden, The Netherlands

M. M. ter Kuile
Department of Psychosomatic Gynecology and Sexology, Leiden University Medical Center, Leiden, The Netherlands

Anwar Moria and Togas Tulandi
Department of Obstetrics and Gynecology, McGill University, Montreal, QC, Canada

Paul PG, Khan Shabnam, Sheetal Avinash Bhosale, Harneet Kaur and Prathap Talwar
Paul's Hospital, Kochi, Kerala, India

Tony Thomas
Walsall Manor Hospital, Walsall, West Midlands, England

P. G. Paul, Shabnam Khan, Prathap Talwar, Harneet Kaur and Sheetal Barsagade
Paul's Hospital, Kochi, Kerala, India

Anil Sakhare Panditrao
Dr.Shankar Rao Chavan, Govt Medical College, Nanded, Maharashtra, India

Jakob Graves Rønk Dinesen, Birgit Hessellund and Lone Kjeld Petersen
Department of Gynecology and Obstetrics, Aarhus University Hospital, 8200 Aarhu Pia Heinonen, Seija Ala-Nissilä, Riikka Aaltonen and Pentti Kiilholma s N, Denmark

Anish Keepanasseril, S. C. Saha, Rashmi Bagga and L. K. Dhaliwal
Department of Obstetrics and Gynecology, Postgraduate Institute of Medical Education and Research (PGIMER), Sector-12, Chandigarh, India 160012

Sameer Vyas
Department of Radiodiagnosis, Postgraduate Institute of Medical Education and Research (PGIMER), Sector-12, Chandigarh, India 160012

S. Motton, F. Vidal, M. Soulé Tholy and J. Hoff
General and Gynecologic Surgery, CHU Rangueil, 1 Avenue Jean Pouilhès, 31059 Toulouse Cedex 9, France

Pierre Lèguevaque
Chirurgie Générale et Gynécologique, CHU Rangueil, 1 Avenue Jean Pouilhès, 31059 Toulouse Cedex 9, France

D. Querleu
Institut Claudius Regaud, Oncological Surgery, 20-24 rue du pont Saint Pierre, 31052 Toulouse Cedex, France

Liselotte Mettler and Thoralf Schollmeyer
Department of Obstetrics and Gynaecology, University Hospitals Schleswig-Holstein, Campus Kiel, Kiel, Germany

Wael Sammur
GMC, Dubai Healthcare City, Dubai, United Arab Emirates

Amir Wiser, Christina A. Holcroft and Haim A. Abenhaim
Department of Obstetrics and Gynecology, McGill University, 687 Pine Avenue West, Montreal, Quebec H3A 1A1, Canada

Togas Tulandi
Centre for Clinical Epidemiology and Community Studies, Jewish General Hospital, Montreal, Quebec, Canada

Malcolm W. Mackenzie and Jeffrey D. Johnson
Department of Obstetrics and Gynecology, Cheshire Medical Center/Dartmouth Hitchcock, Keene, NH, USA
Department of Obstetrics and Gynecology, Mount Auburn Hospital, 330 Mount Auburn St, Cambridge, MA, USA

Jong Woon Bae, Joong Sub Choi, Jung Hun Lee, Chang Eop Son, Seung Wook Jeon and Jin Hwa Hong
Invasive Surgery, Department of Obstetrics and Gynecology, Kangbuk Samsung Hospital, Sungkyunkwan University School of Medicine, 108 Pyung-dong, Jongno-gu, Seoul 110-746, Republic of Korea

Un Suk Jung
Department of Obstetrics and Gynecology, Konyang University Hospital, Konyang University College of Medicine, Daejeon, Republic of Korea

Mark Roberts, Carlota Rosales and Poornima Ranka
Women's Services, Royal Victoria Infirmary, Newcastle upon Tyne NE1 4LP, UK

Olivier Donnez
Department of Gynecology, Cliniques Universitaires de Mont-Godinne, 5530 Yvoir, Belgium

Etienne Marbaix
Department of Anatomopathology, Université Catholique de Louvain, 1200 Brussels, Belgium

Patrick Van Ruyssevelt
Cardiovascular Department, Centre Hospitalier de Jolimont-Lobbes, 7160 Haine-Saint-Paul, Belgium

Sarah Mitri and Jacques Donnez
Department of Gynecology, Université Catholique de Louvain, Cliniques Universitaires St Luc, Avenue Hippocrate 10, 1200 Brussels, Belgium

Virginie Bot-Robin, Jean Philippe Lucot and Géraldine Giraudet
Department of Gynaecologic Surgery, Jeanne de Flandre Hospital, Centre Hospitalier Régional et Universitaire, 59000 Lille, France

Chrystèle Rubod and Michel Cosson
Department of Gynaecologic Surgery, Jeanne de Flandre Hospital, Centre Hospitalier Régional et Universitaire, 59000 Lille, Franc Faculty of Medicine, University of 'Lille Nord de France', 59000 Lille, France

Elisabete Gonçalves, Odete Figueiredo and Fernanda Costa
Division of Gynecology Oncology, Department of Gynecology and Obstetrics of Centro Hospitalar Tâmega e Sousa, Lugar do Tapadinho, Guilhufe, 4564-007 Penafiel, Portugal

Pia Heinonen, Seija Ala-Nissilä, Riikka Aaltonen and Pentti Kiilholma
Department of Obstetrics and Gynecology, University of Turku, 20520 Turku, Finland

Index